Rural Public Health

Jacob C. Warren, PhD, is a behavioral epidemiologist specializing in health disparities research. He is the Rufus C. Harris Endowed Chair in Rural Health and Health Disparities and director of the Center for Rural Health and Health Disparities at Mercer University, where he also serves as associate professor of community medicine. He has been principal investigator or co-investigator on numerous federally funded research and service grants, including funding from the Centers for Disease Control and Prevention, the National Institutes of Health (NIH), the federal Corporation for National and Community Service, and the federal Office of Rural Health Policy within the Health Resources and Services Administration (HRSA). He served as founding co-executive director of the Rural Health Research Institute at Georgia Southern University, co-leading the institute to receive NIH Center of Excellence status in 2012. He has presented his research at numerous national and international conferences, and has published in journals including *Rural and Remote Health, Health and Technology, Drug and Alcohol Dependence, Journal of Ethnicity and Substance Abuse, Pan American Journal of Public Health, AIDS and Behavior,* and *AIDS Education and Prevention.* He also served as co-editor of the book *Rural Mental Health* (2012).

K. Bryant Smalley, PhD, PsyD, is a licensed clinical psychologist with more than a decade of research and practice experience in rural areas. He co-founded and serves as the executive director of the Rural Health Research Institute at Georgia Southern University, a NIH Center of Excellence funded by the National Institute on Minority Health and Health Disparities. The Rural Health Research Institute is an innovative, interdisciplinary hub of research and outreach dedicated to improving health outcomes and reducing health disparities in rural populations. In addition, he is associate professor of psychology and has served as the director of clinical training for the PsyD program at Georgia Southern University, a clinical psychology program focused on preparing mental health practitioners for rural practice. Dr. Smalley currently serves on the Georgia Psychological Association board as the Rural Health Committee Chair. His research has appeared in numerous journals and books, including *Rural and Remote Health, Health and Technology, Psychology of Men and Masculinity, The International Journal of Men's Health,* and *Journal of Clinical Psychology: In Session,* and has been funded by organizations including the NIH, the Office of Rural Health Policy within HRSA, and the federal Corporation for National and Community Service. He also served as the lead editor of the book *Rural Mental Health* (2012).

Rural Public Health

Best Practices and Preventive Models

Jacob C. Warren, PhD
K. Bryant Smalley, PhD, PsyD

Editors

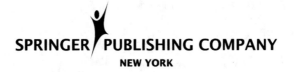

SPRINGER PUBLISHING COMPANY
NEW YORK

Springer Publishing Company, LLC
11 West 42nd Street
New York, NY 10036
www.springerpub.com

Acquisitions Editor: Sheri W. Sussman
Composition: S4Carlisle Publishing Services

ISBN: 978-0-8261-0894-4
e-book ISBN: 978-0-8261-0895-1

15 16 / 5 4 3 2

The author and the publisher of this Work have made every effort to use sources believed to be reliable to provide information that is accurate and compatible with the standards generally accepted at the time of publication. The author and publisher shall not be liable for any special, consequential, or exemplary damages resulting, in whole or in part, from the readers' use of, or reliance on, the information contained in this book. The publisher has no responsibility for the persistence or accuracy of URLs for external or third-party Internet websites referred to in this publication and does not guarantee that any content on such websites is, or will remain, accurate or appropriate.

Library of Congress Cataloging-in-Publication Data

Rural public health : best practices and preventive models / edited by Jacob C. Warren, K. Bryant Smalley.
    p. ; cm.
Includes bibliographical references and index.
ISBN 978-0-8261-0894-4
ISBN 0-8261-0894-6
  I. Warren, Jacob C., editor of compilation.   II. Smalley, K. Bryant, editor of compilation.
  [DNLM: 1. Delivery of Health Care—United States.   2. Rural Health Services—United States.   3. Rural Health—United States.   4. Rural Population—United States.   5. Socioeconomic Factors—United States. WA 390]
  RA445
  362.1—dc23   2013035943

Printed in the United States of America by Gasch Printing.

To my parents, Mark and Rita.

—Jacob

To my parents, Terry and Becky.

—Bryant

Contents

Contributors   *ix*
Preface   *xiii*

INTRODUCTION
1. What Is Rural?   *1*
   Jacob C. Warren and K. Bryant Smalley

SECTION ONE: CHALLENGES AND SOLUTIONS IN RURAL PUBLIC HEALTH
2. Access to Medical Care in Rural America   *11*
   Erika Ziller
3. Public Health Workforce Issues in Rural Areas   *29*
   Suzanne R. Hawley, Shirley A. Orr, and Theresa St. Romain
4. Rural Health Care Ethics   *41*
   Angeline Bushy
5. Rural Church-Based Health Promotion   *55*
   Karen H. Kim Yeary
6. Integrated Care in Rural Areas   *67*
   David Lambert and John A. Gale
7. Mental Health in Rural Areas   *85*
   K. Bryant Smalley and Jacob C. Warren

SECTION TWO: HEALTH ISSUES IN RURAL AREAS
8. Substance Use and Abuse in Rural America   *95*
   Jennifer D. Lenardson, David Hartley, John A. Gale, and Karen B. Pearson
9. Heart Disease in Rural Areas   *115*
   Marylen Rimando, Jacob C. Warren, and K. Bryant Smalley

10. Obesity in Rural America   *139*
    Kimberly Greder, Michelle Ihmels, Janie Burney, and Kimberly Doudna

11. Diabetes in Rural Areas   *155*
    Jacob C. Warren and K. Bryant Smalley

12. HIV Prevention and Treatment Issues in Rural America:
    A Focus on Regional Differences   *169*
    John C. Moring, Timothy F. Page, Anne Bowen, and Julie Angiola

13. Environmental and Occupational Health in Rural Areas   *187*
    Simone M. Charles and Azita K. Cuevas

14. Rural Minority Health: Race, Ethnicity, and Sexual Orientation   *203*
    Jacob C. Warren, K. Bryant Smalley, Marylen Rimando,
    K. Nikki Barefoot, Arthur Hatton, and Kayla LeLeux-LaBarge

15. Migrant Farmworker Health   *227*
    Jennie A. McLaurin

16. Health and Aging in Rural America   *241*
    Bret L. Hicken, Derek Smith, Marilyn Luptak, and Robert D. Hill

CONCLUSION

17. Future Directions in Rural Public Health   *255*
    Jacob C. Warren and K. Bryant Smalley

Index   263

Contributors

Julie Angiola, MS
Graduate Student
Department of Psychology
University of Wyoming
Laramie, WY

K. Nikki Barefoot, MS
Research Associate
Rural Health Research Institute
Georgia Southern University
Statesboro, GA

Anne Bowen, PhD
Professor
Department of Psychology
University of Arizona
Tucson, AZ

Janie Burney, PhD, RD
Professor and Extension Nutrition Specialist
University of Tennessee
Knoxville, TN

Angeline Bushy, PhD, RN, FAAN, PHCNS
Professor and Bert Fish Endowed Chair
College of Nursing
University of Central Florida
Daytona Beach, FL

Simone M. Charles, PhD, MS
Associate Professor of Environmental Health Sciences
Jiann-Ping Hsu College of Public Health
Georgia Southern University
Statesboro, GA

Azita K. Cuevas, PhD, MPH, MS
Senior Research Scientist
Department of Environmental Medicine
New York University School of Medicine
Tuxedo, NY

Kimberly Doudna, MS
Doctoral Student
Department of Human Development and Family Studies
Iowa State University
Ames, IA

John A. Gale, MS
Research Associate
Maine Rural Health Research Center
University of Southern Maine
Portland, ME

Kimberly Greder, PhD
Associate Professor and Human Sciences Extension Specialist
Department of Human Development and Family Studies
Iowa State University
Ames, IA

David Hartley, PhD, MHA
Research Professor and Director
Maine Rural Health Research Center
University of Southern Maine
Portland, ME

Arthur Hatton, MS
Research Assistant
Rural Health Research Institute
Georgia Southern University
Statesboro, GA

Suzanne R. Hawley, PhD, MPH
Chair and Professor
Department of Public Health Sciences
Wichita State University
Wichita, KS

Bret L. Hicken, PhD, MSPH
Health Science Specialist
Veterans Rural Health Resource Center–Western Region
Salt Lake City, UT

Robert D. Hill, PhD
Dean
College of Education and Human Development
University of North Dakota
Grand Forks, ND

Michelle Ihmels, PhD
Affiliate Assistant Professor
Iowa State University
Ames, IA

David Lambert, PhD
Research Associate Professor
Maine Rural Health Research Center
University of Southern Maine
Portland, ME

Kayla LeLeux-LaBarge, MS
Research Assistant
Rural Health Research Institute
Georgia Southern University
Statesboro, GA

Jennifer D. Lenardson, MHS
Research Associate
Maine Rural Health Research Center
University of Southern Maine
Portland, ME

Marilyn Luptak, PhD, MSW
Associate Professor
College of Social Work
University of Utah
Salt Lake City, UT

Jennie A. McLaurin, MD, MPH
Specialist
Child and Migrant Health and Bioethics
Migrant Clinicians Network
Ferndale, WA

John C. Moring, MS
Graduate Assistant
Nightingale Center for Nursing Scholarship
Fay W. Whitney School of Nursing
University of Wyoming
Laramie, WY

Shirley A. Orr, MHS, APRN, NEA-BC
Public Health Consultant
SOCO Consulting
Wichita, KS

Timothy F. Page, PhD
Assistant Professor
Department of Health Policy and Management
Florida International University
Miami, FL

Karen B. Pearson, MLIS, MA
Policy Analyst
Maine Rural Health Research Center
University of Southern Maine
Portland, ME

Marylen Rimando, PhD, MPH, CHES, CPH
Postdoctoral Research Associate
Rural Health Research Institute
Georgia Southern University
Statesboro, GA

K. Bryant Smalley, PhD, PsyD
Executive Director
Rural Health Research Institute
Associate Professor of Psychology
Georgia Southern University
Statesboro, GA

Derek Smith
Graduate Student
Counseling Psychology
University of Utah
Salt Lake City, UT

Theresa St. Romain, MA
Public Health Consultant
Wichita, KS

Jacob C. Warren, PhD
Rufus C. Harris Endowed Chair
Director, Center for Rural Health and Health Disparities
Associate Professor of Community Medicine
Mercer University
Macon, GA

Karen H. Kim Yeary, PhD
Associate Professor
Department of Health Behavior and Health Education
University of Arkansas for Medical Sciences
Little Rock, AR

Erika Ziller, PhD
Senior Research Associate & Deputy Director
Maine Rural Health Research Center
Muskie School of Public Service, University of Southern Maine
Portland, ME

Preface

When we look at the unique health needs that residents of rural areas face, an unfortunate theme begins to emerge: Many people feel that, given the proportion of Americans living in rural areas is the smallest it has ever been, the health problems faced in rural areas must be similarly waning.

Unfortunately, this couldn't be further from the truth.

Despite decades of documentation of the unique public health needs of rural areas, rural groups continue to face challenges in everything from initial access to care to severity of chronic disease sequelae, due to a unique combination of economic, cultural, access to care, and sociodemographic influences. The interrelationship of these factors is complex and difficult to address, and, unfortunately, relatively little attention is paid to rural populations at the highest levels of public health research.

When considering health promotion and intervention, rural residents are much less likely to have access to even basic primary care, are more isolated from hospitals and trauma centers, are more likely to be uninsured, have worse health outcomes in many of the most common chronic conditions (including heart disease and diabetes), and are more likely to live in an area without a robust public health infrastructure. Many rural residents must travel more than 30 minutes to access health care services, and living in a setting where public transportation is not available and poverty is at its peak, travel to prevention and self-management resources can be even more burdensome.

At the same time that rural populations face unique barriers to health, however, they also have unique opportunities and strengths for addressing health needs. For instance, the self-reliance and dependence upon local community, often cited as a barrier to health promotion, can be viewed instead as a strength. Capitalizing on that norm to empower community health workers offers opportunities for intervention that may not exist in the same way in more urban areas. Similarly, the strong presence of groups such as churches can also play an important role in promoting rural health.

In approaching this book, our intent was to create an organized, succinct reference discussing both the current challenges and future directions of rural public health. It is intended for public health practitioners, research-ers, students, and other professionals who work in rural settings or who are interested in learning more about the unique aspects of public health in rural areas. While we wish there were even more literature and evidence-based practices to present, the fact remains that this is still an emerging field due to the paucity of population-level rural health work currently funded and conducted. The book first presents some of the best-established challenges in rural public health, including medical care barriers, workforce issues, and ethics, followed by some of the specific rural-focused solutions that have been developed through faith-based initiatives and integrated care efforts. The book then discusses both the scope and state of prevention for specific health issues in rural settings, including mental health, substance abuse, heart disease, obesity, diabetes, HIV, environmental health, minority health, migrant farmworker health, and elderly health. The text then concludes with a summary of the future directions in rural public health to serve as a road map for moving forward.

We hope the book serves as a means both to document the challenges we face in rural health, as well as to present the current best practices and emerging models for moving the field forward. Rural areas continue to need innovative and cutting-edge programs to address their health needs, and we hope this book can help continue the drive forward for the health of tens of millions of rural Americans.

Jacob C. Warren, PhD
Rufus C. Harris Endowed Chair
Director, Center for Rural Health and Health Disparities
Associate Professor of Community Medicine
Mercer University

K. Bryant Smalley, PhD, PsyD
Executive Director, Rural Health Research Institute
Associate Professor of Psychology
Georgia Southern University

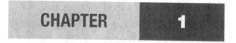

CHAPTER 1

What Is Rural?

Jacob C. Warren and K. Bryant Smalley

The idea of protecting the health of rural populations, or rural public health if you will, is not new. In fact, all societies have roots in rural lifestyles if you go back far enough, so you could almost argue that the bases of all public health lie in rural living. In reality, however, most public health principles and practices are developed, applied, and evaluated in urban settings. It is easy to see how this "urban-centric" approach to public health would have developed: Given that most of public health has its foundation in infectious disease epidemiology and control, it is not surprising that urban models were at the forefront of development. After all, urban areas are the places where risk of contagion is the highest.

As the field of public health grew beyond infectious disease concerns to encompass areas such as maternal and child health, chronic diseases, and mental health, the shift from an urban focus to a more inclusive view of all geographic diversities did not follow, however. Despite its influence in all of our lives from the food we eat to our frequent source of recreational activities, rural areas are remarkably understudied—particularly given the fact that approximately one in five Americans lives in a rural area[1] and 75% of the nation's counties are rural.[2] Although surprisingly limited, the literature does agree, however, that rural areas have unique health considerations that ultimately result in persistent health disparities in outcomes ranging from diabetes to suicide. These disparities occur both when comparing rural groups to urban groups, and when comparing rural subgroups to each other. For example, in many measures of health, rural African Americans and Latinos have even more disparate health outcomes than their Caucasian rural counterparts (see Chapter 9 for an example of this effect in cardiovascular disease). Rural areas have unique health problems, resource shortages, demographic characteristics, cultural behaviors, and economic concerns that combine to impact the health of their residents.

Two of the most pressing challenges faced by rural residents are poverty and access to basic health services. Rural residents are more likely to live below the federal poverty line,[3] with minority rural residents particularly impacted (African Americans, for instance, have poverty rates that are more than double that seen in nonminority rural residents). Rural residents also go longer periods of time without health insurance[4] and are much more likely to live in a health professional shortage area; in fact, 63% of all Health Resources and Services Administration (HRSA)-designated primary care health professional shortage areas are in rural/frontier areas, and it would take more than 4,000 new rural-practicing primary care providers to address this need.

Unfortunately, despite the recognition of the breadth of challenges faced in rural public health, there has been remarkably little progress in eliminating rural health disparities. Much research and action make the assumption that theories, practices, and programs developed in urban settings will be, for the most part, translatable into rural settings. As we will discuss throughout this book, this simply is not the case, although this notion has largely stifled rural-focused research for the better part of at least 50 years.

DEFINING RURALITY

Many researchers agree that one major complication in examining rural health outcomes is the lack of a consistent, objective measure of rurality. When one thinks of rural living, one often calls to mind images of vast, sweeping landscapes, fresh air, and sunshine. Much less frequently called to mind are the unique social, cultural, behavioral, economic, and environmental features that combine to create one of the most challenging settings for establishing and maintaining good health.

The scientific study of these features is significantly impeded by the lack of a clear, consistent definition of what truly constitutes rurality. Definitions vary dramatically across agencies and research groups, and include everything from simple population numbers to complex algorithms that simultaneously examine multiple variables. Even within these types of designations there are variations in the levels of definition—some agencies opt for a rural/urban dichotomy, whereas others rate rurality on a 6-point scale (varying by both population size and proximity to more urbanized areas).

The three leading federal agencies involved in setting rural definitions are (a) the Office of Management and Budget (OMB); (b) the Census Bureau; and (c) the U.S. Department of Agriculture's (USDA) Economic Research Service. Interestingly, the definitions put forth by these agencies do not actually strive to define rurality; they instead typically define urban/metropolitan, with "rural" being functionally defined as any nonmetropolitan area.

The OMB definition focuses on defining counties, and functionally defines rural ("nonmetro") counties as those in which there is neither a city nor urbanized area with 50,000 or more inhabitants. This is useful as a clear-cut, mostly objective definition that can be easily applied (thus its widespread use); however, it focuses only upon population size, ignoring the many other factors of rurality that can influence health outcomes. It also does not take into account the wide variation that can occur within a single county, particularly counties with large geographical areas.

The Census Bureau's definition, on the other hand, identifies urban areas (not counties) as those in which there are 50,000 or more people, and urban clusters as those with at least 2,500 people. Anything that is neither an urban area nor an urban cluster is considered nonurban, applied in practice as rural. However, because the Census Bureau's definition is based largely upon assemblages of census tracts/blocks, the definition is difficult to apply and can lead to seeming "islands" of urbanicity or rurality within the opposite geographic designation.

The USDA has five different ways of classifying rural areas, many of which measure rurality on a continuum, taking into account the diversity that exists within rural settings. Some of these definitions (such as the Frontier and Remote Area codes) even provide suboptions within the definition. The two most commonly used USDA classifications include the Rural-Urban Continuum Codes (RUCCs) and the Rural-Urban Community Areas (RUCAs). The Rural-Urban Continuum Codes classify counties according to a 9-point continuum based upon population size, degree of urbanization, and proximity to metropolitan areas. These codes are defined in Table 1.1.

Table 1.1 Rural-Urban Continuum Codes, With Number of Associated Counties*

		Metro Counties
1	413	Counties in metro areas of 1 million population or more
2	325	Counties in metro areas of 250,000 to 1 million population
3	351	Counties in metro areas of fewer than 250,000 population
		Nonmetro Counties (considered "rural")
4	218	Urban population of 20,000 or more, adjacent to a metro area
5	105	Urban population of 20,000 or more, not adjacent to a metro area
6	609	Urban population of 2,500 to 19,999, adjacent to a metro area
7	450	Urban population of 2,500 to 19,999, not adjacent to a metro area
8	235	Completely rural or less than 2,500 urban population, adjacent to a metro area
9	435	Completely rural or less than 2,500 urban population, not adjacent to a metro area

*www.ers.usda.gov/data-products/rural-urban-continuum-codes/documentation.aspx

The USDA RUCA codes classify census tracts based upon population density, level of urbanization, and the degree to which residents of the area commute to more urbanized areas. The 10-point scale is further subdivided, ultimately resulting in a 33-category classification system. These codes are important from a policy perspective because they are used in combination with the county-level census definition to define eligibility for rural-specific funding administered by HRSA, but are very complex and difficult to both apply and interpret differences found among RUCA areas.

In addition to their individual strengths and weaknesses, attempting to compare across different definitions is very difficult, significantly impeding the ability of researchers and policy makers to compare across individual studies. Just comparing the OMB and census dichotomous definitions high-lights this complexity—when comparing the classification of counties by the two definitions, nearly 20% are classified as rural by one definition, but not the other.[2] Because these definitions are often used to determine eligibility for certain types of funding, these differences in opinion can directly affect millions of rural residents. When considering the multiplicative effect that comes with the plethora of other definitions of rurality, it is easy to see how something that at first may seem simple is in fact quite complex. A compre-hensive examination of the strengths and weaknesses of the OMB, Census Bureau, and USDA classifications can be found in a 2005 article published by Hart, Larson, and Lishner[2] in the *American Journal of Public Health*.

While many of the USDA definitions in particular further subdivide rurality based upon quantitative information, there is also a well-recognized qualitative separation often used when describing rural areas: rural versus frontier. Frontier communities represent the extreme of rurality, with defi-nitions ranging from population densities less than or equal to 6 people per square mile[5] to complex scoring methods that take into account travel time to market centers and medical care.[6-7] Large portions of the western United States and nearly all of Alaska are considered frontier because of their extreme remoteness (many areas of Alaska, for instance, are only accessible via plane or helicopter). Many of the disparities discussed throughout this book are even more pronounced in frontier areas because of their extreme geographic isolation; however, frontier areas are even more understudied than rural areas and the literature is severely limited.

When selecting a particular definition for a study, outreach initiative, or policy decision, it is recommended to select the definition that is most consistent with the intent of the project[2]; for instance, if a project is focusing on decreasing travel distance to a source of care, utilizing a definition of rurality that takes into account provider shortages or actual distance to care could be most beneficial.

SO WHAT IS RURAL?

Overall, the lack of consistency in definition of and within rural areas often leads to conflicting study findings, which partially help to explain why some rural-focused studies seemingly contradict the findings of preceding (or subsequent) studies. Regardless of the definition used, however, rural areas are largely accepted to be those in which population density is lower than a "typical" setting and one in which access to basic services (including health care) is often impeded by sometimes great distances. Beyond these quantifiable characteristics, however, rural areas have a unique cultural background and heritage that can impact health behaviors and outcomes in strong and surprising ways. When thinking of rural residents as a cultural group, it is helpful to consider the fact that there are actually more rural residents than any racial, ethnic, or sexual orientation minority group, representing a large group of individuals being strongly influenced by a culture unto itself that is often not recognized as such.

For rural residents, this culture is shaped by many key factors that include population density and geography, agricultural heritage, economic conditions, religion, behavioral norms, health care stigma, and distance to care. These factors combine to impact not only their potential need for health care, but also the ways in which residents will seek out care (or avoid it). Taking these cultural factors into consideration in the planning, execution, and even evaluation of rural health programs can help ensure public health efforts adequately and appropriately reach rural groups.

Remoteness and Isolation

The most intuitive concepts of rurality stem from ideas of "open land" that are typically associated with rural living—farmlands, fields, prairies, and mountain valleys.[8] As discussed above, many definitions of rurality are in fact based upon similar notions of population size or density; as such, the underlying implication is a dispersed population separated from other residents (sometimes by miles) and other population centers (sometimes by dozens, if not hundreds, of miles).

In addition to the separation this creates from other community members, geographic isolation also contributes to the potentially life-threatening distance to medical and mental health care that is available. A common feature of many rural areas is distance from medical care providers and emergency care,[9-10] likely fostering notions of having to be self-reliant for health issues. Also, because of the increased travel distance associated with seeking health care in rural areas,[11] rural residents likely perceive receiving treatment as even more of an inconvenience and burden to friends and families. For health care providers, this can lead to a perception of noncompliance that is dictated less by choice than by circumstance; exploring the root of failure to complete regimens or inability to attend skill-building workshops may help address core barriers that would otherwise be missed. Because of the increased difficulty in receiving services, it is even more critical for rural health providers and public health programming to be convenient and adaptable, but it is also important to emphasize to rural clients the importance of continuing a program to help ensure they remain motivated throughout the difficult process of commuting to and from the care or program that is frequently many miles away.

This geographic separation from other individuals and from care providers has a distinct influence upon the culture of rural areas. Rural residents are often portrayed as independent and self-sufficient[12,13]—characteristics that stem from necessity when geographically isolated from other groups of people and from service providers. These norms of self-reliance can directly impact an individual's willingness to seek care. For mental health in particular, resistance to therapeutic techniques and to revealing to friends and families the presence of an illness will be amplified in rural settings.

Agriculture

Associated with notions of "wide-open spaces" is the frequent agricultural nature of rural areas. Farming has long been seen as a rural pursuit. In fact, one of the earliest discussions of rurality argued that all of the cultural and economic conditions present in rural areas stem from their direct tie to agriculture.[14] Early sociological reviews on the measurement of rurality proposed that a crude measure of rurality could be constructed using the percentage of residents whose employment is agriculturally based.[15] While not all rural areas are agricultural, there is an undeniable influence of farm living on many rural residents. As with geographic isolation, farm living fosters a sense of independence, strong work ethic, and personal responsibility that will likely spill over into general personality characteristics. It may also influence the view rural residents have on the role of children in supporting a household, as farm families typically rely on children within the family to help operate the farm.

Poverty

As mentioned, rural areas have long been recognized as having high rates of poverty and unemployment that directly impact the health of their populations. Because rural economies often center on agriculture, a highly volatile market,[16-17] economic uncertainty is almost a staple in rural communities. Poverty is also strongly associated with a lack of health insurance, further making affordable health care harder to reach for rural residents.[18] As such, individuals from rural backgrounds may be unable or unwilling to spend limited income on treatment.

The impact of poverty on both physical and mental health status has been well recognized, and poverty has long been one of the largest focuses of social justice movements seeking equality in health for all.[19-20] While publically supported services are sometimes available (but still limited in rural areas), individuals living in poverty have been shown to have a mistrust of public services and a general fear regarding the stigma associated with having to seek public assistance.[21]

Religion

Religion plays an extremely prominent role in rural areas, particularly in the rural South. Rural residents are more likely to regularly attend Church,[22] and many aspects of religious beliefs can impact an individual's approach to and perception of health. Some beliefs can foster a sense of hope for the outcome of treatment, but others may foster a sense of fatalism (that an outcome is "in God's hands"). When considering mental health, rural religious individuals are more likely to believe that the Church can answer life's problems and that psychological problems should be handled within the family or the Church.[23–24] In addition, nearly three fourths of all Americans use their faith as a way to cope with stressful life experiences.[25]

Increasingly, Churches and other religious organizations are being seen as a unique partner and access point for reaching rural populations. Many faith-based and faith-placed initiatives have been developed within rural settings, ranging from basic health screenings to establishing faith-based community health workers. The literature surrounding faith-based public health initiatives is still growing, but it is clear that the connection between health and Churches will continue to grow and will play an important role in addressing the health needs of rural groups. For more details on faith-based initiatives in rural settings, see Chapter 5.

Behavioral Norms

There are many health-related behavioral norms that will also impact mental health treatment (see Chapter 7 for details). Rural residents (and rural youth, in particular) are more likely to engage in alcohol and substance use due partially to permissive cultural norms regarding such use in rural settings. Addressing these cultural norms can be very difficult, but should be considered if working with rural clients with substance abuse concerns. Similar health risk-taking behaviors such as smoking and sedentary lifestyle are also more prevalent in rural settings,[26–27] and may make it even more difficult when working with clients wanting to address these issues.

Prevention and intervention programs for rural groups must take into account these prevailing norms, and find unique ways to address them. For instance, a physical activity program that recommends going to the local high school track may be completely inappropriate for a county with either no track, or potentially even no high school. Taking a critical eye to established programs, or, even more effectively, creating rural-specific programs, will be important to not only shift these norms, but to ensure that programs are adequately addressing barriers to changing those norms.

Stigma

Particularly within the area of mental health, there is generally a negative perception toward those receiving services in rural areas. This stigma has a direct impact on rural residents' likelihood to not only seek care in the first place, but also the likelihood of their continuing care for the recommended course of treatment.[28] Unfortunately, it also impacts rural clients' willingness to share their mental health struggles with others. If social support is needed as a part of the treatment planning process, clients may not be as open to discussing their needs with friends and family members. Practitioners and public health workers focused on psychological outcomes must consider the impact of the culture of mental health stigma in rural regions and be prepared to pursue unique ways of counteracting its effects.

Beyond mental health, the stigma surrounding certain physical health conditions can also impact willingness to both disclose presence of a condition and to receive appropriate care for it—HIV, for instance, is a generally stigmatized health condition for which the stigma is only amplified in rural settings.

CONCLUSION

Although difficult to define, there is no doubt that rurality plays an important role in the health of millions of Americans. From access to care to receptivity of services, living within a rural area is associated with a variety of disparities discussed in more detail throughout this book. By recognizing the socioeconomic and cultural factors unique to rural areas as not only contributing to health disparities (e.g., higher smoking rates) but also as providing avenues for addressing them (e.g., faith-based initiatives), rural public health practitioners can begin to make long-needed progress in protecting the health of one fifth of the U.S. population.

By recognizing the importance of rurality in resources, norms, personal decision making, worldview, and interaction patterns with other people, the helping professions can begin to culturally tailor their messages, approaches, and interventions in a way that will provide maximum impact for rural populations. Public health training programs should incorporate basic knowledge of rural culture into their curriculum—not only within rural-focused programs, but, more importantly, *outside* of such programs where rural competency might not otherwise be acquired.

REFERENCES

1. US Census Bureau. American FactFinder. http://factfinder.census.gov/servlet/DCGeoSelectServlet?ds_name=DEC_2000_SF1_U. 2010.
2. Hart LG, Larson EH, Lishner DM. Rural definitions for health policy and research. *Am J Public Health*. 2005;95(7):1149–1155.
3. Economic Research Service. Rural income, poverty, and welfare: summary of conditions and trends. http://www.ers.usda.gov/Briefing/IncomePovertyWelfare/Overview.htm. 2011.
4. Mueller KJ, Patil K, Ullrich F. Lengthening spells of uninsurance and their consequences. *J Rural Health*. 1997;13(1):29–37.
5. Hewitt ME. *Defining Rural Areas: Impact on Health Care Policy and Research*. Darby, PA: Diane Publishing; 1989.
6. Center for Rural Health. *Defining the Term Frontier Area for Programs Implemented through the Office for the Advancement of Telehealth*. Bismarck, ND: University of North Dakota; 2006.

7. Frontier Education Center. Frontier: a new definition. http://www.frontierus .org/documents/consensus_paper.htm. 2007.

8. Smith BJ, Parvin DW. Defining and measuring rurality. *South J Agricultural Econ.* 1973;5(1):109–113.

9. Connor RA, Kralewski JE, Hillson SD. Measuring geographic access to health care in rural areas. *Med Care Rev.* 1994;51(3):337–377.

10. Weinert C, Boik RJ. MSU rurality index: development and evaluation. *Res Nurs Health.* 1995;18(5):453–464.

11. Health Resources and Services Administration. *Mental Health and Rural America: 1994–2005.* Rockville, MD: Health Resources and Services Administration; 2005.

12. Long KA, Weinert C. Rural nursing: developing the theory base. *Res Theory Nurs Pract.* 1989;3(2):113–127.

13. Weinert C, Long KA. Understanding the health care needs of rural families. *Fam Relations.* 1987;36(4):450–455.

14. Jordan SA, Hargrove DS. Implications of an empirical application of categorical definitions of rural. *J Rural Community Psychol.* 1987;8:14–29.

15. Stewart CT. The urban-rural dichotomy. *Am J Sociol.* 1958;64:52–58.

16. Giot P. The information content of implied volatility in agricultural commodity markets. *J Futures Markets.* 2006;23(5):441–454.

17. Koekebakker S, Lien G. Volatility and price jumps in agricultural futures prices: evidence from wheat options. *Am J Agricultural Econ.* 2004;86(4):1018–1031.

18. DeNavas-Walt C, Proctor BD, Lee CH. *Income, Poverty, and Health Insurance Coverage in the United States: 2005.* Washington, DC: US Census Bureau; 2006.

19. Patrick DL, Stein J, Porta M, Porter CQ, Ricketts TC. Poverty, health services, and health status in rural America. *Milbank Q.* 1988;66(1):105–136.

20. Murali V, Oyebode F. Poverty, social inequality and mental health. *Adv Psychiatr Treat.* 2004;10:216–224.

21. Canvin K, Jones C, Marttila A, Burstöm B, Whitehead M. Can I risk using public services? Perceived consequences of seeking help and health care among households living in poverty: a qualitative study. *J Epidemiol Community Health.* 2007;61(11):984–989.

22. Farley GE, Ruesink DC. Churches. In: Goreham GA, ed. *Encyclopedia of Rural America: The Land and People.* Santa Barbara, CA: ABC-CLIO; 1997: 102–105.

23. Fox J, Merwin E, Blank M. De facto mental health services in the rural south. *J Health Care Poor Underserved.* 1995;6:434–468.

24. Glenna L. Religion. In: Brown DL, Swanson LE, eds. *Challenges for Rural America in the Twenty-First Century.* University Park, PA: The Pennsylvania State University Press; 2003: 262–272.

25. Weaver AJ, Flannelly LT, Garbarino J, Figley CR, Flannelly KJ. A systematic review of research on religion and spirituality in the *Journal of Traumatic Stress: 1990–1999. Ment Health Religion Cult.* 2003;6(3):215–228.

26. Doescher MP, Jackson E, Jerant A, Hart GL. Prevalence and trends in smoking: A national rural study. *J Rural Health.* 2006;22(2):112–118.

27. Tai-Seale T, Chandler C. Nutrition and overweight concerns in rural areas. In: Gamm LD, Dabney B, Dorsey A, eds. *Rural Healthy People 2010: A Companion Document to Healthy People 2010.* Vol 1. College Station, TX: The Texas A&M University System Health Science Center, School of Rural Public Health, Southwest Rural Health Research Center; 2003.

28. Parr H, Philo C. Rural mental health and social geographies of caring. *Soc Cultural Geogr.* 2003;4(4):471–488.

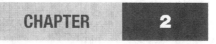

CHAPTER 2

Access to Medical Care in Rural America

Erika Ziller

> Talk with this gentle, wise physician and you, too, may glimpse ...
> counties with mothers but with neither hospitals nor nurses; some
> with no railway, telegraph or telephone. Or you may glimpse the
> mothers in other remote parts, who, to find the doctor, must travel
> 20, 30 or 60 miles.
> —Eleanor Brownson Taylor, *In Behalf of Mothers and*
> *Children: The Story of the U.S. Children's Bureau,* January 1930

Access to medical care is a fundamental factor in a population's health and well-being, yet barriers to optimal care exist for many rural residents. These barriers include a number of economic, social, and geographic factors that may limit a rural person's ability to obtain primary or specialty health care, from preventive health services to treatment for chronic illness. In some cases the barriers experienced by rural people are common to lower-income populations and reflect their higher rates of poverty—including having no health insurance coverage, or being unable to afford care even when insured. Other barriers, such as travel distance or shortages of certain types of medical care providers, are more uniquely rural issues.

Compared to those living in urban areas, the residents of rural communities rank more poorly on many population-based measures of personal health status, chronic disease prevalence, and access to medical care services.[1-3] Individuals living in rural areas are more likely to describe their health as fair or poor, and rates of chronic illness (e.g., diabetes, hypertension, arthritis, heart disease) are higher than among their urban counterparts.[4,5] Yet, despite the higher need for medical care implied by these poor health rankings, those living in rural areas make fewer medical care visits over the course of a year than do their urban counterparts.[6] Residents of rural areas are less likely to receive wellness care, including recommended preventive services such as annual physicals and screenings for high cholesterol, colorectal cancer, and breast and cervical cancer.[4] Possibly because of this poorer access to preventive care, rural people may be diagnosed for cancer at a later stage of disease than those in urban areas.[7]

This chapter provides a conceptual framework for understanding access to medical care and discusses many of the barriers faced by residents of rural communities. While not an exhaustive list of the challenges that rural people face in trying to access medical care, the chapter offers an overview of common barriers and discusses the impact these barriers may have on the health and well-being of rural Americans. Because certain subpopulations of rural residents experience even more pronounced barriers to care, the chapter also includes a section on particularly vulnerable rural populations. In addition to identifying and discussing barriers to care, the chapter presents information on key federal programs that have been created to assist rural and other underserved populations obtain needed medical services. Finally, the chapter highlights innovative programs developed by public health and community-based organizations that have endeavored to promote new medical care delivery models, thereby increasing access for rural residents and improving the health outcomes of those living in rural communities.

UNDERSTANDING BARRIERS TO MEDICAL CARE: THE BEHAVIORAL MODEL OF HEALTH SERVICES USE

Medical care access can be defined as "a broad set of concerns that center on the degree to which individuals and groups are able to obtain needed services from the medical care system."[8] The *Behavioral Model of Health Services Use* is one of the most commonly used conceptual frameworks for understanding the factors that support or impede use of medical care. Developed in the early 1970s by scholars Richard Andersen and Lu Anne Aday, the Behavioral Model describes the ways in which the individual and the health system and other environmental factors interact to predict whether or not an individual will access medical services.[9] The behavioral model conceptualizes three domains of characteristics associated with the use of health care services: *predisposing, enabling*, and *need* factors. In their original article, Aday and Andersen refer to the three domains as "individual" characteristics; however, recent revisions have incorporated community and environmental traits into the behavioral model.

Predisposing characteristics include those aspects of a person that affect his or her propensity to access medical care and exist prior to any need for medical care. These predisposing traits encompass most sociodemographic characteristics such as race and ethnicity, gender, and educational attainment. An individual's views and beliefs about the health care system are also a predisposing characteristic. *Enabling* characteristics are defined as the resources and systems that support a person's efforts to obtain medical care including income, health insurance coverage, availability of child care, and transportation. Community factors such as rural or regional residence, availability of medical providers, and travel time to get services are also enabling factors. As the name suggests, *need* characteristics are those that affect the extent to which an individual requires medical care such as health status, age, and presence of a chronic health condition. Need may be both clinical (e.g., ruptured appendix) and perceptual. Perceptual need may include an individual's assessment about whether he or she is at risk for illness, as well as the individual's views about the utility of a preventive service such as a mammogram or of a treatment for a specified condition.

Since its inception nearly 40 years ago, the Behavioral Model has undergone numerous applications, critiques, and revisions.[10] One revision, the *Behavioral Model for Vulnerable Populations*, made the important point that specific characteristics do not affect all individuals equally, and that some populations may be more vulnerable to the adverse effects of a particular access barrier.[11] Other revisions have described more explicitly the role of community, policy, and other structural characteristics in medical care access in an effort to address criticisms that the original model overemphasized individual characteristics. For example, Andersen and colleague Davidson extend the three domains to what they call "contextual," as well as individual, characteristics.[12] In this model, the contextual predisposing characteristics reflect the sociodemographic composition of a community (e.g., the proportion of individuals that are racial or ethnic minorities, or that live in poverty). Contextual enabling characteristics include organizational, financing, and health policy factors that affect how health care services are structured, delivered, and paid for in a community. Contextual need characteristics are environmental factors, such as proportion of housing with lead-based paint, or community health indices like the obesity rate of a specific town.

Rural residents face a number of barriers to accessing medical care, some of which are a reflection of their sociodemographic composition, and some that are more uniquely related to the places in which they live. The sections that follow describe the characteristics of rural populations that put them at risk for poor medical care access.

MEDICAL CARE NEEDS OF RURAL POPULATIONS

The sociodemographic characteristics of rural residents differ from those of urban populations in ways that may affect their need for medical care. For example, rural residents are, on average, older than urban residents and the proportion of elderly residents that fall into the "oldest old" category (85 or older) is higher in rural areas.[13] Because need for medical care typically increases with aging, rural populations are likely to have greater demand for medical care, yet (as noted previously) studies indicate that they make fewer medical visits throughout the year. Chronic health conditions such as heart disease and diabetes are much more common in elderly populations, and a significant number of adults in this age group have multiple chronic conditions. Among adults of all ages, those living in rural areas are more likely to have a chronic illness and/or to be in fair or poor health compared to individuals living in urban communities.[4]

Part of the poorer health status and higher disease burden among rural residents may be related to poorer health habits. For example, residents of rural communities are more likely than their urban counterparts to smoke cigarettes, and while this is true for both adults and young people, the rural–urban disparity in smoking is particularly pronounced among adolescents.[14] Eighteen percent of rural 12- to 17-year-olds reportedly smoke, compared to only 11% of urban residents in that age group.[14] Obesity is another marker for poor health and higher rates of chronic illness, including diabetes, heart disease, and cancer. Recent evidence based on actual clinical data (versus self-report) indicates that 40% of adults living in rural areas are obese, compared to only 33% of urban adults.[15] This disparity in obesity rates has been attributed to both poorer eating habits among rural residents, as well as increases in sedentary lifestyle as more rural industries have become automated over the years (for additional details on the impact of obesity in rural areas, see Chapter 10). In addition, experts believe that both elevated smoking and obesity rates in rural populations are attributable, at least in part, to poorer access to preventive medical care and evidence-based prevention programs in rural areas.[14]

RURAL RESIDENTS ARE LESS LIKELY TO HAVE RESOURCES THAT ENABLE ACCESS TO MEDICAL CARE

Many of the barriers to rural medical care are fundamentally related to the more limited resources available to rural residents to aid them in achieving access. These resource limitations include financial barriers, as well as the more limited supply of medical professionals practicing in rural areas. In addition to having fewer medical providers available per capita, rural providers are often geographically dispersed, affecting physical accessibility for patients as well as the capacity of providers to offer extended hours, make referrals, and coordinate care. Even when rural residents have a regular medical care provider, they may be unable to obtain care as needed due to other barriers such as lack of transportation, employer support for medical leave, and health literacy.

Health Insurance Coverage

A substantial body of research indicates that individuals without health insurance coverage are at substantially greater risk for poor medical care access and health outcomes. In 2009, only 48% of individuals living in rural (nonmetropolitan) counties had private health insurance coverage, compared to 54% of those living in urban counties (Figure 2.1). One third of all rural residents had public health insurance coverage, including Medicare (the federal program for seniors and persons with disabilities), Medicaid (a program for certain low-income groups), and the Children's Health Insurance Program (CHIP). In contrast, only 29% of urban residents had their health insurance coverage from a public source. About 19% of all persons living in rural areas had no health insurance coverage at all, compared to 17.5% of all urban persons.

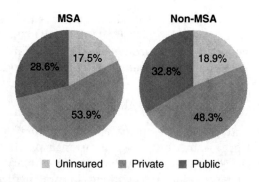

Data: Medical Expenditure Panel Survey, 2009
Source of health insurance different by residence at $p < .01$.
Due to rounding, some characteristics may not total 100 percent.

Figure 2.1 Health insurance coverage in rural and urban America (2009, all ages).
MSA = metropolitan statistical area (urban); Non-MSA = non-metropolitan
statistical area (rural).

These rural–urban differences in insurance coverage reflect the socio-economic and employment characteristics of rural residents. For example, higher rates of public coverage can be attributed to the greater proportion both of rural residents who are over age 65 and qualify for Medicare, and of low-income families that qualify for Medicaid and/or CHIP.[16] Similarly, lower rates of private health insurance coverage can be partly explained by the greater proportion of the rural workforce that is employed by small business and for low wages and consequently has more limited access to employer-sponsored health insurance.[17]

As one would expect, the lack of health insurance coverage is a significant barrier to medical care for rural residents. Across both rural and urban communities, individuals without health insurance coverage are less likely to have a usual source of medical care, must travel farther for care, and face greater barriers to obtaining care from a usual provider after regular office hours. In addition, 8% of uninsured rural residents indicate that they have gone without needed health care because they couldn't afford it, compared to only 1% of those with health insurance coverage.[18] These higher uninsured rates have even been associated with higher rates of death among rural versus urban residents.[19]

Even when rural individuals have health insurance coverage, they may face insurance-related barriers to medical care. For example, while individuals with Medicaid generally have greater access to care than the uninsured, many medical providers are less willing to accept Medicaid as a form of health insurance compared to private coverage.[20] This is due in large part to the fact that Medicaid, and Medicare as well, generally reimburse providers less for the medical services they provide than do private health insurance companies. However, even when rural residents have private health coverage, they are more likely than those living in urban areas to be "underinsured." That is, despite having insurance, they face high out-of-pocket costs relative to their generally lower incomes and may face similar barriers to care as individuals without any health insurance coverage at all.[21] Related to these insurance differences, and the generally lower incomes of rural residents, individuals living in rural areas are more likely to defer needed health services due to cost.[3]

Provider Availability

One of the more intractable access problems facing rural Americans is the relatively lower supply of medical care professionals practicing in rural versus urban settings. While this chapter focuses on primary care and some types of specialty care providers, the shortages in rural medical professionals cut across multiple professional types and impact all areas of medical care, including office and clinic-based care, emergency and trauma care, mental health and substance abuse treatment, dental health services, long-term services and supports, and advanced specialty care.

Primary Care

The more limited supply of health care professionals in rural areas poses unique challenges to health care access. Access to primary care is necessary for maintaining and improving population health as these practitioners provide critical primary and secondary prevention services, including immunizations, well-child and adult checkups, preventive disease screenings and disease management, and health education. Compared to urban areas, rural communities have lower availability of primary care providers, meaning that it can be a particular challenge to obtain needed medical care for some rural residents.[22] Estimates suggest that there are 72 primary care physicians for every 100,000 people living in an urban area, compared to only 55 in rural areas. In small, more isolated rural communities, the number of primary care physicians drops to only 36 per 100,000 people.[22] While these statistics describe averages across the entire country, some regions—most notably the South and Midwest—are particularly disadvantaged. As a result of this uneven distribution of primary care across rural and urban areas, more than three fourths of all rural counties have been designated primary care health professional shortage areas (HPSAs).[22]

   While these shortages of primary care professionals in rural areas affect access to what we think of as "typical" primary care occurring in private medical offices, the ability to provide services through special programs that target the poor and uninsured are also affected. For example, the federal government provides grant funding to community health centers in underserved rural and urban areas to help create a "safety net" for medical care access among people with limited ability to pay for services (this program is described in more detail later in the chapter). However, because proportionally fewer primary care providers practice in rural areas, rural community health centers face greater challenges than their urban counterparts in recruiting primary care physicians. According to one estimate, more than one third of all rural community health centers spent more than 7 months trying to hire a family physician to provide these safety net primary care services.[22]

Local county public health programs are another key player in the medical care safety net, fulfilling one of public health's essential services by providing some basic primary care services (including wellness visits, family planning and sexual health, immunizations, preventive screenings, and treatment for some conditions) to low-income and other vulnerable populations. While the provision of individual-level medical care services is sometimes seen as a deviation from public health's population-based mission, experts note that in some rural counties the local health department is the only source of medical care, especially for those with low incomes. At the same time, however, assessments of the public health infrastructure in rural America have concluded that the competing demands and more limited resources experienced by rural public health departments may make it particularly challenging for them to provide these safety net services (particularly on a continuous basis).[23]

Even when primary care is available to rural residents, issues such as travel distance or hours of operation can be barriers to care. For example, rural residents are much more likely than their urban counterparts to report difficulties reaching their primary care provider after hours or on weekends.[18] Rural primary care providers are much more likely to practice alone or in very small groups, which can make it very difficult to offer extended hours or 24-hour call service. At the same time, rural workers are more likely than those in urban areas to work at low-wage jobs,[16] many of which may not offer time off for medical care appointments. As shown in Figure 2.2, about 14% of nonelderly rural residents have to travel for more than a half hour to reach their usual source of medical care services, compared to only 9% of urban residents. Rural residents are also more likely to report difficulty reaching

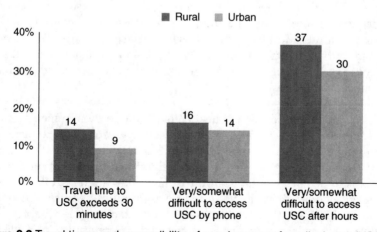

Figure 2.2 Travel times and accessibility of usual source of medical care (USC).
Source: Medical Expenditure Panel Survey, 2009. Access differences by residence significant for travel time and after hours at *p* < .01.

their usual source of care by telephone (16% versus 14% of urban residents). Nearly 40% of all rural residents under age 65 have difficulty getting access to their usual source of care after hours or on weekends, compared to only 30% of urban residents.

Specialty Care

While primary care providers are less available in rural versus urban areas, rural–urban disparities in access to specialty medical care are particularly pronounced.[22] Given the broad range of services that a population may need over its life span, it is clear that few (if any) rural health systems would be able to fully meet the specialty care needs of their communities. Thus, many rural residents may find themselves without local access to needed open-heart surgeons and tertiary hospitals, oncologists and cancer treatment facilities, providers with expertise in HIV treatment, or care for mental illness or substance abuse. In these cases rural residents with more significant health care needs may be referred to regional health systems for care, in some cases at a great distance from home and from local providers and other community support. As a result, the individual may experience a fragmented health care system, with some services provided far away in urban areas and not well coordinated with follow-up care provided more locally.[24]

The travel distance required to obtain specialty care services is often a burden for rural individuals.[25] As a result, many rural residents with complex health care needs will seek care from a local generalist such as their primary care provider, or go without needed treatment.[24] In the former case, the primary care system in rural communities may become even more strained, as rural primary care providers must work to provide care outside their normal scope of services in a context where their typical primary care services are already unable to meet local demand. In the latter case, rural residents may face greater morbidity and mortality as a result of deferred specialty care. Among adults admitted to hospitals for a heart attack, rural residence is associated with higher rates of death.[26] One possible explanation for this disparity could be the smaller proportion of cardiologists and related specialties that practice in rural areas.

One specialty care gap that is commonly filled by rural primary care providers is treatment for mental health conditions, although many lack the expertise to provide these services most effectively. More than 60 percent of rural Americans live in a mental HPSA and may have no provider support available to them in times of mental and emotional duress. In other cases, individuals in need of mental health treatment may not take full advantage of the services that are available in their communities because of concerns about mental illness stigma and other cultural factors (see Chapter 7 for more details).[27] Reflecting this combination of barriers, studies indicate that rural residents enter mental health treatment later, with more severe symptoms and at a greater cost to the medical care system than do their urban counterparts.[28] Given these issues, it is not surprising that state-level health leaders have identified mental health as one of the top unmet rural health needs.[29,30]

VULNERABLE RURAL POPULATIONS

While rural residents in general have been shown to have higher needs and poorer access to medical care, subpopulations of rural residents exhibit even greater disparities in both need and access. In the case of especially vulnerable rural populations (e.g., racial and ethnic minority groups or individuals with disabilities), barriers to medical care are compounded by multiple sources of disparity—including living in a rural area. Referring back to the Andersen and Aday Behavioral Model of Health Services Use, these populations have characteristics that predispose them to experiencing barriers when they need medical care services. These characteristics include sociodemographic factors such as poverty status, lower educational attainment, race/ethnicity, and physical or cognitive limitations. Taken in combination with their residence in rural communities, these subpopulations may experience particularly poor access to medical care, and as a result, have worse health outcomes, including elevated mortality.

Persons With Low Socioeconomic Status

Having low socioeconomic status places individuals at greater risk of experiencing multiple barriers to obtaining needed medical care. The connection between poverty and being uninsured, underinsured, or covered by Medicaid is an obvious example; however, persons in poverty face additional barriers. Individuals with lower income may find it challenging to make and keep medical appointments due to poor/unreliable transportation, no child care, sporadically available telephone access, employers that do not allow time off for medical appointments, or providers that are less experienced or less comfortable serving disadvantaged populations. For example, foregone care or treatment delays have occurred when low-income patients perceived that they would experience provider stigmatization for potentially sensitive conditions.[31] In other cases, providers may perceive that low-income rural patients do not value care, creating barriers on both the patient and provider side.[32]

Intertwined with issues of poverty, individuals with lower educational attainment face challenges in understanding the structure of the medical care system, how to access care, what medical options are available to them, and how to choose the treatment that best meets their needs.[33,34] Given that rural populations are generally poorer and have less formal education than their urban counterparts,[4] these barriers may be particularly common in rural areas. Combined with more global rural challenges of provider supply and health insurance coverage, poor individuals and those with less education that live in rural areas may find it especially challenging to have their medical needs met.

Racial and Ethnic Minority Groups

While rural populations are made up of a higher White, non-Hispanic population than are urban populations, there is still substantial variation in the racial and ethnic composition of rural communities across the country. Among members of racial and ethnic minority groups—and in communities where the concentration of minority populations is high—access to medical care is even worse than among White, non-Hispanic rural residents and communities. We limit the following discussion to the access-related issues faced by rural minorities; a detailed description of individual health outcome disparities faced by these groups is given in Chapter 14.

Racial and ethnic minority populations in rural areas are at high risk of being uninsured, experiencing financial barriers to health services, and having higher rates of chronic conditions and lower rates of service use.[3] Rural communities in which Blacks represent a majority of the population are much more likely than the average rural county to be a HPSA.[35] Black residents of rural areas are at particularly high risk of undetected chronic illness compared to Whites and urban residents and are less likely to obtain preventive care screenings.[35]

Shifting migration patterns in the United States have dramatically increased the size of the Latino population in rural areas. Between 1990 and 2010, the number of Latinos living in small towns and rural areas more than doubled, adding 1.6 million Latino residents to these communities. This growth was predominantly in the midwestern region of the country, although southern rural counties also saw a substantial increase in their Latino residents.[36] Interviews with Latino residents of these small, rural communities suggest that they face multiple barriers to care, including low income and high uninsurance rates. This group also reports difficulties understanding and navigating the country's complex medical care system, and in developing relationships with medical providers because of language and cultural barriers.[37] Although federally funded programs such as community health centers provide at least some primary care services for this population, many gaps remain—including access to specialty services, medications, and chronic disease management. Rural health experts believe that low provider supply in many rural areas particularly exacerbates access for Latino patients, since some providers may be concerned about the resource demands that interpreter services and the inability of some to pay for care may place on their already burdened practices.[38]

Compared to the rest of the U.S. population, American Indians and Alaskan Natives have high rates of morbidity and mortality.[39] At the same time, their access to medical care is affected by unique and sometimes complex service delivery systems. Traditionally covered by the federal programs of the Indian Health Service (IHS), current medical care systems serving American Indians and Alaskan Natives represent a combination of services provided and/or administered by IHS, the tribes and community-based providers.[40] Among all rural racial and ethnic minority groups, American Indians/Alaskan

Natives have the lowest rate of private health insurance coverage and the highest uninsured rate. Not surprisingly, they are also somewhat less likely than other racial–ethnic groups to have any medical care visits in a given year.[35] While most Native Americans and Alaskan Natives have at least some contact with a medical care provider annually, surveys of primary medical care providers for these groups indicate that they face enormous barriers obtaining needed specialty care services and that financial barriers are the primary challenge.[40]

SPECIAL PROGRAMS AND INNOVATIONS FOR RURAL ACCESS

Federal Programs

To address the shortage of health care professionals, the more limited financial resources of rural residents, and the geographic dispersion of rural populations, the federal government has implemented a number of programs aimed at improving access to rural medical care. Some of these programs, such as the State Medicare Rural Hospital Flexibility Program (the program that designates critical access hospitals) and the Rural Health Clinic Program, were designed specifically to maintain or increase access to medical care in rural communities. Other national strategies, such as the Health Resources and Services Administration's Health Center Program (the program that funds the community health centers discussed previously), target both rural and urban areas of the country, but are important sources of health care access for many rural residents, particularly those with limited financial resources.

Critical Access Hospitals and Rural Health Clinics

Established in 1997 as part of the Balanced Budget Act, the State Medicare Rural Hospital Flexibility (Flex) Grant Program is designed to promote the financial viability of small rural hospitals and ensure access to at least some basic hospital services for rural residents, particularly emergency room access. The flex program allows states to designate certain small rural hospitals (no more than 25 inpatient beds) as critical access hospitals because no other hospital is within a reasonable driving distance (generally 35 miles), or because the hospital is otherwise essential to medical care access for that community. The flex program was created in response to a large number of rural hospital closures in the late 1980s and early 1990s following a shift in the Medicare program (and later private insurance) away from paying hospitals' actual costs and to paying predefined rates based on a list of specific conditions and services (called diagnostic related groups, or DRGs). Many small, particularly rural, hospitals lacked the necessary economic efficiency to respond to these new payments and subsequently closed. Under the flex program, however, critical access hospitals can bill Medicare (and in many states Medicaid)[41] for the actual cost of a hospital stay, within reason, plus an additional 1% above these costs. In addition, physicians (including psychiatrists) that provide services through critical access hospitals that are located in HPSAs are eligible for bonus payments for these services. As of September 2012, there were 1,330 critical access hospitals in the United States.[42]

In an effort to address the limited availability of primary care in rural areas, the federal government established the Rural Health Clinics Program in 1977 as an amendment to the Social Security Act. Unlike community health centers created by the Health Center Act (described in the following section), rural health clinics do not receive grant funds to cover uninsured or underinsured rural residents. However, like critical access hospitals, rural health clinics are entitled to enhanced reimbursement through Medicare and Medicaid for the primary care services that they provide to rural residents. In order to be established as a rural health clinic, a primary care provider (ranging from solo physician practice to hospital-owned primary care provider group practice) must be located in a rural area that is also categorized as a "medically underserved" community by the federal government. In addition to these criteria, rural health clinics are required to employ at least one midlevel medical care practitioner such as a physician's assistant or nurse practitioner. These "physician extender" providers are an important component of the rural primary care infrastructure and some studies suggest that they are more willing than physicians to practice in rural and underserved communities.[43]

Community Health Centers

Established in 1975 under Section 330 of the federal *Public Health Services Act*, the Health Center Program provides grant support to public or private nonprofit community organizations that provide primary medical care and other services to low-income and medically underserved populations. More recently, funding for community health centers has been substantially increased under the federal Affordable Care Act of 2010 (health care reform). Also known as federally qualified health centers (FQHCs), these organizations must demonstrate that they serve geographic areas of high poverty and low medical provider availability. As a result, most FQHCs are located in poor, inner-city urban and rural communities. Unlike critical access hospitals and rural health clinics that stem from explicitly rural programs, FQHCs are part of a broader federal effort to improve access to medical care in both urban and rural areas. Yet, because of the relatively greater proportion of rural areas that are poor and medically underserved, estimates suggest that nearly 30% of FQHCs are located in a rural county (compared to roughly 20% of the U.S. population overall).[44] In addition, some medical centers created under the Health Center Program target special populations, including migrant and seasonal farm workers. Given the rural connection to agriculture, migrant health centers have a large rural presence in many parts of the country. However, the distribution of FQHCs in rural areas varies substantially among states due to differing rates of participation in the program—for example, in 2008 Alaska had more than 130 rural FQHCs, while Wyoming had only 5.[22]

Private and Community-Based Efforts to Promote Rural Access

In addition to formal programs developed by the government to improve access to medical care in rural and other underserved areas, hundreds of small-scale innovations have emerged from local medical care and community-based organizations to better meet the needs of rural populations. These interventions range from allowing different medical professionals to practice with greater professional flexibility, to bringing more care into rural areas through mobile and technology-based distance strategies such as telehealth (see Chapter 17). While further study is needed to fully understand how these programs may improve the medical care access and health status of rural populations, they offer new ways of thinking about how to serve hard-to-reach populations in resource-poor environments.

Creative Deployment of Medical Professionals

In some respects the medical care sector has been characterized by clear scopes of practice and strong adherence to traditional roles of different professional types. In trying to creatively meet the medical needs of underserved populations, rural communities have sometimes led the way in promoting greater role flexibility and allowing paraprofessionals to deliver services that might be outside their normal scopes of practice. For example, in 2006, the Livingston Help for Seniors program was developed out of recognition that isolation and limited contact with medical providers are a great risk to the health and safety of rural seniors. In response, this program began using emergency medical technicians (EMTs) to screen rural-dwelling older adults for depression, medication-related problems, and falls when they respond to an emergency call. A case manager reviews the screening results and contacts at-risk individuals to schedule a free home visit that includes a psychosocial assessment and referrals to needed medical and social services. While mental health and medication screenings are not typically within the professional purview of EMT/first responders, evaluations of the program suggest that it has enhanced access to these services for at-risk, rural-dwelling older adults and has generated high levels of satisfaction among those served.[45]

In a similarly creative model, the Improving Health Among Rural Montanans program was established in 2002 to incorporate existing medical professionals and students into new ways of delivering care in rural areas. The program operates in rural and frontier communities to identify and train pharmacists and students from various disciplines on how to administer screening tests for osteoporosis, diabetes, hyperlipidemia, hypertension, and lung function. The program then transports screening equipment to these areas to be used during screening clinics that are held for low-income and underserved populations. By redeploying pharmacy professionals and taking advantage of the skill sets possessed by students in various medical professions, the program has enhanced access to health care screenings, identified unmet health needs, and increased the number of trained professionals in remote locations.[45]

Mobile Services

Given that brick and mortar facilities such as hospitals and medical care offices and clinics are costly and slow to develop, multiple rural communities have relied on mobile health services as a way of reaching underserved rural populations for certain basic primary care services. For example, a Maine-based program has used a mobile van to conduct hypertension and diabetes screenings throughout rural areas of the state. Data from this program suggest that it was an effective tool for increasing the rate of disease screening services available to rural residents.[46] In a similar model, follow-up to clinic-based comprehensive care has been provided successfully to rural veterans in southwestern Virginia through a mobile health and wellness program.[47] Mobile health clinics staffed by teams of multidisciplined medical professionals, students, and lay community advisors have been used to provide culturally appropriate, accessible care to Latino immigrant populations.[48]

Distance and Telehealth Programs

Models of delivering care via telephone or other telecommunication medium such as video "telehealth" have been promoted as options to increase access to medical care in rural communities. While research to date has been limited on the quality and effectiveness of these distance methods of providing medical care, there is some evidence that they may improve access and outcomes for rural populations. For example, a behavioral weight loss program delivered by phone to groups of rural Kansas women appeared to be cost effective and result in measurable weight loss.[49] Telemedicine innovations like videoconferencing, telephone, secure messaging (e-mail), and the Internet have been used successfully to provide medical consultation to rural primary care patients receiving services for depression and other mental health issues.[50] First implemented in 2006, the Michigan Stroke Network uses telemedicine to enable round-the-clock access to stroke specialists in 30 hospitals and one freestanding emergency department throughout the state. Since its inception, the program has assessed more than nearly 1,000 patients and has assisted hospitals in expediting patient transfers to stroke centers for comprehensive stroke treatment and management.[45] For additional details on telehealth procedures and effective telehealth programs, please see Chapter 17.

CONCLUSION

Rural residents face many barriers to accessing appropriate medical care, including lower income, lower rates of private health insurance coverage, and lower supply of primary and specialty medical care providers. They must often try to coordinate care across long distances with few supportive resources. Taken in combination with rural residence, certain characteristics such as poverty and racial or ethnic minority status may place a rural person at particularly heightened risk of not receiving adequate preventive screenings or treatment for acute or chronic conditions. As a result of these barriers, the health and well-being of rural populations may be compromised. In recognition of the challenges that rural areas face in terms of medical care access, multiple federal agencies have targeted rural residents as a "priority" population and programs such as critical access hospitals, rural health clinics, and community health centers/FQHCs exist to augment the medical care infrastructure of rural communities. Other strategies aimed at using mobile vans and technology to reduce the geographic distance between rural areas and better-resourced urban and suburban areas show some promise and should be investigated further.

REFERENCES

1. Eberhardt MS, Ingram DD, Makuc DM, et al. *Urban and Rural Health Chartbook. Health United States, 2001* (PHS 01-1232). Hyattsville, MD: National Center for Health Statistics; August 2001.
2. Hartley D. Rural health disparities, population health, and rural culture. *Am J Public Health.* 2004;94(10):1675–1678.
3. Bennett KJ, Olatosi B, Probst JC. *Health Disparities: A Rural-Urban Chartbook.* Columbia, SC: South Carolina Rural Health Research Center; 2008. http://rhr.sph.sc.edu/report/(7-3)%20Health%20Disparities%20A%20Rural%20Urban%20Chartbook%20%20Distribution%20Copy.pdf.
4. Ziller EC, Coburn AF, Loux SL, et al. *Health Insurance Coverage in Rural America: A Chartbook.* Washington, DC: Kaiser Commission on Medicaid and the Uninsured; 2003. http://www.kff.org/uninsured/4093.cfm.
5. Pleis JR, Lethbridge-Cejku M. Summary health statistics for U.S. adults: National Health Interview Survey, 2006. *Vital Health Stat 10.* 2007;(235):1–153.
6. Larson SL, Fleishman JA. Rural-urban differences in usual source of care and ambulatory service use: analyses of national data using Urban Influence Codes. *Med Care.* 2003;41(7 suppl):III65–III74.
7. Higginbotham JC, Moulder J, Currier M. Rural v. urban aspects of cancer: first-year data from the Mississippi Central Cancer Registry. *Fam Community Health.* 2001;24(2):1–9.
8. Institute of Medicine, Committee on Monitoring Access to Personal Health Care Services; Millman M, ed. *Access to Health Care in America.* Washington, DC: National Academy Press; 1993.
9. Aday LA, Andersen R. A framework for the study of access to medical care. *Health Serv Res.* 1974;9(3):208-220.
10. Andersen RM. Revisiting the behavioral model and access to medical care: does it matter? *J Health Soc Behav.* 1995;36(1):1–10.
11. Gelberg L, Andersen RM, Leake BD. The behavioral model for vulnerable populations: application to medical care use and outcomes for homeless people. *Health Serv Res.* 2000;34(6):1273–1302.
12. Andersen RM, Davidson PL. Improving access to care in America: individual and contextual indicators. In: Andersen RM, Rice TH, Kominski GF, eds. *Changing the U.S. Health Care System.* 2nd ed. San Francisco, CA: Jossey-Bass; 2001:3–30.
13. United States Administration on Aging. *Statistics on the Aging Population.* Washington, DC: US Administration on Aging; 2007.
14. Eberhardt M, Ingram D, Makuc D, et al. *Health, United States, 2001: Urban and Rural Chartbook.* Hyattsville, MD: National Center for Health Statistics; 2001.

15. Befort CA, Nazir N, Perri MG. Prevalence of obesity among adults from rural and urban areas of the United States: findings from NHANES (2005–2008). *J Rural Health*. 2012;28:392–397.

16. Lenardson JD, Ziller EC, Coburn AF, et al. *Profile of Rural Health Insurance Coverage: A Chartbook*. Portland, ME: University of Southern Maine, Muskie School of Public Service, Maine Rural Health Research Center; 2009. http://muskie.usm .maine.edu/Publications/rural/Rural-Health-Insurance-Chartbook-2009.pdf.

17. Coburn AF, Kilbreth EH, Long SH, Marquis MS. Urban-rural differences in employer-based health insurance coverage of workers. *Med Care Res Rev*. 1998;55(4):484–496.

18. Ziller EC, Lenardson JD, Coburn AF. Health care access and use among the rural uninsured. *J Health Care Poor Underserved*. 2012;23(3):1327–1345.

19. Probst JC, Bellinger JD, Walsemann KM, Hardin J, Glover SH. Higher risk of death in rural Blacks and Whites than urbanites is related to lower incomes, education, and health coverage. *Health Aff (Millwood)*. 2011;30(10):1872–1879. http://content .healthaffairs.org/content/30/10/1872.abstract.

20. Bisgaier J, Rhodes KV. Auditing access to specialty care for children with public insurance. *N Engl J Med*. 2011;364:2324–2333.

21. Ziller EC, Coburn AF, Yousefian AE. Out-of-pocket health spending and the rural underinsured. *Health Aff (Millwood)*. 2006;25(6):1688–1699. http://content .healthaffairs.org/cgi/content/abstract/25/6/1688.

22. Fordyce MA, Chen FM, Doescher MP, et al. *2005 Physician Supply and Distribution in Rural Areas of the United States* (Final Report #116). Seattle, WA: WWAMI Rural Health Research Center; 2007. http://depts.washington.edu/uwrhrc/uploads/ RHRC%20FR116%20Fordyce.pdf.

23. National Advisory Committee on Rural Health and Human Services. *Rural Public Health: Issues and Considerations, A Report to the Secretary, U.S. Dept. of Health and Human Services*. Rockville, MD: Department of Health and Human Services; February 2000.

24. Jones CA, Parker TS, Ahearn M. Taking the pulse of rural health care: new health information technologies hold promise for improving health care in remote areas. *Amber Waves*. 2009;7(3):10–15. http://webarchives.cdlib.org/sw1vh5dg3r/ http://ers.usda.gov/AmberWaves/September09/PDF/RuralHealth.pdf.

25. Hart LG, Salsberg E, Phillips DM, Lishner DM. Rural health care providers in the United States. *J Rural Health*. 2002;18:211–231.

26. Agency for Healthcare Quality and Research. *2006 National Health Disparities Report* (AHRQ Publication No. 07-0012). Rockville, MD: US Department of Health and Human Services; 2006.

27. Gamm L, Hutchison L, Dabney B, Dorsey A, eds. *Rural Healthy People 2010: A Companion Document to Healthy People 2010*. College Station, TX: Texas A&M University System Health Science Center, School of Rural Health, Southwest Rural Health Research Center; 2004:3.

28. Mohatt D. *Rural Mental Health: Challenges and Opportunities Caring for the Country*. Presentation at the All Programs Meeting Conference, Federal Office of Rural Health Policy; August 21, 2003; Rockville, MD.

29. O'Grady MJ, Mueller CD, Wilensky GR. Essential research issues in rural health: the state rural health directors' perspective. *Policy Anal Brief W Ser*. 2002; 5(1):1–4.

30. Gamm L, Hutchinson L. Rural health priorities in America: where you stand depends on where you sit. *J Rural Health*. 2003;19(3):209–213.

31. Jesse DE, Dolbier CL, Blanchard A. Barriers to seeking help and treatment suggestions for prenatal depressive symptoms: focus groups with rural low-income women. *Issues Ment Health Nurs.* 2008;29(1):3–19.

32. Shell R, Tudiver F. Barriers to cancer screening by rural Appalachian primary care providers. *J Rural Health.* 2004;20(4):368–373.

33. Pirisi A. Low health literacy prevents equal access to care. *Lancet.* 2000;356 (9244):1828.

34. Merriman B, Ades T, Seffrin JR. Health literacy in the information age: communicating cancer information to patients and families. *CA Cancer J Clin.* 2002;52(3): 130–133.

35. Probst JC, Moore CG, Glover SH, Samuels ME. Person and place: the compounding effects of race/ethnicity and rurality on health. *Am J Public Health.* 2004;94(10):1695–1703.

36. *Author Tabulations From U.S. Census 1990 and 2010 SF-1 Files.* 2012. U.S. Bureau of the Census. http://www2.census.gov/census_2010/04-Summary_File_1/National; http://www2.census.gov/census_2000/datasets/Summary_File_1/0Final_ National

37. Blewett LA, Smaida SA, Fuentes C, Zuehlke EU. Health care needs of the growing Latino population in rural America: focus group findings in one midwestern state. 2003;19:33–41.

38. Casey MM, Blewett LA, Call KT. Providing health care to Latino immigrants: community-based efforts in the rural midwest. *Am J Public Health.* 2004;94(10):1709–1711.

39. Roubideaux Y, Dixon M. *Promises to Keep: Public Health Policy for American Indians and Alaska Natives in the 21st Century.* Washington, DC: American Public Health Association.

40. Baldwin L-M, Hollow WB, Casey S, et al. Access to specialty health care for rural American Indians in two states. *J Rural Health.* 2008;24:269–278.

41. Radford A, Hamon M, Nelligan C. *States' Use of Cost-Based Reimbursement for Medicaid Services at Critical Access Hospitals* (Findings Brief 94). UNC-Chapel Hill, Cecil G. Sheps Center for Health Services Research, North Carolina Rural Health Research Policy Analysis Center; April 2010. http://www.shepscenter.unc.edu/ rural/pubs/finding_brief/FB94.pdf.

42. Flex Monitoring Team. *CAH Information* [Web Page]. September 30, 2012. Accessed October 30, 2012. http://www.flexmonitoring.org/cahlistRA.cgi

43. Dehn RW. The distribution of physicians, advanced practice nurses, and physician assistants in Iowa. *J Physician Assist Educ.* 2006;17(1):36–38.

44. Hartley D, Gale J, Leighton A, et al. *Safety Net Activities of Independent Rural Health Clinics* (Working Paper No. 44). Portland, ME: University of Southern Maine, Muskie School of Public Service, Maine Rural Health Research Center; September 2010. http://muskie.usm.maine.edu/Publications/rural/WP43/Rural-Health-Clinics-Safety-Net.pdf.

45. Agency for Healthcare Research and Quality. *AHRQ Health Care Innovations Exchange* [Web Page]. October 10, 2012. Accessed October 23, 2012. http://www .innovations.ahrq.gov/content.aspx?id=2260

46. Harris DE, Hamel L, Aboueissa AM, Johnson D. A cardiovascular disease risk factor screening program designed to reach rural residents of Maine, USA. *Rural Remote Health.* 2011;11(3):1–15.

47. Therien J. Establishing a mobile health and wellness program for rural veterans. *Nurs Clin North Am.* 2000;35(2):499–505.

48. Sherrill W, Crew L, Mayo RB, et al. Educational and health services innovation to improve care for rural Hispanic communities in the USA. *Rural Remote Health.* 2005;5(4):402.
49. Befort CA, Donnelly JE, Sullivan DK, Ellerbeck EF, Perri MG. Group versus individual phone-based obesity treatment for rural women. *Eat Behav.* 2010;11(1):11–17.
50. Hilty DM, Yellowlees PM, Cobb HC, et al. Models of telepsychiatric consultation: liaison service to rural primary care. *Psychosomatics.* 2006;47(2):152–157.

CHAPTER 3

Public Health Workforce Issues in Rural Areas

Suzanne R. Hawley, Shirley A. Orr, and
Theresa St. Romain

In a 2002 study of rural public health policy and capacity issues, authors Berkowitz, Ivory, and Morris identified several areas of shortfall that could "impact . . . the responsiveness of the rural public health system to emerging threats to health."[1, p. 187] Noting fragmented financing, inconsistent clinical services, limited information technology capacity, and the exclusion of rural public health leaders from statewide policy making, the authors conclude that "these issues can be characterized as system deficits and have serious consequences for population health."[1, p. 187]

More than 10 years later, the rural public health workforce has seen significant progress in technology and, supported by the national public health accreditation movement, in the uniformity of services provided. However, each change brings new consequences and responsibilities. This chapter provides an overview of the rural public health workforce and its present challenges; aspects of present-day practice, including competency development, training, and social capital; and strategies for sustaining the rural public health workforce in this era of rapid transformation.

OVERVIEW AND PRESENT CHALLENGES OF THE RURAL PUBLIC HEALTH WORKFORCE

The rural public health workforce faces many constraints—the first of which is simply identifying its composition and scope. Enumeration of the public health workforce as a whole proves difficult due to the diversity of agencies and occupations that contribute to public health. Still, it is clear that work-force shortages exist, with rural shortages being the most severe. The rural work environment is distinct from that of urban public health practice, and the workers themselves have less access to local professional support networks as well as education and training opportunities. These disparities have implications for recruitment and retention, two ongoing challenges faced by rural public health agencies.

Enumerating the Rural Public Health Workforce

The rural public health workforce is significant from a national perspective; two-thirds of the nation's local health departments (LHDs) serve fewer than 50,000 people.[2] The diversity of the public health workforce makes enumeration of these rural workers difficult, but nonetheless essential. In 2000, the Health Resources and Services Administration (HRSA) conducted the first nationwide enumeration in 20 years, and the last to date. Since the 1980 enumeration, HRSA found "an apparent erosion of public health capacity," though "the absence of a clear national policy on definitions complicates the process." As a result, HRSA concluded that "analysis of trends is virtually impossible."[3, pp. 273, 271] Approximately 34% of the total public health work-force in 2000 served the public at the local level; a further 33% worked at state-level agencies, 19% federal, and 14% at other agencies related to public health, such as university programs.[3]

Not surprisingly, these workers were unevenly geographically distributed. Though the national average is 156 public health workers to 100,000 population members, regions tended to be far over or under this average. The Midwest—the 16 states of regions V, VII, and VIII—had the lowest proportion of public health workers nationwide.[3] Though the federal report did not isolate rural data, a cross reference with state-level data indicates that 13 of those 16 understaffed states also have higher-than-average percentages of nonmetropolitan (i.e., rural) inhabitants.[4] In states with a decentralized public health system, such as the state of Kansas, shortages are exacerbated, since LHDs have historically relied on local agency-level staffing. Declining rural populations result in decreasing tax bases for funding public services, while growing percentages of aging residents result in increased demand for services (see Chapter 16 for a more detailed discussion of the impact of the aging population on rural health demands).

Statewide averages can suppress workforce trends that are unique to rural areas. Even in states with no *overall* shortage of workers, rural areas of the state still tend to experience regional or local staffing shortages, while urban areas possess a surplus.[5,6] A county-level study in Nebraska found that the number of actively employed registered nurses exceeded need in the state's urban areas almost every year, while the most remote areas experienced the greatest gap between workforce and need. Vacancies accounted for only one-third of the estimated gap, demonstrating how workforce needs can be consistently underestimated.[5] In an environment of constant understaffing, rural workers could be expected to experience greater job stress and concerns about patient safety than their urban counterparts—factors leading to turnover and exacerbating the shortfall, especially considering that rural vacancies were found to take 60% longer to fill.[5] Since nurses are the largest single professional group within the public health workforce,[2,3] tracking nursing shortages would provide helpful evidence of rural—and potentially urban—areas suffering from public health staffing shortages.

Characteristics of the Rural Public Health Workforce

Just as the rural work environment differs from urban public health practice settings, so in some ways do the workers themselves. While the rural health workforce is no less diverse than the public health workforce as a whole, this subset does possess some distinct characteristics. Rural public health workers are more likely to be part-time and less likely to have a background in public health.[2] Small/rural LHDs are more often led by nurses, compared to the physicians or administrators that lead larger/urban LHDs.[7] Nurse leadership has historically been found to be associated with a greater breadth of service and direct patient care (as one would expect in a clinical-service–oriented rural agency), but less environmental health or regulatory activity (which is usually performed by dedicated employees that may simply not be a part of rural agencies).[7]

The population served may contribute to the distinct culture of rural public health practice. Previous research has identified a set of rural values that include an emphasis on self-reliance and an association of health with productivity.[8] Nurses that work alone in rural and remote offices have been found to display significantly higher competency in the Community Dimensions of Practice public health competency domain.[9] However, rural public health workers may feel deprived of a support network, experiencing isolation and role diffusion.[8]

Recruiting and Retaining Rural Public Health Workers

Rural public health staffing is an ongoing challenge, but of great importance amidst the growing effort to offer the essential services of public health.[10] As has already been seen, staffing shortages may be ingrained in the rural public health system, which affects not only the quality of service provided, but also the recruitment and retention of providers.[5] One study found that health worker retention is the same in health professional shortage areas (HPSAs) and non-HPSAs, indicating that shortages come from less successful recruitment strategies.[11] However, so-called "coercive" recruitment measures, such as J-1 waivers, loan forgiveness, or other financial incentives for workers who elect to practice in underserved areas, have also been connected to lowered retention.[12–14]

One possible reason for this low retention following recruitment is unsatisfactory integration of the provider into the community.[14] If rural health workers are encouraged to think of their positions primarily in economic terms, then they may view their years in rural practice as a career stepping stone, leaving to practice in a larger (and more lucrative) community when the contracted term is over. In addition, the coercive aspect in and of itself implies that rural practice is undesirable and that workers who choose rural practice must be rewarded. While such incentives are indeed critical to addressing workforce disparities, economic orientations may unknowingly diminish or ignore community of practice/quality of life issues in a rural setting. Not surprisingly, research has found job satisfaction to be the most important factor in retention, but this satisfaction is rooted in employee support rather than direct compensation.[15] Workplace daycare and tuition reimbursement, for example, contribute greatly to job satisfaction and are only indirectly related to salary.[15] It is clear that the rural public health workforce requires a support system—and also that the recruitment and retention practices of the urban workforce may not be best suited for their rural counterparts.

ASPECTS OF RURAL HEALTH PRACTICE

In its 2003 publication *Who Will Keep the Public Healthy?: Educating Public Health Professionals for the 21st Century*, the Institute of Medicine concluded that a well-educated public health workforce is the key to ensuring that public health services are effective.[16] Education and training underpin the primary concerns of public health agencies today, since besides providing the 10 essential services they must also be well poised for accreditation and the related concepts of capacity development and quality improvement. In this section, those issues will be considered within the context of rural health practice, which requires unique resources and methods—and therefore a different model for education and training.

Providing Essential Services: Expectations of the Rural Public Health Workforce

In September 2011, the Public Health Accreditation Board began nationwide voluntary accreditation of state, local, and tribal health departments. Intended as a means of ensuring performance standards regardless of agency size or population served, accreditation "demonstrates the capacity of the public health department to deliver the three core functions and the ten essential services of public health."[17, p. 5] In an atmosphere of declining financial and staff resources, performance standards and quality improvement become more essential as well as potentially more difficult to attain. Some rural LHDs collaborated to meet goals jointly, a process known as "regionalization," after successfully using this method to meet emergency preparedness standards[18] or provide workforce training.[19]

Regionalization represents only one potential type of collaboration that is needed. Academic-practice partnerships are also important collaborations, bringing together the research strengths of the former with the rich data of the latter.[20] Because academic centers tend to be in urban areas, such partnerships tend also to be urban–rural partnerships, allowing programs for rural health workers and students to be continuously reevaluated and fine-tuned.[20–22] To support rural agencies in both their day-to-day function and the accreditation process, trainings for current workers as well as educational programs have become increasingly competency oriented. Tracking of competency—that is, knowledge, skill, or ability—has become a standard method of showing pre-/postimprovement, which is the quantifiable evidence of success needed by funders and administrators, as well as a necessary step in the accreditation process.

Training and Educating the Rural Health Workforce

The shared purpose of training and education, at its heart, is to ensure that workers have the necessary competency to provide the core functions and essential services of public health. General job training, program-specific training, and continuing education for licensure are needs for all public health workers, but rural workers experience significant barriers in access to such training.[19] These include limited budgets for training costs, prohibitive travel time, or lack of staff to cover shifts during worker trainings.[8] Even if the same resources are available to urban and rural public health workers, those in the rural environment tend to be more widely spread.[13]

As a result, rural public health workers might be tempted to complete training and continuing education that is convenient or inexpensive, instead of choosing courses that best fit their needs. The broad-based skill of information retrieval may be a rural health worker's best tool,[8] and one that could be developed through academic-practice partnerships. One such academic-practice partnership, the Kansas Public Health Leadership Institute, included a mixed-method competency-based structure intended to minimize travel for rural participants. In this environment, rural workers in Kansas experienced significantly greater competency increases in several domains than their urban counterparts, indicating a pent-up need for relevant competency-based training among rural public health workers.[23]

Leadership training is of particular importance for rural workers, because rural health practice is so autonomous that most workers will serve in a leadership role at some point. According to Berkowitz et al., "Leadership is particularly important to efforts designed to pull community health, managed care, and public health in rural America into a more interactive system."[1, p. 195] A key aspect of public health leadership training, and a concept highly relevant to the rural public health workforce, is that of *social capital*. Social capital is commonly defined by Putnam as "connections among individuals," or "social networks and the norms of reciprocity and trustworthiness that arise from them."[24, p. 19]

In the rural environment, connections and collaborations are less likely to occur organically; a community-level study of Kansas social capital found that rural communities reported significantly lower levels of social capital than urban communities on 9 of 11 indicators.[25] However, training intended to develop collaborations and linkages between workers from different agencies—such as statewide public health leadership training—has been found to significantly increase characteristic indicators of social capital.[26] In applied practice, too, drawing on social capital for a participatory research approach to survey-taking greatly increased participant response rate.[27] Because rural health workers function as an integral part of their community of practice,[28] the value of intangible social capital connections may far exceed the economic resources available.

KEEPING THE RURAL PUBLIC HEALTHY: SUSTAINING THE RURAL WORKFORCE

A healthy public requires a healthy workforce, and in an atmosphere of worker shortages and limited training opportunities, it may seem as though the rural public health system is ailing. However, recent educational developments offer hope, as interdisciplinary collaboratives have created a pipeline of students better prepared for rural practice. Such programs also provide a larger professional connection to others in the field. Worker retention has traditionally been considered an economic issue, but in rural communities, quality of life issues and professional networks are at least as important. The rural public health workforce is not simply a scaled-down version of the urban workforce; the difference is one of culture.

Collaborative Education: Building a Strong Pipeline for the Future Workforce

There is some indication that "culture shock" might strike urban-educated students sent to practice in rural areas.[29] When educational programs intentionally prepare students for rural practice, though, employment outcomes improve. Designing a program specifically to prepare nursing, medical, and public health students for rural practice has been shown to result in significantly higher rates of rural practice and retention.[21] Since participation in the study program was elective, it is likely that the study population was more interested in rural practice to begin with; however, the opportunity for pre-job learning about rural practice was certainly beneficial. More than other health care workers, rural health providers need collaborative as well as clinical skills. For isolated rural employees, community connections are a necessary part of practice[9]—not only for improved patient care and outcomes, but for greater collegial support and job satisfaction.

Increasingly, educational programs intended to prepare students for rural health practice have incorporated collaborative, interdisciplinary components that foster characteristics of social capital.[21,30,31] For example, when interdisciplinary training was incorporated into a quality improvement course on rural health care, post-course follow-up found significantly improved attitudes toward interdisciplinary collaboration.[30] By entering the rural public health workforce already aware of the need for a support system, as well as how to develop one, these students will be well poised to practice effectively within the unique rural public health system.

Such specialized educational programs focus on fit between provider and practice—a sort of prerecruitment for the rural public health system. Successful rural recruitment seems to result from these "normative" policies rather than "coercive" economic incentives, though a combination of incentives and supportive structures (such as Area Health Education Centers [AHECs]) may encourage retention.[13] The National Health Service Corps places primary care physicians in rural areas[32]; many of these physicians will serve as county public health officers while simultaneously developing private practices. Due to this intersection between allopathic medicine and public health, further integration of public health education within medical and allied health educational training programs is recommended.

Rural Work, Rural Life: The Connection Between Career and Community

In rural practice, a community's and a provider's needs often become closely intertwined. The rural value of self-reliance discourages clients from seeking services from a stranger, but supports interaction with a trusted neighbor.[8] The more a practitioner is integrated into a community, therefore, the better service he or she will be able to provide to that community. Positive caregiving experiences frequently result in "positive gossip" through closely knit rural communities, which further increase trust in the provider.[28]

To a much greater degree than their urban counterparts, rural health workers occupy positions of status and respect in their communities. In a city with dozens of doctors, a nurse practitioner may garner little professional respect; in a rural community, the same worker is likely to serve in a leadership role as health department administrator or as a major provider of clinical services.[28] Such professional respect is an important contributor to job satisfaction, as well as to overall quality of life—key factors in a health worker's decision to remain in a rural community.[28,33,34] While compensation may be lower in rural areas, health workers also enjoy greater autonomy and are recognized as community assets.[28]

This close connection between worker and community can have its drawbacks, however. Role diffusion, or the blurring of personal and professional roles, can occur, and the desirable aspects of autonomy can sometimes transform into feelings of professional isolation.[8,35] Though the struggle for personal and professional balance is hardly unique to rural health providers, these downsides may be ameliorated through familiarity with the realities of rural life. For instance, a survey of rural female physicians found that 7 of 10 came from a rural background themselves.[35] Training "homegrown" health workers may, in fact, be rural public health's greatest option for sustainability and growth. Community colleges represent an important avenue for early professional education; health courses could offer rural "success stories" and connect students with resources for mentorships.[8,28] On a national level, the

National Rural Health Association (NHRA) maintains a networking site called NRHA Connect.[36] Other resources are unique to a region, state, or even county. The Southern Rural Access Program serves as a resource clearinghouse and grant-making entity for eight largely rural Southern states.[37] In Kansas, the Kansas Association of Local Health Departments serves as a unifying nonprofit for the state's 100 independent LHDs,[38] while the state health department maintains a Bureau of Community Health Systems with further rural health resources.[39] Additionally, the Kansas Public Health Association (KPHA) brings together researchers, health service providers, administrators, teachers, and other health workers from all areas of the state in a unique, multidisciplinary environment of professional exchange, study, and action.[40] A key role for mentors could be helping students or early career workers navigate the complex network of resources.

In a study of rural health agency sustainability, Wright found four key contributing factors: physician advocates, innovative practices, organizational flexibility, and community integration.[41] In other words, a well-trained workforce, rich in connections between health disciplines, is a vital component of a sustainable system. This goal is by no means out of reach for the rural public health workforce. Rural educational collaboratives, community incentives, and competency-oriented training programs are already in place. Innovations such as mobile health clinics and telehealth, emerging organizational structures such as multi-county rural public health regions, and governmental policies like water fluoridation can also support the public health workforce—and, in turn, the health of the rural public in the future.[42]

The challenge, as always, is locating and retrieving available resources. Increasing the resources available is unlikely in an environment of shrinking budgets and heightened preparedness and quality improvement responsibilities. Instead, a priority should be increasing awareness of and access to existing resources, as well as cross-jurisdictional sharing of resources, for the growth and development of collective capacity among professionals and agencies serving rural communities. In addition, alternative sources of funding, such as foundations, are critical to ongoing sustainability as federal funding sources have declined.

CONCLUSION

The rural public health workforce is diverse and isolated by nature, yet conversely, rural health workers tend to flourish when they are closely knit with their community of practice. A rural worker's access to training is far more limited than that of an urban worker, and perhaps because of this, the rural worker is likely to benefit more when given relevant training. Such seeming contradictions are evidence that the practice of rural public health is distinct from that of urban public health.

Current trends in public health, including accreditation and the aging population, have drawn increased attention to the rural health workforce. Articles of interest on enumeration include recent methodology studies led by Gebbie,[43,44] as well as state-level surveys that provide detailed workforce information.[5,27] In Kansas, an academic-practice team has overseen the development of competency-based leadership training that has not only increased participant competency and social capital,[20,23,26] but also has fostered 170 practice-based research projects as of April 2012. Participants have offered compelling feedback that the supportive professional network developed through training has had a positive impact on their careers. To their increased competency and social capital, they attribute increased retention in the public health workforce and greatly improved morale in the midst of shrinking resources. There is great potential in collaboration across organizations and professional disciplines, an approach to education and practice that will best leverage the needs of a diverse and challenged rural public health workforce.

REFERENCES

1. Berkowitz B, Ivory J, Morris T. Rural public health: policy and research opportunities. *J Rural Health*. 2002;18(suppl):186–196.
2. Rosenblatt RA, Casey S, Richardson M. Rural-urban differences in the public health workforce: local health departments in 3 rural Western states. *Am J Public Health*. 2002;92(7):1102–1105.
3. Health Resources and Services Administration. *The Public Health Workforce Enumeration 2000*. In: US Department of Health and Human Services, ed. Washington, DC: 2000.
4. Kaiser Family Foundation. Population distribution by metropolitan status, states (2009–2010), U.S. (2010). n.d. http://statehealthfacts.org/comparemapdetail.jsp?ind=18&cat=1&sub=4&yr=252&typ=2. Accessed April 9, 2012.
5. Cramer M, Nienaber J, Helget P, Agrawal S. Comparative analysis of urban and rural nursing workforce shortages in Nebraska hospitals. *Policy Polit Nurs Pract*. 2006;7(4):248–260.
6. O'Grady MJ, Mueller CD, Wilensky GR. Essential research issues in rural health: the state rural health directors' perspective. *Policy Anal Brief W Ser*. 2002;5(1):1–4.
7. Bekemeier B, Jones M. Relationships between local public health agency functions and agency leadership and staffing: a look at nurses. *J Public Health Manag Pract*. 2010;16(2):E8–E16.
8. McCoy C. Professional development in rural nursing: challenges and opportunities. *J Contin Educ Nurs*. 2009;40(3):128–131.
9. Bigbee JL, Gehrke P, Otterness N. Public health nurses in rural/frontier one-nurse offices. *Rural Remote Health*. 2009;9(4):1282.
10. Centers for Disease Control and Prevention. National Public Health Performance Standards Program (NPHPSP): 10 essential public health services. 2010. http://www.cdc.gov/nphpsp/essentialServices.html. Accessed April 6, 2012.
11. Pathman DE, Konrad TR, Dann R, Koch G. Retention of primary care physicians in rural health professional shortage areas. *Am J Public Health*. 2004;94(10):1723–1729.
12. Bauer K. Distributive justice and rural healthcare: a case for e-health. *Int J Appl Philos*. 2003;17(2):241–252.
13. Ricketts TC. Workforce issues in rural areas: a focus on policy equity. *Am J Public Health*. 2005;95(1):42–48.
14. Crouse BJ, Munson RL. The effect of the physician J-1 visa waiver on rural Wisconsin. *WMJ*. 2006;105(67):16–20.

15. Stratton TD, Dunkin JW, Juhl N, Geller JM. Retainment incentives in three rural practice settings: variations in job satisfaction among staff registered nurses. *Appl Nurs Res.* 1995;8(2):73–80.

16. Gebbie K, Rosenstock L, Hernandez LM, eds. *Who Will Keep the Public Healthy?: Educating Public Health Professionals for the 21st Century.* Washington, DC: National Academies Press; 2003.

17. Public Health Accreditation Board. *Guide to National Public Health Department Accreditation, Version 1.0.* Alexandria, VA: 2011.

18. Wetta-Hall R, Berg-Copas GM, Ablah E, et al. Regionalization: collateral benefits of emergency preparedness activities. *J Public Health Manag Pract.* 2007;13(5):469–475.

19. Hajat A, Stewart K, Hayes KL. The local public health workforce in rural communities. *J Public Health Manag Pract.* 2003;9(6):481–488.

20. Hawley SR, Molgaard CA, Ablah E, Orr SA, Oler-Manske JE, St Romain T. Academic-practice partnerships for community health workforce development. *J Community Health Nurs.* 2007;24(3):155–165.

21. Florence JA, Goodrow B, Wachs J, Grover S, Olive KE. Rural health professions education at East Tennessee State University: survey of graduates from the first decade of the community partnership program. *J Rural Health.* 2007;23(1):77–83.

22. Taren DL, Varela F, Dotson JA, et al. Developing a university-workforce partnership to address rural and frontier MCH training needs: the Rocky Mountain Public Health Education Consortium (RMPHEC). *Matern Child Health J.* 2011;15(7):845–850.

23. Hawley SR, St Romain T, Orr SA, Molgaard CA, Kabler BS. Competency-based impact of a statewide public health leadership training program. *Health Promot Pract.* 2011;12(2):202–208.

24. Putnam RD. *Bowling Alone: The Collapse and Revival of American Community.* New York, NY: Simon & Schuster; 2000.

25. Easterling D, Foy CG, Fothergill K, Leonard L, Holtgrave DR. Assessing social capital in Kansas: findings from quantitative and qualitative studies. *J Kansas Civic Leadership Devel.* 2009;1(1):23–35.

26. Hawley SR, St Romain T, Rempel SL, Orr SA, Molgaard CA. Generating social capital through public health leadership training: a six-year assessment. *Health Educ Res.* 2012; 27(4):671–679.

27. Alejos A, Weingartner A, Scharff DP, et al. Ensuring the success of local public health workforce assessments: using a participatory-based research approach with a rural population. *Public Health.* 2008;122(12):1447–1455.

28. Rempel SL. *Building a Conceptual Anthropological Framework of Rural American Medicine: Understanding the Culture of Rural Physicians and Factors Influencing Retention.* St Louis, MO: Department of Anthopology, Washington University; 2012.

29. Muecke A, Lenthall S, Lindeman M. Culture shock and healthcare workers in remote indigenous communities of Australia: what do we know and how can we measure it? *Rural Remote Health.* 2011;11(2):1607.

30. Lennon-Dearing R, Florence J, Garrett L, Click IA, Abercrombie S. A rural community-based interdisciplinary curriculum: a social work perspective. *Soc Work Health Care.* 2008;47(2):93–107.

31. Vanleit B, Cubra J. Student-developed problem-based learning cases: preparing for rural healthcare practice. *Rural Remote Health.* 2005;5(4):399.

32. US Department of Health & Human Services. National Health Service Corps. n.d. http://nhsc.hrsa.gov. Accessed April 25, 2012.

33. Henderson Betkus M, MacLeod ML. Retaining public health nurses in rural British Columbia: the influence of job and community satisfaction. *Can J Public Health*. 2004;95(1):54–58.
34. Kelley ML, Kuluski K, Brownlee K, Snow S. Physician satisfaction and practice intentions in Northwestern Ontario. *Can J Rural Med*. 2008;13(3):129–135.
35. Kimball EB, Crouse BJ. Perspectives of female physicians practicing in rural Wisconsin. *WMJ*. 2007;106(5):256–259.
36. National Rural Health Association. NRHA Connect. n.d.; http://connect .nrharural.org/Home. Accessed April 24, 2012.
37. Southern Rural Access Program. Our history. n.d. http://www.srap.org/about-history.html. Accessed April 24, 2012.
38. Kansas Association of Local Health Departments. Home. 2003–2012; http:// kalhd.org. Accessed April 24, 2012.
39. Kansas Department of Health and Environment. Community health systems. 1996–2012; http://www.kdheks.gov/olrh/index.html. Accessed April 24, 2012.
40. Kansas Public Health Association. About KPHA. n.d. http://www.kpha.camp8 .org/aboutkpha. Accessed April 27, 2012.
41. Wright DB. Care in the country: a historical case study of long-term sustainability in 4 rural health centers. *Am J Public Health*. 2009;99(9):1612–1618.
42. Skillman SM, Doescher MP, Mouradian WE, et al. The challenge to delivering oral health services in rural America. *J Public Health Dent*. 2010;70(suppl 1):S49–S57.
43. Gebbie K, Merrill J, Sanders L, et al. Public health workforce enumeration: beware the quick fix. *J Public Health Manag Pract*. 2007;13(1):72–79.
44. Gebbie KM, Raziano A, Elliott S. Public health workforce enumeration. *Am J Public Health*. 2009;99(5):786–787.

CHAPTER 4

Rural Health Care Ethics

Angeline Bushy

Approximately one fifth of the U.S. population resides in areas that are defined as rural, dispersed over nearly three quarters of our nation's total land mass. As discussed throughout this book, rural residents often must contend with limited access to public health, primary care, and specialty health care services. Access to care for rural residents is often hampered by geographical and climatic conditions coupled with social, cultural, and economic factors. The burden of illness for rural populations can be considerable, placing even greater demands on a resource-poor health care system. Consequently, rural residents are increasingly being recognized as an underserved population. Attaining an appropriate standard of care for ruralities has emerged as a major concern in the national discussion of health disparities.[1,2]

There is wide diversity among rural communities; however, *rural context* generally implies great(er) geographic distances, low(er) population density, and the social dynamics that occur among residents in small close knit towns. An often overlooked factor in the dynamics of rural public health is the fact that these features can also create unique ethical challenges and opportunities for rural health care providers.[3] Essentially, rural ethical situations can be impacted by:

- Limited access to health care and social service resources
- Overlapping professional and personal relationships that contribute to conflicting roles and altered therapeutic boundaries
- Local cultural values and care-seeking preferences
- Threats to client confidentiality and privacy
- Unique stresses that confront health professionals in rural practice

These contextual features can be contributing factors in an ethical issue, and definitely must be considered when resolving an ethical conflict that occurs in a rural setting. Health professionals (clinicians) and administrators of public health agencies need to recognize and attempt to prevent real and potential ethics conflicts. This chapter highlights contextual attributes that can impact bioethical situations that arise in rural practice settings, and provides rural considerations for several ethical situations that are more likely to present in public health.

BIOETHICS: THE RURAL PERSPECTIVE

The *Encyclopedia of Bioethics* notes four overlapping areas of ethical inquiry: (a) theoretical ethics; (b) clinical ethics; (c) regulatory and policy ethics; and (d) cultural health care ethics.[4] Theoretical health care ethics focuses on the underlying foundations of moral reasoning that are applied to various health care topics. Clinical ethics refers to specific questions or uncertainty related to client care. Regulatory and policy health care ethics refers to the organizational and legal focus of health care-related ethics questions. Cultural health care ethics systematically relates health care ethics to the cultural, ethnic, religious, and social context in which ethics conflicts arise.

In health care ethics, one cultural subgroup of inquiry is *rural*, given its unique contextual characteristics. There is an emerging body of information, albeit much of it anecdotal in nature, specifically focusing on rural-focused bioethics.[5] Rural health care professionals reiterate concerns regarding their discipline's *professional codes of ethics* and *ethical standards of practice*, as these do not adequately address ethical situations that present in small communities. Formal professional ethics documents are deemed to be most applicable to ethical events that occur in resource-rich, less interdependent, and more densely populated urban settings.[6,7] The information deficit is even more of a concern given that rural clinicians have less access to ethics committees, ethics consultants, and ethics-related continuing education offerings. The following *Rural Research Agenda* was put forth in an effort to help resolve the information deficit, and highlights the areas of broadest concern within rural health ethics (pp. 137–138)[8]:

* Develop a clear understanding of what constitutes the scope of rural health care ethics
* Increase awareness and understanding of rural health care ethics issues, including the contextual nature of the ethical issues and how the issues are different from nonrural settings
* Increase awareness and understanding of rural health care ethics decision making, including how living and working in rural communities affects the response to ethical issues
* In collaboration with rural health care professionals, draft guidelines for addressing common ethical conflicts
* Explore, assess, and propose models for "doing ethics" in small rural health facilities

- Develop training curricula and other educational resources for and with rural clinicians, administrators, and policymakers
- Provide an ethics perspective, supported by empirical data, to administrators and policymakers who are charged with allocating health care resources
- Foster a dialogue with the general health care ethics community regarding the unique contextual nature of rural ethical issues

Those who are entrusted with providing competent and ethically sound clinical care have further noted an urgent need for resources that can offer guiding principles to health professionals in rural settings.[3,9] Enveloping rural ethical challenges are contextual realities of the rural environment. In reality, context is what rural bioethics is all about. Rural health care ethics entails application of an ethics framework and ethical standards to bioethical issues that occur in more austere environments, as is the case for most rural settings. Rural ethics tends not to be concerned with more commonly encountered ethical domains, such as conflicts about end-of-life decision making or issues associated with threats to privacy and confidentiality. These particular ethics challenges can occur in any setting and are not unique to rural practice. What is unique is the manner in which rural contextual features can shape and weave into the dynamics surrounding ethical uncertainty as well as responses to the challenge.[10,11]

Regardless of the setting, every community has unique demographic, economic, and sociocultural features. However, there are some general contextual characteristics that influence most ethics situations that present in a rural community. More specifically, there are often limited health care resources, including medical specialists and ethics experts.[12-14] Public health clinicians often work in more isolated practice settings with less immediate access to professional colleagues. Then, too, there are geographic barriers that must be taken into consideration to access and deliver services such as travel challenges associated with roads and weather conditions, along with limited (if any) public transportation. Regardless of the setting, moral distress (sometimes even legal and ethical situations) can arise for a health professional when stigma is associated with a client's diagnosis or situation events such as interpersonal violence, substance abuse, behavioral mental health conditions, sexually transmitted diseases, and refusal to adhere to recommendations of the health professional to treat the condition. These concerns become even more pronounced in rural settings, in which it is more likely that the clinician is not only aware of others who are potentially impacted (e.g., sexual partners in the case of an STD diagnosis), but also possibly personally knows the individuals at potential risk.

Moral Distress

Moral distress, an underpinning of many ethical conflicts, occurs when an individual knows the ethically appropriate action to take, but situational or contextual constraints make it nearly impossible to pursue this course of action.[15-17] Clinicians may experience moral distress when confronted with chosen treatment options that they believe are not in the best interest of the client, do not mesh with their innate sense of right and wrong, and/or do not represent the known highest standard of care. Sources of moral distress may be personal, interpersonal, and/or environmental in nature. Moral distress can lead to burnout and is a contributing factor of employees' intentions to leave a position, high turnover rates, defensiveness, and lack of collaboration among employees. Essentially, moral distress occurs when the clinician acts in a manner that is contrary to personal and/or professional values, ultimately undermining personal integrity.

The practice template by which most health professionals are educated may not take into consideration rural context. This approach often becomes a source of moral distress for health professionals who practice in rural settings, and provides a framework by which to examine the most frequent ethical challenges faced in rural contexts. The remainder of this chapter will discuss predominate rural contextual features that contribute to moral distress and ethical situations in that setting, specifically (a) health status and health care resources; (b) overlapping personal and professional boundaries; (c) variance in cultural perspectives; (d) threats to confidentiality and privacy; and (e) professional practice expectations.

Health Status and Health Care Resources

A professional in public health practice should always be aware of the community's health status and the resources that are available to address local health care needs. Such information can be critical when planning and implementing client-centered care. However, community-specific data may not be what urban-educated providers are accustomed to obtaining, understanding, or much less using in their practice, but may be key in preventing and recognizing potential ethical situations unique to rural contexts.[1,18] A serious gap exists in the health-status data of vulnerable and at-risk populations in rural areas; however, some characteristics have emerged in the literature. As for overall health status, rural residents are more likely to report fair to poor health status and are more likely to have experienced a limitation of activity caused by chronic conditions compared to urban counterparts. Rural residents also have a higher prevalence of long-term health problems compared to urban residents. This finding is attributable to a higher proportion of poor and elderly residents, coupled with higher rates of accidents and trauma occurring among rural residents. Yet rural residents have relatively low mortality in light of their high rate of chronic illnesses. As discussed in more detail in Chapter 7, behavioral and mental health needs are particularly significant in rural settings where residents struggle with a significant disproportion of substance dependence, mental illnesses, and psychiatric–medical comorbidity.[17,19-21] Suicide rates in rural areas have surpassed urban suicide rates for several decades. Despite these known risks and increased health problems, an austere provider network, lack of adequate and affordable health care insurance coverage, and access to quality care are factors in rural health status and are often associated with moral distress among caregivers in rural practice.

Economic and financial factors mitigate care-seeking behaviors among local residents. More specifically, in rural communities, compared to those in more populated cities, employment opportunities are limited, salaries are often lower, and employees are less likely to have health insurance benefits. The economic climate is a driving force in the growing number of uninsured and underinsured families, and there is a higher proportion of working poor in rural areas. As a result, cost of health care is a major deterrent to seeking medical care in rural settings. In turn, rural-based health care professionals regularly encounter situations where they must decide whether or not to provide essential care with little or no reimbursement. Obviously, these practice realities can be a source of uncertainty for the health professional, and could lead to unresolved ethical or sometimes even legal situations.[12,22,23] Fundamentally, providers can face an ethical conundrum: Do I see the patient whom I know is unable to pay for my services (thus impacting my own and my family's financial well-being), or do I refuse to see the patient despite knowing I am the only medical provider in town?

Economic infrastructure is another contextual feature that often becomes a consideration in ethical discussions regardless of setting, be it urban or rural. For instance, in many rural counties, the health care system is one of the (if not the) largest employers. Given the tenuous fiscal condition of many small hospitals, financial stressors experienced by these institutions will significantly impact the broader community and vice versa. More specifically, the closure of a small hospital can have a dramatic ripple effect on the economic status of the local community, as a high proportion of locals may have been employed in that facility.[24-26]

As an example of the types of ethical situations that may emerge surrounding hospital closures, such closures are often due to the lack of a physician. For instance, when a small town's only physician departs, this could mean the local hospital must close even if there are other health professionals from other disciplines living in the area. Out of desperation, a health professional (most often a physician) who has a questionable background or practice patterns could be recruited into the community simply because of a lack of alternatives that would readily present in a more urban setting. At the cost of losing their jobs, other health professionals may be reluctant to report the unprofessional activity. Ultimately, this secrecy can create moral distress and pose an ethical conflict for the other health professionals, impacting the quality of rendered services and unfortunately potentially having dire consequences for patients. While we are not saying this is the case for all rural hospital staffing situations, the likelihood of such situations occurring is much greater in rural settings where the decision is between hiring someone with a potentially questionable background or closing the only care access point in the community. Such decisions may seem unrealistic or overly hypothetical from an urban standpoint, but can be a distinct reality in rural settings.

Overlapping Professional and Personal Boundaries

One of the most often-cited reasons for moral distress among caregivers that can foster ethical conflicts is associated with overlapping relationships between clinicians and clients.[1,13,14] Associated with social dynamics among residents in small towns, health care providers interact with clients and their extended family in a multitude of settings. For instance, the local public health nurse may serve on the local school board along with one or more patients who seek services in the county health department. Similarly, the children of the only physician in town would likely be in classes with the children of the physician's patients, or the social worker in the local mental health clinic may be an active member of a congregation where clients under his or her immediate care are often encountered. It is not unusual for rural professionals to live and work in the same community where most residents are acquainted or related. Certainly nearly everyone in the county knows the physicians and nurses who work in the local hospital, health department, or clinic. For caregivers, such chance encounters with clients and their extended family and friends make it difficult to escape the professional role even outside of office or hospital. Overlapping professional roles and boundaries can both enhance and complicate the clinician–client relationship.[25,26]

On the one hand, informal chance client interactions within the community allow the clinician to have ongoing contact with a client and his or her family that is unlikely to occur in more populated settings. In other words, the client–provider relationship is formed and cultivated in both the examining room and in the grocery store or post office. Informal interpersonal exchanges can enhance rapport and sometimes even be beneficial for treatment outcomes. Rural clinicians have a unique opportunity to understand their clients in depth, including their values, perspectives, preferences, and broader cultural context.

On the other hand, diffuse personal–professional boundaries can be a source of significant discomfort and stress for someone not accustomed to dealing with these types of client interactions.[1,23,27,28] Residents (clients) in a rural community may judge the health care provider's ability based on these informal encounters. A clinician's personal life and family will also be much more visible to patients, potentially raising concerns over not only perceptions, but personal safety as well. In addition, these overlapping relationships can create ethical dilemmas surrounding patient confidentiality: If a physician sees a patient in an informal setting, should the physician even acknowledge the individual? If the patient does acknowledge the physician, how should the physician react when a family member or friend asks how he or she knows the individual? While such scenarios are possible in urban settings, they are both more likely and more frequently recurring in rural areas. More details on similar confidentiality-related concerns are discussed in the following section.

Threats to Confidentiality and Privacy

Closely related to overlapping relationships are threats to confidentiality and privacy. Breaches in confidentiality and privacy can be both intentional and unintentional, due to the close-knit nature of rural social structures.[1,2,9] For instance, it is not unusual for a resident in a small town to report there is no one that he or she can trust to discuss problems of a personal nature. This perception is partly attributable to residents in small towns having a genuine interest in the lives and well-being of neighbors, friends, and relatives; however, it nonetheless creates a system in which patients feel less confidentiality even seeking care. Regardless of the setting, it can be devastating when a personal problem becomes public knowledge. Informal social structures—for example, extended family or a faith community—may impose restrictions or perhaps even sanctions to seeking professional help for certain conditions having moral overtones such as substance abuse, behavioral problems, unplanned pregnancy, sexuality issues, interpersonal violence, or mental illness.

Maintaining client confidentiality can be challenging, particularly when a clinic or agency is located within a public facility, such as the county courthouse. It is not unusual for the waiting room to be located in a common hallway, or to have a reception area in which clients are likely to be recognized. In a "semipublic" setting such as this, conversations occur about not only medical issues, but also personal and family issues, and can be overheard by others in the area. Then, too, announcements of specialty services or programs such as prenatal or family planning clinics; HIV testing; the Women, Infants and Children (WIC) nutrition program; and immunization clinics often are publicized in the local media (newspaper, church bulletins, radio, television) and sometimes posted in public places such as a grocery store, laundromat, service station, or grain elevator. Individuals may be less likely to not only seek such services, but also to even take information regarding them because of concerns over what others may discover.

When the family planning clinic is scheduled on Friday mornings, for example, assumptions may be made by local residents about anyone seen parking in front of the building, even if it is not to attend the clinic. People in small towns often are recognized by the car they drive; thus, even parking lots can jeopardize confidentiality. Leaks in confidentiality can result from such observations and quickly become public knowledge via the local rumor mill. Maintaining confidentiality must always be a consideration in the rural context. For example, prenatal or family planning clinics could be scheduled to coincide with an immunization clinic, or STD clinics and HIV testing might be offered on a walk-in basis or within another health facility such as a multi-physician clinic, and so on. Innovative approaches are required on the part of clinicians in rural practice to address the community's concerns surrounding anonymity and confidentiality, which, ultimately, if not addressed, could become ethical or legal situations.[17,20,24]

Variance in Professional–Client Cultural Perspectives
Individuals hold different views of the etiologic explanations for sickness, tolerance of illness and pain, care-seeking behaviors, and self-care practices for health promotion and illness prevention. Generally these beliefs

are culturally based and sanctioned by the community. However, when pervasive community values about illness and appropriate treatment for the condition differ from the ethos of clinicians, it is more likely that client–professional conflicts can arise. For instance, health and illness are defined in various ways and are influenced by individuals' cultural backgrounds. Among some rural residents, health is defined as the ability to work, to do what needs to be done. Thus, a client with this perspective may not seek "formal" health care until he or she is too ill to do the expected work.[1,22,23]

Along with economics, time-related factors, travel conditions, and employment conditions often determine when, or even if, an individual or family seeks medical care. For instance, in more remote settings a family may combine visiting the health department for immunizations or WIC services with some other work or family activity requiring a trip to "town." Thus, appointments may not be kept, or immunizations may not be current, and caregivers may determine this to be "noncompliance." Client–professional conflicts may occur when a caregiver demonstrates inappropriate respect for community economic realities or cultural preferences in deeming a patient to be noncompliant. Recognizing community values and openly communicating with clients when these differ from conventional health care are critical to prevent and resolve actual or potential ethical and sometimes legal conflicts.[12,27,28] For example, rather than being transported to a large tertiary hospital located in a more distant urban area, a local value may be that an individual nearing death be allowed to remain at home with extended family, friends, and neighbors supporting the immediate family during this life event. When such local customs conflict with a provider's own set of values, ethical conflicts can occur that have no clear outcome or course of action.

Cultural insensitivity can exacerbate a client's mistrust of a clinician. In turn, this individual perspective will likely be shared with other locals via the main street grapevine.[26] The clinician's perceived attitude can also impact the health outcome of a client who may be embarrassed about health problems. For instance, a patient may minimize the symptoms of an illness or not acknowledge culturally based self-care practices to a health care provider. These behaviors can result in misdiagnosing a condition or delaying treatment until there is an acute emergency. To diminish risks for potential ethical issues created by professional–community cultural variances, professional education programs should expose students to the rural context and sociocultural values among residents in small towns. For example, a rural-focused elective course could promote cultural and linguistic sensitivity to the health care preferences of rural communities. Rural-based clinical student experiences can facilitate mutual sensitivity and trust between clinicians and clients to prevent bioethical situations from occurring or, perhaps, early recognition of potential ethical situations. Likewise, clinicians in rural practice should develop approaches to client care that integrate community values with their professional standards of practice, and proactively consider the types of internal ethical conflicts that may arise to avoid having to make a decision in the midst of a challenging situation.

Professional Practice Expectations

Stress, sometimes even moral distress, for rural health care providers is often associated with community expectations, an overwhelming workload, professional isolation, or a combination thereof.[2,25,26] A clinician in the rural context is expected to function as a generalist who is able to care for individuals across the life span who have a variety of health-related or medical conditions.[22,23] It is not unusual, for example, on one shift at a 15-bed critical access hospital (CAH), for a nurse or a physician to be expected to care for an obstetrical family (mother and newborn infant), a middle-aged adult transferred from a medical center with postoperative complications from recent surgery, a child with a serious upper respiratory infection, and an elderly person with life-threatening comorbid chronic illnesses. Or, in a very small county health department, the nurse may function as the sanitation and nuisance officer; set and empty mosquito traps; and offer sexuality education, immunizations, and screenings in all of the schools in the county. In other words, the health professional in the rural context is an *expert* generalist. This role expectation is perceived as a positive experience by some but for others can be a source of intense stress, perhaps even moral distress. Given the scarcity of health care providers in some rural regions, professional isolation and high demands for health, a physician, nurse, or public health official may be *on call* 24/7 for weeks or months without professional backup. An individual clinician's own personal needs are then put into conflict with individual patient needs; if the only nurse in the clinic needs to take time off to attend to personal issues, it may result in numerous patients not being able to receive needed care. Needless to say, such community- and work-related expectations take a personal and professional toll on health professionals as well as their families. One must also question if these expectations impact quality of care that is rendered by the provider and how this can influence ethical events.

Availability, accessibility, and acceptability of health care services, or lack thereof, almost always impinge on rural ethics situations.[1,3,12] Lack of services and specialists, such as public and mental health professionals, creates situations where the general practitioner may need to provide specialized mental health care. Again, the tension arises regarding preparedness—an individual may not feel particularly well trained in the area, but for lack of another available option must assume that role despite potential personal/ethical reservations. Other health care professionals, including nurses and social workers, may become the de facto primary care provider in settings with limited resources. Many rural communities have no hospitals, yet travel to the large, distant medical centers can create significant burdens on both the client as well as the provider. For example, a client may need to travel long distances over challenging roads to find needed emergency care or specialized oncology treatments. However, the client does not choose this option; rather, the client prefers to receive treatment in his or her own community. Situations such as this place significant burden on rural primary care clinicians who ultimately may be forced to provide care that is beyond their level of expertise. Together, limited availability, accessibility, and acceptability of service converge, resulting in a heightened risk for errors and for rendering quality care, and definitely shape ethical discussions encountered by rural clinicians.

When a potential or actual bioethical event occurs in small towns it may not be possible to remediate it using professional guidelines that were, in most cases, developed and applied in urban-based and resource-rich medical centers.[3,17] The rural clinician's response to ethical conflict is based not only on his or her education, experience, and professional ethics guidelines, but also on the community's values regarding health, illness, and care-seeking preferences. The social, economic, and cultural characteristics of small communities reflect the values of their residents. Understanding health care ethics conflicts that have occurred in the past in rural communities can provide insights to clinicians, enabling them to more effectively respond to ethical conflicts and to anticipate potential conflicts.[28–30]

RURAL PUBLIC HEALTH ETHICAL CONSIDERATIONS

Information specifically addressing rural public health ethics is lacking. However, the ethical situations that occur in rural public health are likely similar to those that occur in urban-based settings, such as allocation of scarce resources, screening, dealing with incompetent health care professionals, case finding, and access to an institutional review board and ethics committee.[4] By no means is this a comprehensive discussion that details the various ethical principles pertaining to each of these issues, and the reader is referred to a bioethics textbook for those details. Rather, for each of these domains, a few comments will offer a rural perspective. After all, as mentioned previously in this chapter, rural ethics is about context, that is to say, the social dynamics and values that characterize small communities.

Allocation of Scarce Resources

Health departments in rural counties or regions generally have a small professional staff with extremely limited financial resources associated with low local tax revenue.[4,31] Likewise, in rural counties the decision makers may not see funding for public health as a priority compared to maintaining roads, bridges, or public utility infrastructures. An austere economic reality, coupled with the high proportion of vulnerable, uninsured, and professionally underserved residents, can be a source of extreme stress for administrators and professional staff. Prioritizing and allocating scarce resources, particularly in a disaster event, can lead to significant moral distress. When faced with the potential decision between closing the immunization clinic or stopping the WIC program, not only must the administrator emotionally deal with his or her own "best guess" based on the information that is available at a given time, he or she is never out of the limelight with local residents in the small community, be it in the agency office, the Walmart parking lot, a service station, or a church. Making these decisions can be extremely difficult and stressful; however, dealing with community residents can be devastatingly stressful for the administrator as well as his or her family members.[2,24]

Screening and Case Finding

The ethical issues that envelop screening and case finding are extensively discussed in the public health literature and space constraints limit extensive debate in this chapter.[4,32,33] In respect to rural regions, confidentiality, community values, and financial constraints are important considerations when planning and implementing a screening initiative, especially in situations where there may be stigma associated with the condition, such as obesity or certain types of disability. One of the most debated considerations is what intervention will or can be offered to those who require it. Given the high number of underinsured and uninsured, what other alternatives (if any) are there to pay for the care needs that may be identified through screening programs? Then, too, there are the access challenges (travel, room/board, child care, etc.) to obtain the intervention by a specialist in an urban-based setting. Conversely, how does one manage the care of a client who has a positive screen but refuses treatment, even though the health care provider believes treatment would lead to a favorable outcome?[12-14]

Case finding in a small, tightly knit community can present overwhelming challenges related to diffuse professional–client boundaries and threats to client confidentiality.[2,9,24-26] Case finding contacts associated with someone having a diagnosis with stigma can be devastating, especially if the case finder is a local resident. Sometimes the only solution is to have an outsider to the community involved in these epidemiologic investigations, or for the person with the condition to seek care in an urban-based setting where he or she is less likely to personally know or be related to personnel who are employed in the agency.

Dealing With Incompetent Providers

In previous paragraphs the topic of incompetent providers was alluded to, along with the personal stress this can impose on other employees in that institution. Administrators in particular have a moral responsibility to deal with these issues and to carefully listen to such reports by employees as well as clients. Taking appropriate action (be it within the agency or at a higher level such as the state Board of Medicine) can be extremely difficult given the health professional shortages in the community. Reporting and pursuing issues may in turn result in a complete disruption of care provision for an entire county; however, not doing so can lead to more serious consequences such as a serious medical error or dissatisfaction among local residents who then are forced to travel elsewhere for care.

Limited Ethics Resources

To prevent, identify, and effectively respond to ethics situations, rural clinicians must be aware of both the formal and informal resources that make up the local health care system. They also need to understand how the two interface locally, and what it takes to connect a client with these resources.

Unlike their urban counterparts, many rural facilities and health care professionals have limited access to ethics resources to help them address ethics conflicts. As a result of limited access to an ethics committee, bioethicists, and rural-focused ethics publications, there is a need for educational offerings that integrate rural culture and values into ethical reflection and decision making. Various strategies have been developed to address the ethical information deficit, but there is still significant work to be done in this area.[26,34–36]

One important step for rural providers is to identify and connect with an existing ethics committee (even one that is urban based) that could provide consultation or education. For instance, a local critical access hospital may be part of a large health care network that has a system-wide ethics committee, an ethics consultant, and continuing education opportunities for participating members. Rural clinicians should ask and become informed about what is available to system members. Other small communities within a given geographical setting have combined resources and developed their own health care ethics committees and educational resources. In some cases, health care providers in small communities have partnered with institutions of higher learning to educate local health professionals about ethical principles and decision making.[26,32]

Educational programs for health professionals are generally located in urban areas, and most clinical experiences occur there.[12,37] Subsequently, students are not exposed to rural clients and rural health care systems, and thus have no idea about the contextual realities of this practice setting. To modify this traditional education pattern, rural clinicians in public health must become proactive and educate urban-based educators about rural contextual features that can impact ethical situations occurring in more remote environments. Arranging with faculty to have students in a rural public health agency for a practicum or internship can provide very valuable exposure. Also, collaboration with faculty on research projects having a rural focus or measuring program outcomes can increase exposure to rural context. Most rural health care institutions do not have an institutional review board (IRB) that can ensure protection of human subjects; therefore, administrators from the various health care institutions in a community could work together to develop an IRB that reviews and approves research proposals that include local residents.

Education of health professionals and the community on ethical content is perhaps the most important strategy to create ethics awareness.[12,37] Two rural-focused web-based ethics publications are available at no cost and are a wonderful resource for clinicians, educators, administrators, and ethicists. These two publications by Nelson et al. (2009) were specifically designed for use in the continuing education of health professionals, and include a variety of specialty-centered learning modules, with supplementary case studies, background information, and supporting resources. Generally, in a rural setting, one individual must take the initiative to "get the ball rolling" locally. Often interest is spurred after an ethical event presents within the institution or agency. Eventually, an interested group of individuals can organize to foster ethics awareness among local health professionals as well as among the community as a whole. Another objective could be to develop educational offerings that target professionals from various agencies and institutions in the community.

Finally, there is a critical need for information in the literature about best practice ethics models in rural health care institutions in general, and in rural public health agencies in particular. Needed even more is information about ethical situations related to public health programs and ethical resources in the most remote and usually underserved frontier areas having fewer than six persons per square mile. The field of rural public health ethics is still relatively new; however, it is nonetheless important to expand.

REFERENCES

1. Bushy A. Nursing in rural and frontier areas: issues, challenges and opportunities. *Harv Health Policy Rev.* 2006;9(1):17–27.
2. Cook A, Hoas H. No secrets on main Street. *Am J Nursing.* 2000;101(8):67, 69–71.
3. Nelson W. The challenges of rural health care. In: Klugman CM, Dalinis PM, eds. *Ethical Issues in Rural Health Care.* Baltimore, MD: Johns Hopkins University Press; 2008:34–59.
4. Reich W, ed. *Encyclopedia of Bioethics.* 3rd ed. New York, NY: Simon & Schuster Macmillan; 2003.
5. Nelson W, Greene M, West A. Rural health care ethics: no longer the forgotten quarter of medical ethics. *Cambridge Q Healthcare Ethics.* 2010;19(4):510–517.
6. Nelson W, Lushkov G, Pomerantz A, Weeks W. Rural health care ethics: is there a literature? *Am J Bioethics.* 2006;6(2):44–50.
7. Nelson W, Schmidek J. Rural healthcare ethics. In: Singer PA, Viens AM, eds. *The Cambridge Textbook of Bioethics.* New York, NY: Cambridge University Press; 2008:289–298.
8. Nelson B, Pomerantz A, Howard K, Bushy A. A proposed rural health care ethics agenda. *Am J Medical Ethics.* 2007;33:136–139.
9. Klugman C, Dalinis P, eds. *Ethical Issues in Rural Health Care.* Baltimore, MD: Johns Hopkins University Press; 2008.
10. Cook A, Hoas H. Where the rubber hits the road: implications for organizational and clinical ethics in rural healthcare settings. *HEC Forum.* 2000;12(4):331–340.
11. Cook A, Hoas H. Ethics and rural healthcare: what really happens, what might help? *Am J Bioethics.* 2008;8(4):52–56.
12. Nelson W, ed. *Handbook for Rural Health Care Ethics: A Practical Guide for Health Professionals.* Lebanon, NH: University Press of New England; 2009.http://dms.dartmouth.edu/cfm/resources/ethics/chapter-00.pdf. Accessed May 1, 2012.
13. Nelson W. Health care ethics and rural life: stigma, privacy, boundary conflicts raise concerns. *Health Prog.* 2010;9(15):50–54.
14. Nelson W. Boundary issues in rural America. *Healthcare Executive.* 2010;25(2):54–57.
15. Austin W, Lemermeyer G, Goldberg L, Bergum V, Johnson MS. Moral distress in healthcare practice: the situation of nurses. *HEC Forum.* 2005;17(1):33–48.
16. Austin W, Rankel M, Kagan L, Bergum, V, Lemermeyer G. To stay or to go, to speak or stay silent, to act or not to act: moral distress as experience by psychologists. *Ethics & Behav.* 2005;15(3):197–212.
17. Stiffman A, Freedenthal P, Ostmann E, Osborne V, Silmere H. Ethical challenges of mental health clinicians in rural and frontier areas. *Psychiatr Serv.* 2006;57(3):1185–1191.

18. Braveman P, Kumanyika S, Fielding J, LaVeist T, Borrell L, Mandershied R. Health disparities and health equity: the issue is justice. *Am J Public Health.* 2011;101(1):S149–S155.

19. Roberts L, Battaglia J, Epstein R. Frontier ethics: mental health care needs and ethical dilemmas in rural communities. *Psychiatr Serv.* 1999;50(4):497–503.

20. Roberts L, Johnson M, Berms C, Warner T. Ethical disparities: challenges encountered by multidisciplinary providers in fulfilling ethical standards in the care of rural and minority people. *J Rural Health.* 2007;23(suppl):89–97.

21. Malone J. Ethical professional practice: exploring the issues for health services to rural Aboriginal communities. *Rural and Remote Health: The International Electronic Journal of Rural and Remote Health Research, Education, Practice and Policy.* 2012: http://www.rrh.org.au/publishedarticles/article_print_1891.pdf Accessed May 1, 2012.

22. Davis D, Droes N. Community health nursing in rural and frontier counties. *Nursing Clin North Am.* 1993;28(1):159–169.

23. Case T. Work stressors of community health nurses in Oklahoma. In: Bushy A, ed. *Rural Nursing.* Vol. 2. Newbury Park, CA: Sage; 1991:220–232.

24. Larson K, Elliot R. The emotional impact of malpractice. *Nephrol Nurs J.* 2010; 37(2):153–155.

25. Roberts L, Battaglia J, Smithpeter M, Epstein R. An office on main street: health care dilemmas in small communities. *Hastings Cent Rep.* 1999;29(4):28–37.

26. Molinari D, Bushy A, eds. *The Rural Nurse: Transition to Practice.* New York, NY: Springer; 2012.

27. Simpson C, McDonald F. 'Any body is better than nobody?' Ethical questions around recruiting and/or retaining health professionals in rural areas. *Rural and Remote Health.* 2011. http://www.rrh.org.au/publishedarticles/article_print_1867.pdf. Accessed May 1, 2012.

28. Pavlish C, Brown-Saltzman K, Hersh M, et al. Early indicators and risk factors for ethical issues in clinical practice. *J Nursing Scholarship.* 2011;43(1):13–21.

29. Nelson W, Rosenberg M, Mackenzie T, Weeks W. The presence of ethics programs in critical access hospitals. *HealthCare Ethics Committee Forum.* 2010;22(4):267–274.

30. Schlairet M. Bioethics mediation: the role and importance of nurse advocacy. *Nursing Outlook.* 2009;77:185–193.

31. DeBruin D, Liaschenko J, Marshall M. Social justice in pandemic preparedness. *Am J Public Health.* 2012;102(4):586–590.

32. Cook A, Hoas H. Protecting research subjects: IRBs in changing research landscape. *Hastings Cent IRB: Ethics Hum Res.* 2011;33(2):14–19.

33. Lee L, Helig D, White A. Ethical justification for conducting public health surveillance without patient consent. *Am J Public Health.* 2012;102(1):38–44.

34. Jameton A. *Nursing Practice: The Ethical Issues.* Englewood Cliffs, NJ: Prentice Hall; 1984.

35. Grady C, Danis M, Farrar A, et al. Does ethics education influence the moral action of practicing nurses and social workers? *Am J Bioethics.* 2008;8(4):4–11.

36. Rural Assistance Center. Frontier frequently asked questions: what is the definition of frontier? 2012. http://www.raconline.org/topics/frontier/frontierfaq.php

37. Nelson W, Schifferdecker K. Rural health care ethics: a manual for trainers. 2009. http://dms.dartmouth.edu/cfm/resources/manual/manual.pdf. Accessed May 1, 2012.

CHAPTER 5

Rural Church-Based Health Promotion

Karen H. Kim Yeary

Religion continues to play an important role in the United States, with 62% of the population reporting membership in a church or synagogue, 44% reporting attending church almost every week or every week, and 56% reporting that religion is very important in their own lives.[1] Religion's enduring influence is particularly prominent in Americans living in rural communities, who have the highest levels of overall religiosity in the nation compared to urban and suburban communities.[2] Given the relevance of religion in rural America, churches are essential partners in promoting health in rural areas.

Churches offer unique advantages for health promotion. They often play a pivotal role in the social welfare, service, and education of their communities, particularly in communities with limited resources, such as rural, low-income, and minority communities.[3,4] Churches are also widely located and have deep community ties that facilitate their ability to reach those that other organizations or agencies have not been able to reach,[5,6] including persons in rural areas.[7] Churches commonly have well-established social networks that can reinforce health programs.[5,8] Churches' history of volunteerism may also reinforce health programs that are instituted in churches by increasing program participation. In addition, their involvement of multiple generations encourages the instigation and maintenance of healthy behavior changes in all age groups.[5] Churches and public health also embody a similar set of ethos in respect to health by placing value on service, education, and behavioral change.[8] Some religious groups even use health behaviors as identifiers to distinguish their communities from others: Judaism has

The author thanks Brooke Montgomery for her helpful comments on an earlier draft of the book chapter.

Kosher food regulations,[9] Islam uses Halal food guidelines,[9] Seventh-Day Adventists encourage a lacto-ovo vegetarian diet,[10] and the Church of Latter Day Saints (Mormon) prescribes a balanced diet and discourages excess meat intake.[11] General religiosity in the United States also encompasses theological teachings about the body as a temple where God resides.[12] Thus churches are important partners in health promotion, particularly in rural and other underserved populations.

This chapter provides a narrative review of church-based health promotion programs in U.S. rural areas. The chapter builds upon previous reviews of church-based health promotion programs[13–15] by extracting only those programs from the reviews that were conducted in rural areas as defined by the U.S. Census Bureau definition.[16] In addition to extracting studies from previous reviews, relevant articles from 2009 to 2012 were identified utilizing a similar methodology as DeHaven et al.[14] Inclusion criteria included a health program or intervention that directly connected with attempting to change a health outcome, and the program being conducted in a rural area. A total of 19 interventions were identified and addressed general health, cancer, cardiovascular disease, diabetes, obesity, sexually transmitted diseases, smoking, nutrition, and physical activity. These are discussed in the following section in hopes of providing a meaningful resource for individuals wishing to engage in faith-based health promotion in rural communities.

RURAL CHURCH-BASED HEALTH PROMOTION

General Health

One program addressing general health was identified. A church-based health promotion intervention that addressed heart disease, hypertension, stroke, cancer, substance abuse, arthritis, nutrition, exercise, smoking, stress, obesity, and access to care was developed for rural African American older adults in Northern Florida.[17] Four churches participated in the program through the formation of church health committees that implemented health activities. Health activities included newsletters, community-wide health screenings, and the development of learning resource materials such as exercise videos. There were significant changes from baseline to follow-up in weight and blood pressure within some churches. Participants in each church reported higher levels of perceived overall health and health status.

Cancer

Five studies addressed cancer prevention. Three of the studies focused on screening practices (fecal occult blood test, breast self-examination, mammography), whereas two focused on changing dietary behaviors, particularly fruit and vegetable intake. Diverse groups were engaged among the screening interventions, including African Americans, Native Hawaiians, and Latinas. The nutrition interventions worked with African American churches only.

Cancer Screening

The *Wellness for African Americans Through Churches* (WATCH) *Project* was a randomized trial that engaged 12 rural African American North Carolina churches (participant $n = 587$) to test the comparative effectiveness of a tailored print and video intervention with a lay health advisor intervention to increase colorectal cancer screening through fecal occult blood testing.[18] The tailored print and video intervention consisted of personalized messages by demographic, psychosocial, behavioral, church, and community-specific factors. Participants in the print and video intervention received tailored newsletters and videotapes. In the lay health advisor intervention, church members were trained to build upon their natural helping and support skills to support colorectal cancer screening, healthy eating, and physical activity. Those in the tailored print and video intervention significantly increased fruit and vegetable consumption (0.6 servings) and recreational physical activity (2.5 metabolic task equivalents per hour). Among those 50 and older, there was a 15% increase in fecal occult blood testing from baseline to 12-month follow-up ($p = 0.08$).

The *Tepeyac Project* was a 6-year study that used a community-based participatory approach to compare the effectiveness of a culturally targeted print intervention with a *promotora* intervention to increase breast cancer screening among Latinas in Colorado.[19,20] A total of 209 churches participated in the print intervention arm, and 4 churches participated in the *promotora* arm, where *promotoras* spoke personally with women about breast health. Mammography claim rates from Medicaid and five insurance plans were used to examine the comparative effectiveness of the two arms. In women enrolled in public or private insurance plans, there were no significant changes in mammography rates from baseline to follow-up in both intervention arms. Women in the *promotora* arm had a significantly higher increase in biennial mammograms compared to the print intervention (generalized estimating equation [GEE] parameter estimate of .24 [± .11]; $p = 0.03$).[19] Among Latinas enrolled in Medicaid, there were no significant changes in mammography rates from baseline to follow-up in both intervention arms. Those in the *promotora* intervention had a marginally higher increase in biennial mammograms compared to the print intervention ($p = 0.07$).[20]

The *Witness Project* is a community-based program designed to increase breast self-examination and mammography through the African American church.[21] Local African American women talk about their own experiences as cancer survivors and the importance of screening. The program also includes education about breast self-examination and navigation to receive free and reduced-cost mammography. In a quasi-experimental design that compared two treatment counties with two control counties, Witness Project participants significantly increased their practice of breast self-examination and mammography compared to controls. Spirituality played an important role in the program by serving as a conduit to provide meaningful cancer education messages.[22]

Partially informed by the Witness Project, *ka lei mano'olana (KLM)* was a culturally targeted intervention designed to increase intent to seek routine mammography among Native American women.[23] The project used a participatory approach and included spiritual messages that were consistent with the faith-based orientation of the population. The program consisted of testimonials from breast cancer survivors, a 90-minute educational session, print materials, and screening reminders. Using a randomized, two-group pre-/post-control group comparison design, the study was conducted in 12 churches (participant $n = 198$). Women receiving the intervention reported greater intent to seek yearly mammograms compared to women in the control arm. The program was also feasible in terms of acceptability, recruitment, retention, and data collection.

Nutrition and Cancer

Two church-based nutrition interventions designed to decrease cancer risk were identified. The *Black Churches United for Better Health Project* was a multilevel intervention designed to increase fruit and vegetable intake in rural African American adults.[24] Conducted in 50 Black churches (participant $n = 2519$) in 10 rural North Carolina counties, the 20-month intervention consisted of individual-level, tailored bulletins for each participant; church-level activities such as educational sessions, printed materials to be distributed at the church, cookbook and recipe tasting, lay health advisors, and pastor support; and community-level activities including grocer-vendor involvement and community coalitions. At 2-year follow-up, the intervention group reported greater fruit and vegetable intake (0.85 more servings; standard error [*SE*] = 0.12) compared to the delayed intervention group.

The most efficacious components of the *Black Churches United for Better Health Project* and an urban church-based nutrition project that had the greatest potential for dissemination were combined to create *Body and Soul*.[25] *Body and Soul* was a randomized effectiveness trial designed to understand the "real-world" effectiveness of previously developed dietary interventions for African Americans. Conducted in 16 churches (participant $n = 854$) across the nation—including rural areas—Body and Soul consisted of church-wide events, environmental changes, and motivational interviewing for individuals to change dietary intake to decrease cancer risk. At 6-month follow-up, participants in the treatment group reported significantly higher servings of fruit and vegetable intake compared to participants in the control group. After adjusting for controls, intervention participants had 1.4 greater servings of fruit and vegetables. The intervention group also reported modest and salubrious changes in percent of calories from fat and in psychosocial variables.

Cardiovascular Disease

A total of three church-based interventions addressed cardiovascular disease. One was a large randomized trial across the state of Rhode Island that addressed multiple cardiovascular disease risk factors. The other two programs focused on changing awareness and knowledge of cardiovascular disease and worked exclusively with African American churches.

The *Health and Religion Project (HARP)* was a 5-year randomized trial of 20 churches across Rhode Island.[26] The cardiovascular disease risk reduction intervention trained church members to deliver the intervention, which consisted of separate programs in smoking cessation, blood pressure control, nutrition, weight loss, and physical activity. The nutrition program adapted the Pawtucket Heart Health Program and provided trained church members with a manual and structured outlines for each 1-hour intervention session, which was delivered weekly over 7 weeks.[27] A total of 64 participants completed the intervention. Compared to a comparison group, those in the treatment group reported more frequently reading nutrition labels, limiting salt intake, limiting cholesterol and saturated fat intake, and selecting or adapting recipes to reduce fat and salt intake from baseline to 12-month follow-up. The weight loss program used a behavioral approach and included 8 weekly 1-hour sessions, followed by 3 biweekly maintenance sessions.[28] A total of 97 completed the lay health advisor-led behavioral weight loss intervention. The mean weight loss of program participants was 6.78 (standard deviation [SD] = 5.55) pounds from the first session to the last session. At 12-month follow-up, program participants gained an average of 2.59 (SD = 6.50) pounds compared to the 0.64 (SD = 5.86) pounds gained in the comparison group; the difference in weight loss at 12 months between the treatment and comparison groups was not statistically significant.

Practitioners worked with a council of local church leaders to develop a cardiovascular disease prevention intervention for four African American churches in Northern Florida.[29] The purpose of the program was to increase cardiovascular awareness and change cardiovascular-related behavioral outcomes (e.g., blood pressure, nutrition, physical activity) from 1991 to 1992. Churches were provided monthly training workshops to develop intervention activities, which included media campaigns, physical activity, healthy cooking demonstrations, health fairs, and access to educational resources. Approximately 294 churches participated in 1991 and 343 participated in 1992. Significant changes in cardiovascular outcomes (decreased systolic pressure, increased diastolic pressure, lower salt intake) were reported from 1991 to 1992.

The *BLESS Project* was a stroke risk-reduction intervention that was implemented in one African American church in North Carolina.[30] Program activities were characterized as "faith-placed" (churches as sites for intervention only) and "faith-based" (engaging faith practices in health promotion activities) and included print materials about stroke prevention and risk factor reduction, quarterly health screenings, opportunity to participate in Weight Watchers®, exercise classes, lay health advisor training, and a special Sunday service about health. At the end of the intervention, approximately half of the congregation members demonstrated knowledge about stroke and about 60% had been screened for stroke risk factors.

Diabetes

Three church-based interventions addressing diabetes in rural groups were identified. All worked with African American adult congregations. One used a randomized controlled design.

A New DAWN: Diabetes Awareness and Wellness Network was a 12-month culturally appropriate church-based intervention for African American adults with type 2 diabetes.[31] The self-management program consisted of an 8-month intensive stage (which included an individual counseling visit, group sessions, postcard messages, and telephone calls), followed by a 4-month reinforcement stage. A total of 24 churches participated in the 2-year randomized controlled trial (participant $n = 201$). Controlling for potential confounders, participants in the treatment arm had 0.5% (95% confidence interval, 0.2–0.7; $p < .001$) lower mean A1c levels at 8-month follow-up. At 12-month follow-up, there were no significant differences between the treatment and control groups.[32]

A church-based diabetes prevention program designed for African American adults was developed by adapting a segment of the Diabetes Prevention Program.[33] The 6-session intervention was modified to accommodate a group format and was led by a volunteer health care professional. A prayer began and ended each session. The feasibility of the intervention was tested in one African American church (participant $n = 10$). Mean body weight decreased from 231 ± 55.7 pounds to 224.5 ± 60 pounds at 6-month follow-up, and to 220.4 ± 34.7 pounds at 12-month follow-up.

The 6-session diabetes prevention intervention described above was examined in conjunction with a Diabetes Prevention Program translated into a 16-session version in 5 African American Baptist churches in rural Georgia (participant $n = 37$).[34] The project team modified the Diabetes Prevention Program to accommodate a group-based design, including encouragement of group interaction. Prayer was also implemented in the beginning and end of each session. There were no significant differences in outcomes between the 6- and 16-session intervention arms. Combining the data from participants in the 6- and 16-session intervention arms, there was statistically significant decreases in fasting glucose, weight, and body mass index. Mean fasting blood glucose decreased from 108.1 ± 6.4 to 101.7 ± 6.4 from baseline to program completion; this decrease in fasting blood glucose was maintained at 6- and 12-month follow-up. Body mass index decreased from 33.2 ± 6.2 to 32.6 ± 6.0 from baseline to program completion; however, the magnitude of the change diminished at 6- (32.9 ± 6.6) and 12- (32.9 ± 6.5) month follow-up.

Obesity

Two weight-loss interventions for rural faith populations were identified. Both projects worked with African American churches using a participatory approach, shared similar programmatic aspects, and incorporated faith beliefs throughout the curriculum.

In the *Wholeness, Oneness, Righteousness, Deliverance* (WORD) projects in North Carolina[35] and Arkansas,[36] a community-based participatory research approach was used to design a culturally appropriate weight-loss intervention for rural African American adults. The WORD in Arkansas adapted materials and methods from the Diabetes Prevention Program and conducted a feasibility pilot in three churches (single group design), whereas the WORD in North Carolina conducted a quasi-experimental pilot in four churches, with two churches in the treatment group and two in the control group. Both projects trained church members to deliver the intervention, and both incorporated faith beliefs and practices. In the WORD in North Carolina, there was significant weight loss from baseline to 8-week follow-up, with 3.60 ± 0.64 pounds mean weight loss in the treatment group compared to 0.59 ± 0.59 pounds mean weight loss in the control group. In the WORD in Arkansas, participants lost an average of 5.16 (SD = 5.46) pounds (from baseline to 16-week follow-up, for a mean weight change of –2.7% (SD = 5.78%). In both WORD projects, participants and church members who delivered the intervention reported that the faith elements of the interventions were well received and encouraged participants to change their health behaviors.

Sexually Transmitted Diseases

The *Columbia-Union Faith-Based Adolescent STI/HIV Prevention Project* was conducted in collaboration with 43 African American churches in rural North Florida.[37] The intervention included trained adults and adolescents to deliver four abstinence-based intervention sessions to prevent sexually transmitted diseases (including HIV) for adolescents aged 13 through 19. Intervention content included HIV/AIDS statistics, group discussions, interactive activities, and educational videos. Adult-led intervention sessions were compared to peer-led intervention sessions. A total of 143 persons participated in the program; pretest and posttest data were collected from 101 participants. A significant increase in knowledge and self-perceived risk of HIV was reported in only the adult-led group.

Smoking

One smoking intervention for rural churches was identified. The *Alliance of Black Churches Health Project* was a smoking cessation intervention for African Americans.[38] Based on community empowerment, the project held county-wide events, distributed self-help materials, and trained church members to deliver one-on-one counseling. The effect of the intervention was tested through assessing baseline and 18-month smoking prevalence, smoking cessation, and other relevant variables across two counties, one treatment and one control. At follow-up, the smoking cessation rate (1 month continuous abstinence) was higher in the treatment county (9.6%) compared to the control county (5.4%), with those attending church more frequently reporting higher quit rates (10.5%) compared to less frequent attenders (5.9%); however, these differences were not significant ($p = 0.18, 0.20$, respectively).

Nutrition and Physical Activity

One study with the primary outcome of nutrition and physical activity was identified. *Guide to Health* was an intervention to increase healthy nutrition and physical activity in African Americans and Whites attending Baptist or United Methodist churches.[39] The intervention consisted of an Internet component (12 modules to increase physical activity; to increase fruit, vegetable, and fiber intake; and to decrease fat intake) and church-based supports (e.g., reminders from the pulpit, church bulletins, and newsletters). A total of 14 churches (participant $n = 1071$) were randomized to one of three arms: internet only, Internet plus church-based support, or wait-list control. Participants in the Internet-only arm and the Internet plus church-based support arm significantly increased fiber intake (approximately 3.00 g/1000 kcal), and fruit and vegetable intake (approximately 3.30 g/1000 kcal) compared to control churches from baseline to postintervention. There were no differences among the treatment groups. There was a statistical trend toward decreased fat intake in the Internet plus church-based support group. Compared to the control group, those in the Internet plus church-based support group arm lost weight (2.43 pounds) and increased physical activity (2.20 steps/day) from baseline to postintervention. Changes in fiber intake, fruit and vegetable intake, fat intake, and physical activity remained at 6-month follow-up.

DISCUSSION

Few Church-Based Health Promotion Programs in Rural Areas

Although a large number of church-based health promotion programs have been conducted, a relatively small number of these programs have been conducted in rural areas.[13,14,40] This is surprising given the greater religiosity of rural residents.[2] To have a large enough sample size to test for intervention efficacy, some studies have purposly worked with larger churches (e.g., some studies have required minimum church memberships of 100).[14] Since smaller churches are more likely to be prevalent in rural areas, previous church-based health interventions may have inadvertently overlooked rural churches. Future studies may consider combining small churches in a way to meet sample size requirements so small churches can be included (e.g., two similar small churches could be considered one church in statistical analysis). For example, in the WORD projects,[35,36] each church was asked to recruit an intervention group of 10 participants. To allow smaller churches to participate, the program was designed to welcome members from other churches to join an intervention group sponsored by a participating church. In some cases, members from other churches may not feel comfortable attending an intervention group held at another church; in these cases, the intervention group can be advertised as being sponsored by a number of churches, and the intervention held in a local community center.

Success of Rural Faith Health Promotion

Given the limited number of church-based programs in rural areas, the success of rural faith health promotion is unclear (the evidence base being limited by the lack of studies assessing their impact). There is strong evidence for engaging rural churches to change health behaviors to prevent cancer, particularly fruit and vegetable intake and breast and colorectal cancer screening in African American adults. There is some evidence for church-based health promotion to prevent chronic disease and its risk factors, although the number of studies that have been conducted in rural areas is too limited to make definitive conclusions. There was no evidence for church-based rural mental health, as no interventions were identified, although this topic has been addressed through churches in nonrural areas.[41] In general, there is a significant stigma against mental health treatment. Thus, maintaining participant confidentiality in receiving treatment is an important factor. Given that rural communities tend to have tight social networks that make the maintenance of confidentiality more challenging, rural residents may be more hesitant to participate in mental health interventions.[42,43] Faith-based approaches to this and other particularly stigmatized outcomes should consider innovative ways of minimizing stigma (e.g., packaging as part of a larger health intervention or using creative naming).

Despite data from church-based health studies in nonrural areas for the efficacy of church-based health promotion, future studies examining these interventions in rural areas are sorely needed. Rural areas have a distinctive culture that necessitates programs for this unique population.[4] The relative paucity of faith-based rural health promotion coupled with religion's greater salience in rural populations illustrates great potential for future work in this area.

Future Directions for Church-Based Health Promotion in Rural Areas

The future directions for church-based rural health initiatives largely parallel the growing consensus regarding the future directions of church-based health promotion in general.[13,14] There is some evidence that church-based health promotion programs are effective in changing health behaviors, but more scientifically rigorous studies are needed to establish the efficacy of rural church-based health promotion. Given that the majority of rural church-based interventions have been conducted in African American adults, future work is needed to establish the efficacy of church-based health promotion in other racial and age groups, including children. Building on the strengths of the church—including faith beliefs and values—has also been argued to produce more culturally sensitive interventions to improve program impact.[13] Different terminology (e.g., faith-based vs. faith-placed[13]; collaborative[14];

Lasater's levels I–IV[44]) has been used to categorize the degree to which the church and the larger community are involved in the creation of the intervention. Placing church-based health programs in a spiritual context may be particularly salient to churches in rural areas, which have higher levels of religiosity compared to nonrural areas.[2] Collaborative approaches to intervention development would help ensure that church-based interventions build upon these and other strengths of the rural church.[13]

Persons living in rural areas face considerable challenges to good health. The poorer health outcomes in rural areas are well documented,[4] in addition to the myriad of factors that contribute to these disparities.[45]Although more work needs to be done in the area of church-based rural health promotion to establish efficacy, there is preliminary evidence for the effectiveness of church-based interventions to change health behaviors. Given the salience of faith in rural areas, church-based health promotion has great potential to address rural health disparities, particularly those interventions that build upon the strengths of faith communities through a participatory approach.

REFERENCES

1. Gallup Poll G. United States: The Roper Center for Public Opinion Research; 2007.
2. Gallup Poll G. United States: The Roper Center for Public Opinion Research; 2002.
3. Olson LM, Reis J, Murphy L, Gehm JH. The religious community as a partner in health care. *J Community Health.* 1988;13(4):249–257.
4. Hartley D. Rural health disparities, population health, and rural culture. *Am J Public Health.* 2004;94(10):1675–1678.
5. Lapane KL, Lasater TM, Allan C, Carleton RA. Religion and cardiovascular disease risk. *J Religion and Health.* 1997;36(2):155–163.
6. Lasater TM, Carleton RA, Wells BL. Religious organizations and large-scale health related lifestyle change programs. *J Health Educ.* 1991;22(4):233–239.
7. Eberhardt MS, Ingram DD, Makuc DM, et al. *Urban and Rural Health Chartbook.* Hyattsville, MD: National Center for Health Statistics; 2001.
8. Chatters LM, Levin JS, Ellison CG. Public health and health education in faith communities. *Health Educ Behav.* 1998;25(6):689–699.
9. Regenstein JM, Chaudry MM. Kosher and Halal laws with an emphasis on important issues when considering fruit and vegetable coating. In: Gennadios A, ed. *Protein-Based Films and Coatings.* Boca Raton, FL: CRC Press; 2003:601–620.
10. Fraser GE. Diet as primordial prevention in seventh-day adventists. *Preventive Med.* 1999;29(6, pt 2):S18–S23.
11. Shatenstein B, Ghadirian P. Influences on diet, health behaviours and their outcome in select ethnocultural and religious groups. *Nutrition.* 1998;14(2): 223–230.
12. Kim KH, Sobal J. Religion, social support, fat intake, and physical activity. *Public Health Nutr.* 2004;7:773–781.
13. Campbell MK, Hudson MA, Resnicow K, Blakeney N, Paxton A, Baskin M. Church-based health promotion interventions: evidence and lessons learned. *Annual Rev Public Health.* 2007;28:213–234.
14. DeHaven MJ, Hunter IB, Wilder L, Walton JW, Berry J. Health programs in faith-based organizations: are they effective? *Am J Public Health.* 2004;94(6):1030–1036.

15. Yeary KH, Klos LA, Linnan L. The examination of process evaluation use in church-based health interventions: a systematic review. *Health Promot Pract.* 2012;13(4):524–534.
16. Coburn AF, MacKinney AC, McBride TD, Mueller KJ, Slifkin RT, Wakefield MK. *Choosing Rural Definitions: Implications for Health Policy.* Columbia, MO: Rural Policy Research Institute Health Panel; 2007.
17. Cowart ME, Sutherland M, Harris GJ. Health promotion for older rural African Americans: implications for social and public policy. *J Appl Gerontol.* 1995;14(1):33–46.
18. Campbell MK, James A, Hudson MA, et al. Improving multiple behaviors for colorectal cancer prevention among African American church members. *Health Psychol.* 2004;23(5):492–502.
19. Sauaia A, Min SJ, Lack D, et al. Church-based breast cancer screening education: impact of two approaches on Latinas enrolled in public and private health insurance plans. *Prev Chronic Dis.* 2007;4(4):A99.
20. Welsh AL, Sauaia A, Jacobellis J, Min SJ, Byers T. The effect of two church-based interventions on breast cancer screening rates among Medicaid-insured Latinas. *Prev Chronic Dis.* 2005;2(4):A07.
21. Erwin DO, Spatz TS, Stotts RC, Hollenberg JA. Increasing mammography practice by African American women. *Cancer Prac.* 1999;7(2):78–85.
22. Erwin DO. Cancer education takes on a spiritual focus for the African American faith community. *J Cancer Educ.* 2002;17(1):46–49.
23. Ka'opua LS, Park SH, Ward ME, Braun KL. Testing the feasibility of a culturally tailored breast cancer screening intervention with native Hawaiian women in rural churches. *Health Soc Work.* 2011;36(1):55–65.
24. Campbell MK, Demark-Wahnefried W, Symons M, et al. Fruit and vegetable consumption and prevention of cancer: the Black Churches United for better health project. *Am J Public Health.* 1999;89(9):1390–1396.
25. Resnicow K, Campbell MK, Carr C, et al. Body and soul. A dietary intervention conducted through African-American churches. *Am J Prev Med.* 2004;27(2):97–105.
26. Lasater TM, Wells BL, Carleton RA, Elder JP. The role of churches in disease prevention research studies. *Public Health Rep.* 1986;101(2):125–131.
27. Lasater TM, DePue J, Wells BL, Gans KM, Bellis J, Carleton RA. The effectiveness and feasibility of delivering nutrition education programs through religious organizations. *Health Promot Int.* 1990;5(4):253–257.
28. Wells BL, DePue J, Lasater TM, Carleton RA. A report on church site weight control. *Health Educ Res.* 1988;3(3):305–316.
29. Turner LW, Sutherland M, Harris GJ, Barber M. Cardiovascular health promotion in North Florida African-American churches. *Health Values.* 1995;19(2):3–9.
30. Williamson W, Kautz DD. "Let's get moving: let's get praising:" Promoting health and hope in the African American church. *ABNF J.* 2009;20(4):102–105.
31. Samuel-Hodge CD, Keyserling TC, France R, et al. A church-based diabetes self-management education program for African Americans with type 2 diabetes. *Prev Chronic Dis.* 2006;3(3):A93.
32. Samuel-Hodge C, Keyserling TC, Park S, Johnston LF, Gizlice Z, Bangdiwala SI. A randomized trial of a church-based diabetes self-management program for African Americans with type 2 diabetes. *The Diabetes Educator.* 2009;35(3):439–454.
33. Davis-Smith M. Implementing a diabetes prevention program in a rural African-American church. *J Natl Med Assoc.* 2007;99(4):440–446.

34. Boltri JM, Davis-Smith M, Okosun IS, Seale JP, Foster B. Translation of the National Institutes of Health Diabetes Prevention Program in African American churches. *J Natl Med Assoc.* 2011;103(3):194–202.
35. Kim KH, Linnan L, Campbell MK, Brooks C, Koenig HG, Wiesen C. The WORD (Wholeness, Oneness, Righteousness, Deliverance): a faith-based weight loss program utilizing a participatory approach. *Health Educ Behav.* 2008;35(5):634–650.
36. Yeary KHK, Cornell CE, Turner J, et al. Feasibility test of an evidence-based weight loss intervention translated for a faith-based, rural, African American population. *Prev Chronic Dis.* 2011;8(6):1–12.
37. Baldwin JA, Daley E, Brown EJ, et al. Knowledge and perception of STI/HIV risk among rural African American youth: lessons learned in a faith-based pilot program. *J HIV/AIDS Prev Child Youth.* 2008;9(1):97–114.
38. Schorling JB, Roach J, Siegel M, et al. A trial of church-based smoking cessation interventions for rural African Americans. *Prev Med.* 1997;26(1):92–101.
39. Winett RA, Anderson ES, Wojcik JR, Winett SG, Bowden T. Guide to health: nutrition and physical activity outcomes of a group-randomized trial of an Internet-based intervention in churches. *Ann Behav Med.* 2007;33(3):251–261.
40. Yeary KH, Klos LA, Linnan L. The examination of process evaluation use in church-based health interventions: a systematic review. *Health Promot Pract.* 2012;13(4):524–534.
41. Hankerson SH, Weissman MM. Church-based health programs for mental disorders among African Americans: a review. *Psychiatr Serv.* 2012;63(3):243–249.
42. Corrigan PW, River LP, Lundin RK, et al. Three strategies for changing attributions about severe mental illness. *Schizophr Bull.* 2001;27(2):187–195.
43. Rost K, Fortney J, Fischer E, Smith J. Use, quality, and outcomes of care for mental health: the rural perspective. *Med Care Res Rev.* 2002;59(3):231–265; discussion 266–271.
44. Lasater TM, Becker DM, Hill MN, Gans KM. Synthesis of findings and issues from religious-based cardiovascular disease prevention trials. *Ann Epidemiol.* 1997;7(57):S47–S53.
45. USDA Economic Research Service. Rural Poverty at a Glance. http://www.ers .usda.gov/publications/rdrr100/rdrr100.pdf. 2005.

CHAPTER 6

Integrated Care in Rural Areas

David Lambert and John A. Gale

Over the past decade there has been a substantial push within our health care system to integrate physical and mental health care. One impetus for integration is that the traditional separation of general health and mental health services may hinder a holistic medical approach necessary to treat effectively what are often comorbid health problems. Another impetus is that there are simply not enough mental health clinicians to treat all the persons with a mental health problem or illness. In addition, many individuals prefer receiving mental health care in a primary care setting, for reasons to be presented in this chapter. In fact, more persons with a mental health problem or illness are treated by a primary care provider than by a specialty mental health care provider.[1,2]

Efforts to integrate primary and mental health care came early to rural America. There was simply no choice—more than 80% of psychiatrists and doctoral-level psychologists reside in urban areas, and this distribution has remained essentially unchanged for decades.[3] There is rich experience to draw on in designing and sustaining integrated programs in rural areas. This same experience suggests that there are also significant and persistent barriers to rural integration. Successful rural integrated programs are increasing, but they often require adapting to the local infrastructure and community context and understanding the changing policy environment.

This chapter is presented in six sections. Following this overview, the second section presents the background for integration, including definitions, models, barriers, and evidence from the general integration literature. Section three describes the history of integration in rural areas, while the fourth section takes a closer look at current and best practices of integrating care in rural areas and highlights several exemplary programs. Section five takes a look at the road ahead for integrating care in rural areas, including an analysis of current policy initiatives—parity, person-centered medical homes, and health care reform—that will inevitably affect this road. Section six presents practical strategies for integrating care in rural areas.

BACKGROUND

There is widespread support for the "idea" of integration—that is, people's physical and mental health problems should be coordinated and not treated separately or in isolation from each other. Seminal reports have endorsed the importance of integration, including the Surgeon General's Report on Mental Health,[4] the President's New Freedom Commission on Mental Health,[3] and the Institute of Medicine's *Improving the Quality of Health Care for Mental and Substance-Use Conditions.*[5] Comprehensive health care policy initiatives, such as the Bureau of Primary Health Care's New Access Initiative,[6] which expands the role and reach of community health centers[7] and the current development and promotion of the patient-centered medical home, include an important place for integration.

Despite widespread support for the idea of integration, there is less agreement about what integration means, how it should work, and what it has accomplished. Below is presented the current state of discussion and understanding of definitions, specific integrated care models, and evidence for integrated care.

Definition of Integration

A number of definitions of integration are found within the literature, usually reflecting the specific clinical settings and the health care providers being studied or described. In their review of this literature, the federal Agency for Healthcare Research and Quality (AHRQ) posits a simple but robust definition of integration: "Integrated care occurs when mental health specialty and general medical care providers work together to address both the physical and mental health needs of their patients."[8] The AHRQ paper notes that integration can work in two ways: integrating specialty mental health care into primary care or integrating primary care into specialty mental health care. AHRQ further emphasizes that it is important to consider at least two dimensions: integration of providers and integration of processes of care. Making a similar distinction, Gale and Lambert note that it is important to move beyond the question of *where* care is provided and by whom to the question of *how* care is provided.[9] It is important to move beyond the *structure* of integration to the *function* of integration. This distinction is particularly important in understanding and improving integrated care in rural areas.

Models of Integration

A number of different approaches and models of integration have been developed. An important foundational model for much of this work is the Four Quadrant Clinical Integration Model, first introduced in 1998 to depict treatment options for persons with co-occurring mental health and substance abuse disorders.[10] The model characterizes clients by the severity of their mental health/substance abuse problems and their physical health problems to determine the most appropriate treatment setting. In 2003, the National Council for Community Behavioral Healthcare issued a paper that argued that integration had become "stuck" at the policy idea level and required support at the policy, training, and clinical levels to move forward.[11] The report adapted the Four Quadrant Model to classify the level of integration and clinical competencies needed to treat persons with differing behavioral health (BH) and physical health (PH) complexity. The resulting four quadrants are: (a) low BH, low PH; (b) high BH, low PH; (c) low BH, high PH; and (d) high BH, high PH. The Four Quadrant Model continues to be adapted and used in policy discussions, including the rationale and need to include behavioral health in the patient-centered medical home.[12]

As mentioned, depictions of integration models have evolved from the question of *where* care is provided (general health care or specialty health care) to *how* care is provided. Schemes such as Wagner's Chronic Care Model,[13] anchored by a care manager, and Strosahl's model,[14] in which mid-level behavioral health specialists help engage primary care patients, have gathered significant support. In general, there is a preference within the literature for more highly integrated models. However, this preference tacitly assumes that sufficient infrastructure and resources are available to support full integration. This is often not the case in many urban areas and is rarely the case in rural areas. Doherty, McDaniel, and Baird capture these issues in a five-level classification of integration: (a) separate systems and facilities, (b) basic collaboration from a distance, (c) basic collaboration on site, (d) close collaboration in a partially integrated system, and (e) a fully integrated system.[15] This model allows for practices to adapt the level of integration most suitable to their resources and needs and to move to higher levels of integration as needs and resources allow.

Barriers to Integration

Efforts to develop and sustain integrated programs face substantial barriers that are well documented and described in the literature.[8,16,17] Gale and Lambert summarize this literature in terms of five levels:[18]

National and system-level barriers include the limited supply of specialty behavioral health providers and their maldistribution relative to need; the separation of funding streams for general and behavioral health care services; and the lack of parity between coverage for general medical and behavioral health conditions.

Regulatory barriers include state-level licensure laws governing the requirements for a professional title; the scope of practice (specific activities persons meeting these requirements are permitted to perform); and facility licensure governing the provision of services by behavioral health agencies.

Reimbursement barriers include lack of reimbursement for integrative and preventive services; variation in reimbursement rules across third-party payers; different coding and billing classifications by setting and payer; and mental health carve-outs (in which payment and management of mental health care is separated from physical health care).

Practice and cultural barriers between primary and mental health practice include different practice styles, culture, language, and administration. Differences include methods used to reach a diagnosis, lengths, and content of typical visits; the use of separate patient records; and approaches to charting, record keeping, and communication with other providers. The lack of integration of information technology, both within and across practices, compounds these barriers.

Patient-level barriers include poor access to behavioral health services; limitations on coverage and reimbursement by third-party payers; impact of high deductibles and co-pays on use of services; complexity of authorization and utilization review; and patient perception of stigma in receiving behavioral health care.

Evidence for Integration

In their evidentiary review of the integration literature, AHRQ identified 33 clinical trials of integrated programs that fit their screening criteria and differentiated them according to level of provider integration and level of processes of care.[8] Integrated care programs tended to have positive outcomes for symptom severity, treatment response, and remission compared to usual care. However, there was wide variation in levels of provider integration and integrated processes of care, but this variation was not related to outcome. This led the authors to characterize the evidence on the effectiveness on integrated care as being a choice of viewing the glass as half empty or half full, cautioning that "while there is much to be optimistic about there is also little to suggest adherence to strict orthodoxy in defining and adhering to what an effective integrated care program might be."[8]

INTEGRATED CARE IN RURAL AREAS

Efforts to integrate care in rural areas extend back over 40 years and can be traced to major federal initiatives to expand access to health care. Legislation creating community and migrant health centers in 1967 required these entities to offer basic mental health services.[19] During the late 1970s and early 1980s, programs such as the Rural Health Initiative, the Health Underserved

Rural Areas grants, the Rural Mental Health Demonstration Program, and the Linkage Initiative Program provided incentives to link primary care and mental health in rural areas. The creation in 1989 of FQHCs that could be reimbursed on a cost basis by Medicare and Medicaid introduced additional resources to linking care in rural areas. However, by the early 1990s, it was not clear to what extent there were sustained integrated care programs in rural areas. Evaluations of the earlier demonstration programs suggested that while they were initially effective, the programs and their services did not last once their funding ended. It was also not clear to what extent FQHCs were able to provide mental health services in rural areas. To better understand the scope and nature of integrated care in rural areas, the Maine Rural Health Research Center conducted a national survey of 53 primary care programs in rural areas that provided or coordinated mental health care.[20] They found that rural primary care providers used four different strategies or models to integrate care:

- *Diversification*: Care provided onsite directly with a center's own mental health staff
- *Linkage/co-location*: Care provided onsite by a noncenter staff health worker
- *Referral*: Care provided off-site by noncenter staff under a formal agreement
- *Enhancement*: Primary care practitioners are trained to provide mental health care onsite

At the time the survey was conducted, rural community health centers and other primary care providers had relatively limited information to help them develop and provide mental health services. In the ensuing decade, a variety of screening tools and guidelines were developed for identifying mental health problems and linking and integrating care. In 2004, the National Rural Health Association asked the Maine Rural Health Research Center to revisit their earlier study and to assess whether rural primary care providers were using approaches similar to or different from a decade earlier to integrate care and to assess what challenges rural providers faced in integrating care. To examine these issues, the Maine Rural Health Research Center conducted case studies of community health centers in Colorado, Montana, New Hampshire, North Carolina, Pennsylvania, and South Dakota.[21]

The case studies found that rural community health centers were more likely in 2004 than in the 10 years before to provide mental health care using staff employed by the health centers (diversification model). The authors described two key components of care delivered in these settings—integrative activities and direct care services—that create a synergy that contributes to the success of integrated programs. Integrative activities were usually performed by the mental health clinician and include patient screening and engagement, consulting with primary care staff (in formal meetings and "hallway consults"), "warm handoffs" to introduce patients to the mental health clinicians, and responding to patient and staff questions. Warm handoffs are particularly useful to enhance the trust and rapport developed between the primary care provider and the patient, and to improve the likelihood that the patient will follow through with mental health treatment. Integrative activities help to reduce demands on primary care staff and allow them to see more patients, but are usually not directly reimbursable services.

Direct care services include medication management by the primary care physician and counseling and therapy provided by the mental health (licensed counselor) staff using appropriate behavioral health codes. Direct services, when delivered by an appropriately licensed clinician, as defined by state law and/or third-party payer policies, are usually reimbursable by third-party payers.

Five of the six centers used a standardized screening tool (usually the PHQ-9) with most patients as a mechanism for identifying depression. The PHQ-9 is the nine-question depression module of the Patient Health Questionnaire, a self-administered diagnostic tool, containing five modules covering anxiety and somatoform, alcohol, and eating disorders, developed by Robert L. Spitzer, MD, Janet B. W. Williams, DSW, and Kurt Kroenke, MD. Medication management and obtaining psychiatric consultations to support the primary care providers in prescribing psychotropic medications remained an ongoing challenge for most centers. Depression is the most common mental health condition identified and treated in rural primary care centers and many primary care clinicians are comfortable prescribing frontline antidepressants. The challenge emerges when these medications are not effective or comorbidities are present without a readily accessible mental health specialist with whom to consult. A confounding problem is the increased complexity and severity of mental health problems of patients turning to rural primary care providers for care. Two factors have contributed to this trend: (a) decreased funding for specialty mental health care in nearly every state; and (b) specialty mental health providers and agencies, unlike community health centers, are not funded to be safety-net providers (i.e., to serve low-income, uninsured, and underinsured clients).

The study found that rural community health centers were more likely to provide mental health care than a decade earlier, which was consistent with policy expectations. As the authors observe, the question facing rural community health centers had largely shifted from *whether* to *how* to provide mental health care: "The primary questions rural CHCs [community health centers] face are how to treat these problems in an acute care setting with very limited options for psychiatric consultation and referral and how to improve the functioning of their clinical team. CHCs must determine how many patients and what conditions they can treat."[21]

CURRENT AND BEST PRACTICES IN RURAL INTEGRATION

There is no single best way to integrate care in rural areas.[16,21,22] Rather, a variety of approaches can and do work. What seems to be important is that providers first understand what their goals are and prioritize them. Is their goal to expand access to mental health services for all persons in their community or to those whom they are already treating for physical health conditions (i.e., current patients of their practice)? What behavioral health conditions will patients have? How severe and complex are these conditions likely to be? Given these considerations, what role and function do they envision for their primary care staff and how will they work with behavioral health clinicians? What resources for referral and/or consultation are available in the community? How will the program be reimbursed? Are resources available to support nonreimbursable services, typically the integrative component of the program? When rural providers understand their integration goals, it is possible to start modestly and evolve and expand with experience?

Case Studies of Integrated Care in Rural Communities

This section reviews the experience and lessons learned by four rural primary care providers who have successfully integrated care. One rural federally qualified health center (FQHC), Community Health Partners in Livingston, Montana, strategically chose to add mental health services incrementally. Another FQHC, the Open Door Community Health Centers in northwest California, added tele-mental health to enhance its integration approach. The DIAMOND (Depression Improvement Across Minnesota Offering a New Direction) Program, a collaborative initiative involving third-party payers, the Minnesota Department of Human Services, and providers, developed an integrated model and reimbursement mechanisms to treat Medicaid beneficiaries with depression. The fourth program, Cherokee Health Care System in eastern Tennessee, is a well-resourced and organized care system that integrates community health and community mental health centers and is widely touted as a model of rural mental health and primary care integration. These rural providers have been selected because they vary in size, approach, and funding, yet have all been successful. Their variety of approaches and funding illustrates a key point of this chapter: Providers should choose models and approaches for which there is evidence and that fit their needs, experience, and resources.

Community Health Partners (CHP) is a small network of FQHCs in south-central Montana.[21] The primary site was established in Livingston in 1997 and a second site was opened in Bozeman in 2002. The population served by CHP includes a significant percentage of persons in poverty as well as high-income persons attracted to the state's natural resources. Specialty mental health services were not readily available to CHP's clients, prompting CHP in the early 2000s to develop mental health services.

CHP chose to adopt Kirk Strosahl's model of integration. In this model, primary care providers screen for behavioral health problems during patient exams.[14] If the screen is positive, the patient is encouraged to meet that day with an onsite clinical counselor, who tries to engage the patient in treatment. During this brief initial behavioral health encounter (15–30 minutes), the counselor undertakes an initial assessment and begins the development of a treatment plan. The PHQ-9 is administered to screen more fully for depression and to assess functionality. Motivational interviewing is used to encourage the patient to identify stressors and additional counseling visits are scheduled as necessary. To accommodate "same-day referrals,"counselors leave half of their daily schedules open.

The Strosahl model fits well with CHP's strategic needs and organizational culture, which includes a relatively young, highly motivated staff. Counselors provide an important consulting resource to the primary care staff in addition to direct service responsibilities.[21] A psychiatrist is available onsite one afternoon a month for consultation. Approximately 60% of CHP's funding is supported by its Section 330 federal grant, 10% by Medicaid, 10% by private insurance, and 20% by private pay patients and other grants. Section 330 of the Public Health Service Act defines federal grant funding opportunities for organizations to provide care to underserved populations. Types of organizations that may receive 330 grants include: FQHCs/ community health centers, migrant health centers, health care for the homeless programs, and public housing primary care programs.

Open Door Community Health Centers (Open Door) has nine sites and a mobile dental unit serving primarily low-income persons over a very large rural area in northwest California, including Humboldt and Del Norte Counties and portions of Trinity and Siskiyou Counties.[23,24] Started in 1971 as a small local clinic staffed largely by volunteers, Open Door has expanded its staff services and locations over the past four decades. Today its staff includes 37 full-time equivalent (FTE) medical staff, 9 FTE dental staff, and 9 FTE behavioral health practitioners, and offers a wide array of services including family practice, pediatrics, women's health, prenatal and birth, family planning, geriatrics, dental care, urgent care, mental and behavioral health, STD testing and counseling, HIV/AIDS care, alternative medicine, health education, and smoking cessation. Open Door earned FQHC status in 1999, making it eligible for Section 330 grant funding to support care for the uninsured as well as enhanced Medicare and Medi-Cal (California's Medicaid program) reimbursement.

Although Open Door found it difficult to recruit and retain specialist providers, it was able to hire a psychiatrist in 2004 to rotate among several clinic locations. While this hire enhanced the center's ability to provide behavioral health services, the significant travel demands of up to several hours a day (also known as "windshield time" among providers) led the psychiatrist to leave Open Door after a year. Excessive travel demands were experienced by Open Door's patients as well. A 2005 survey conducted by Open Door found that its patients, on average, traveled 558 miles and 12 hours to see a specialist.[24]

These issues led the Open Door to expand its current use of telehealth to provide specialty services to remote locations. Open Door first used telehealth in the late 1990s (working with the California Telemedicine and eHealth Center and sponsored by Blue Cross of California) to provide specialty consultation using a large computer screen, a video camera, and a keyboard. The heaviest demand was for dermatology and psychiatry. To provide tele-mental health services, Open Door worked with a group of psychiatrists in Santa Rosa (200 miles south of the Center). Limited telehealth reimbursement ultimately limited the use of these psychiatrists and the service despite the relatively high demand for psychiatric services by Open Door's patients.

To enhance its telehealth services, Open Door opened the Telehealth and Visiting Specialist Center (TVSC) in 2006. TVSC is housed in its own building with significantly improved equipment (a Polycom VSX 5000 video conferencing unit) supported by foundation funding. TVSC enabled Open Door to centralize (and thus spread) the costs related to its telehealth programs, including connectivity, training, support staff, and equipment.

Open Door also received funding from the Health Resources and Services Administration (HRSA) to expand the scope of its services, including those now provided through the TVSC. This allowed Open Door to charge a higher reimbursement that included the costs of the TVSC computer. In addition to providing services to its own clients through the TVSC, Open Door contracts to provide specialty services using telehealth to other organizations across California, thus working as both a "hub" as well as a "spoke" of telehealth services. In 2009, Open Door provided nearly 1,000 telehealth visits, including 158 pediatric, 132 psychiatric, and 40 pediatric behavioral health visits.[23]

Open Door's experience suggests that telehealth can be used effectively to complement existing onsite mental health to persons spread over a very large rural area. However, Open Door's experience also suggests that the service must be large enough to incorporate other health services (in addition to mental health) in order to spread the costs of staff, equipment, and space across a wider array of services.

In 2003, the Minnesota Council of Health plans and the Minnesota Department of Human Services created the Minnesota Mental Health Action Group (MMHAG) to promote public–private partnerships and initiatives to improve access to quality mental health services. In 2007, the Governor's Mental Health Initiative built on the work of the MMHAG to: (a) develop a comprehensive mental health benefit for proven treatment across public and private plans; (b) integrate mental health and physical health services; and (c) make significant investments in mental health infrastructure.[25] Work on integration focused on developing integrated service networks that would receive reimbursement for providing integrated care under a "preferred integrated network" status. This effort resulted in the *DIAMOND Initiative* (Depression Improvement Across Minnesota Offering a New Direction), which was created in 2008. Under the DIAMOND initiative, 10 primary care clinics across the state screen adult primary care patients for depression (via the PHQ-9) using a care management model. The integrative care management service is provided by a care manager for which the clinics receive a periodic depression care fee payment from the participating third-party payers. Support for the care manager is not time limited as it was under earlier demonstrations, and the specific payment details are negotiated between each health plan and medical clinic. Minnesota is developing a bonus program to pay primary care physicians for providing quality depression care under a pilot program involving a coalition of the state's 40 largest employers.[26]

Minnesota has taken a strategic path to integrating primary and behavioral health care that started with facilitating discussions among key players and later evolved to implement focused regulatory and reimbursement changes. Noteworthy from a policy perspective are the development and continued use of viable public-private partnerships. Noteworthy from a practice perspective is the decision to reimburse for the integrative services provided by care managers. These services are not usually considered reimbursable services by many third-party payers. If they are covered, it is usually paid for as part of a demonstration project, which has proved to be a barrier to maintaining integration over time.

Cherokee Health Systems (CHS) spans 22 sites in 15 eastern Tennessee counties and is a frequently cited example of the integration of primary and behavioral health care in a rural setting.[27,28] The agency started as a single-site mental health center in 1960 and changed its name in 1973 to the Cherokee Guidance Center to destigmatize mental illness. School-based psychology services were established in 1970 and outreach to primary care began in 1980. CHS's involvement in primary care increased in 1984 when it established its first primary care clinic. In 1989, CHS was designated as the mental health carve-out provider in eastern Tennessee by HealthSource, a behavioral health management company that contracted with third-party payers to manage mental health benefits. In 1994, CHS was designated as the Behavioral Health Organization under the mental health program component of TennCare, Tennessee's Medicaid care program established under a Medicaid Waiver. CHS continued to add clinical services and locations, assisted by a series of Health Resources and Services Administration grants including a 2002 Rural Health Outreach grant (to provide outreach and services to the growing Hispanic population in Grainger, Hamblen, and Jefferson Counties) and a 2003 Bureau of Primary Health Care (BPHC) grant to support the evolution of a number of sites into comprehensive community health centers.[27] In 2005, CHS received BPHC designation as a migrant health center. In 2009, the Tennessee Legislature and Board of Pharmacy approved Cherokee to operate a telepharmacy program at two locations.[28]

Twelve of CHS's 22 sites are fully integrated with a licensed behavioral health specialist embedded within each primary care team through the use of a shared electronic health record. Primary care providers conduct the initial physical assessments, which include screening for behavioral health issues. For appropriate patients, the primary care providers do "warm handoffs" to the behavioral health consultants who provide brief targeted interventions and arrange for follow-up services as needed. Visits with the behavioral health consultants typically last between 15 and 25 minutes instead of the 45 to 50 minute visits that are common in traditional mental health settings. These consultants routinely see patients for a limited duration of time (one to three visits) instead of five or more visits as in traditional settings. This practice improves the behavioral health consultants' productivity and improves access to care. A psychiatrist is available for consultation either by telephone or tele-health technology. CHS also participates in the 340B Drug Pricing Program, which provides access to reduced-price psychiatric medications for patients.

RURAL INTEGRATION IN A CHANGING POLICY ENVIRONMENT: THE ROAD AHEAD

As this chapter is written, a number of national trends and policy initiatives are likely to influence access to rural mental health care in the years ahead. While these trends and initiatives will evolve and change over time, they will almost certainly increase the demand for integrated behavioral and physical health care. In this last section, emerging trends and initiatives are described and suggestions are made for next steps that rural providers should consider in developing integrated services.

State Fiscal Pressures

As a result of the economic downturn, nearly all states were experiencing significant budget shortfalls and fiscal distress in 2010.[29] In response, most states significantly reduced their general fund obligations, including funds committed to the state Medicaid match. Currently, state Medicaid programs are supported by a match of state and federal funds. Medicaid financing rules require states to spend their own funds to receive a federal financial match for Medicaid services. Each state dollar draws down an equal or higher number of federal dollars. As a result, many states have decreased reimbursement to community mental health providers and have increased or renewed the use of managed care programs to control state Medicaid spending for mental health services. This has contributed to a significant downsizing and consolidation of community mental health systems and reduced the supply of mental health clinicians and access to their services. As access to care in community mental health systems has declined, more persons with mental health and emotional issues have turned to integrated behavioral health programs for care. These persons are likely to have more serious and complex needs than in the past, and there are fewer specialty mental health providers to consult with primary care providers.

At the same time that fiscal pressures constrain availability of specialty mental health services, the Paul Wellstone and Pete Domenici Mental Health Parity and Addiction Equity Act of 2008 [30] and the Patient Protection and Affordable Care Act (ACA)[31] have increased legal and regulatory pressure to expand access to mental health care and for insurers to provide benefits equivalent to those provided for physical health services. Providers and service systems are being asked to do more with less. As previously noted, this is likely to result in more persons with more complex and severe mental health conditions seeking care through primary care providers. While this trend is not new, the extent to which this may be occurring is.

Another trend likely to increase the demand for service integration is the increasing policy focus on development of patient-centered medical homes (PCMHs). The basic concept is that all patients, but particularly those with chronic and complicated conditions, should have a primary medical home where their medical conditions and health can be managed and coordinated. At the core of the PCMH model is care management and support for the patient, and an increased role for patients to direct their care in partnership with interdisciplinary teams of providers, typically directed by a physician. A number of states, including Maine and North Carolina, have implemented medical home pilot programs that call for the increased integration of behavioral and physical health services in their pilot sites.[18,32]

The ACA also included an option and resources for state Medicaid programs to provide chronic disease management to targeted Medicaid beneficiaries through health homes. States choosing this option must describe in their state plan amendments how the behavioral health needs of health home beneficiaries will be met. An important question is to what extent behavioral health will be included and integrated within medical homes, within Medicaid and elsewhere. The case for including behavioral health in medical homes is compelling; however, medical homes may very well run into the same workforce and financial barriers in including behavioral health that other programs and initiatives have.[18]

Another trend is the promotion by the specialty mental health sector of integrating primary care into behavioral health sites (sometimes referred to as "reverse integration"). The case for this is compelling on clinical grounds. Persons with a serious mental illness die, on average, 25 years younger than persons without a serious mental illness,[33] suffer from higher rates of chronic illnesses, and routinely do not receive recommended courses of primary and preventive care. In addition, routine physical health screening is often not conducted in behavioral health settings (even if medications are being prescribed). To address this gap, the National Council for Community Behavioral Healthcare (NCCBH) has recommended that behavioral health providers ensure regular physical health screening and tracking at the time of psychiatric visits for persons receiving psychotropic medications, including blood pressure, glucose and lipid levels, and body mass index.[12] The NCCBH currently serves as the Coordinating Center for the Substance Abuse and Mental Health Services Administration's Primary Care-Mental Health Initiative, which promotes integration of behavioral health into primary care settings and integration of primary care into behavioral health settings. Until recently, the vast majority of integration efforts have involved the former rather than the latter despite the compelling need for both.

The Road Ahead

In the past, much of the impetus and energy behind integration originated at the policy level, particularly the development and promotion of different models. While the policy level will remain very important, integration will ultimately succeed or fail at the clinical level. Changes occurring at the clinical level are unlikely to go away, regardless of the specific path that health care reform or PCMHs take.

Primary care clinicians will increasingly be asked to screen for a range of behavioral health problems and to treat or refer those patients as necessary. Given the shortage of specialty mental health services in rural areas, this is a role that will heavily impact rural primary care providers. In addition to direct care services, mid-level behavioral health providers will increasingly assume the role of a care manager for a range of behavioral and physical health issues. As described in the discussions of community health partners in Montana and the CHS in Tennessee, behavioral health specialists will be called on to see a greater number of patients but for shorter periods of time. They will also be asked to maintain the flexibility to see and engage patients as the need arises and to consult with the primary care team. Integrative skills will be as important as direct service clinical skills. While it is hoped that reimbursement policies will change to help support this new role, it is not clear if reimbursement levels will be adequate to support this expanded behavioral health role.

PRACTICAL STEPS TO GETTING STARTED

Given this picture, how might rural primary care and behavioral health providers begin to undertake the development of integrated care programs? First, they should decide what their goals are and prioritize them. Do they want to expand access to mental health services within the general community, or address the needs of patients within their clinics and settings? Are they focused on integrating services within their clinic (i.e., vertical integration) or improving the integration of services across practices within the community (i.e., horizontal integration)? Do they want to provide direct care or consultative services for primary care practitioners? Is their major focus on increasing the productivity of primary care providers or improving the coordination of care?

Next, providers should determine the best way to achieve each goal within the context of their practice settings and available resources. Recall that the evidence indicates that integrated care achieved positive outcomes, but that improvements in outcomes did not increase as levels of provider integration or integrated process of care increased.[8] This suggests that no single model of care integration is right for all settings. It is often best to view integration at the provider level as a "work in progress" by starting simply. This would involve assessing the practice's current readiness for integration and implementing an appropriate model of integration that is consistent with the clinic's capacity, resources, and patient needs. With experience, clinics can move further along the continuum of integration, as appropriate.

It is important to understand the functional elements of integration: Clinical, administrative, and structural aspects of the care process can be managed to improve access, quality, patient and provider satisfaction, and efficiency. These structural components are important considerations as they drive how care is delivered and coordinated, how the patient is served, how information is shared, and where patients access the service. From a clinical standpoint, the functional issues that must be considered include the extent to which the practice and all providers use a shared medical/health record; share clinical decision making; engage in regular communications in staff and clinical meetings; use common treatment plans and models; use critical pathways or practice guidelines; and refer patients among the services within the clinic. From an administrative/structural standpoint, the key issues are where the behavioral health services are located; the extent to which the behavioral health service is fully integrated into the clinic (i.e., the service is owned by the clinic and the behavioral health staff are employees of the practice) or a subcontracted service in which space is provided to external behavioral health staff to care for patients; the extent to which medical records, billing, and scheduling are shared by all services; and the extent to which the risk for the success of the service is shared by all parties.

It is also important for providers to avoid unnecessary competition for scarce resources within their organizations and communities. Unless a new provider is recruited to the community, expansion of services through hiring of clinicians in one setting will come at the expense of other clinics or agencies. At the very least, this may negatively impact the relationship between agencies and existing referral patterns and service capacity.

It is very important to be clear about what services are being offered and how they fit the needs of patients. Is the service designed to expand access to traditional mental health services to address the needs of patients with episodic or chronic depression, anxiety, or mood disorders? Will the service target the needs of specific populations such as the elderly and/or children? Will the service target the behavioral health issues of individuals with chronic illnesses such as diabetes, obesity, and hypertension? These different types of behavioral health services are not fully interchangeable from the perspective of providers, patients, and third-party payers.

It is also very important to review and understand mental health reimbursement policies across the range of third-party payers covering the practice's patient populations. Procedure and diagnostic coding expertise is a skill that can heavily influence the success of an integrated service. The primary categories of procedure codes that may be used in integrated settings include:

* Evaluation and management codes used for the delivery of office, inpatient, and nursing home services to new and existing patients
* Health and behavioral assessment codes used for the delivery of services provided to patients not diagnosed with a psychiatric problem, but whose cognitive, emotional, social, or behavioral functioning affects prevention, treatment, or management of a physical health problem
* Psychiatric codes used for the delivery of specific psychiatric services, including initial psychological diagnostic interview exams, medication management, individual or group psychotherapy, and so on

Third-party payers have different policies regarding which types of clinical providers can use each of these codes. It is important to check with individual programs and insurance carriers to verify their billing policies prior to developing specific services. It is also important to understand the managed care requirements (e.g., prior authorization, limits on number of visits) implemented by third-party carriers, as this will influence levels of coverage and how services can be delivered. Providers can use this information to develop and implement an integrated service that best meets the needs of their practice and patients.

Developing integrated physical and behavioral health services can be a significant undertaking for providers, particularly in rural areas, as reflected in the examples provided in this chapter. Despite the challenges, it can also be a rewarding activity that improves the range and quality of services provided to patients and can enhance the satisfaction of providers practicing in rural integrated settings. Finally, evidence suggests that integration improves patient satisfaction, which enhances patient loyalty and retention.

REFERENCES

1. Reiger D, Goldberg I, Taube C. The de facto US mental health services system: a public health perspective. *Arch Gen Psychiatry*. 1978;35:685–693.
2. Regier DA, Narrow WE, Rae DS, Manderscheid RW, Locke BZ, Goodwin FK. The de facto US mental and addictive disorders service system. Epidemiologic catchment area prospective 1-year prevalence rates of disorders and services. *Arch Gen Psychiatry*. 1993;50(2):85–94.
3. New Freedom Commission on Mental Health. *Achieving the Promise: Transforming Mental Health Care in America* (DHHS Publication No. SMA-03-3832). Rockville, MD: US Department of Health and Human Services; 2003.
4. National Institute of Mental Health. *Mental Health: A Report of the Surgeon General*. Rockville, MD: US Department of Health and Human Services; 1999.
5. Institute of Medicine, Committee on Crossing the Quality Chasm: Adaptation to Mental Health and Addictive Disorders. *Improving the Quality of Health Care for Mental and Substance-use Conditions: Quality Chasm Series*. Washington, DC: National Academies Press; 2006.
6. Bureau of Primary Health Care. Program information notice 2003–03: Opportunities for health centers to expand/improve access to mental health and substance abuse, oral health, pharmacy services, and quality management services during fiscal year 2003. ftp://ftp.hrsa.gov/bphc/docs/2003pins/2003-03.pdf; 2003.
7. Proser M, Cox L. *Health Centers' Role in Addressing the Behavioral Health Needs of the Medically Underserved*. Washington, DC: National Association of Community Health Centers, Inc; 2004.
8. Butler M, Kane R, McAlpine D, et al. *Integration of Mental Health/Substance Abuse and Primary Care, No. 173* (AHRQ Publication No. 09-E003). Rockville, MD: Agency for Healthcare Research and Quality; 2008.
9. Gale J, Lambert D. *Maine Barriers to Integration Study: Environmental Scan*. Portland, Maine: University of Southern Maine, Muskie School of Public Service; 2008.
10. National Association of State Mental Health Program Directors and National Association of State Alcohol and Drug Abuse Directors. *National Dialogue on Co-occurring Mental Health and Substance Abuse Disorders*. Alexandria, VA: Author; 1998.

11. Mauer B. *Behavioral Health/Primary Care Integration, Models, Competencies, and Infrastructure*. Rockville, MD: National Council for Community Behavioral Healthcare; 2003.

12. Mauer B. *Behavioral Health/Primary Care Integration and the Person-centered Healthcare Home*. Rockville, MD: National Council for Community Behavioral Healthcare; 2009.

13. Wagner E. Chronic disease management: what will it take to improve care for chronic illness? *Effective Clin Pract*. 1998;1:2–4.

14. Strosahl K. Integrating behavioral health and primary care services: The primary mental health model. In: Blount E, ed. *Integrated Primary Care: The Future of Medical and Social Mental Health Collaboration*. New York, NY: W.W. Norton & Company; 1998:136–166.

15. Doherty W, McDaniel S, Baird M. Five levels of primary care/behavioral healthcare collaboration. *Behav Healthc Tomorrow*. 1996;5:25–27.

16. Lambert D, Hartley D. Linking primary care and mental health: where have we been? where are we going? *Psychiatr Serv*. 1998;49(7):965–967.

17. Institute of Medicine, Committee on Crossing the Quality Chasm. *Quality Through Collaboration: The Future of Rural Health*. Washington, DC: National Academies Press; 2005.

18. Gale J, Lambert D. *Maine Barriers to Integration Study: The View from Maine on the Barriers to Integrated Care and Recommendations for Moving Forward*. Portland, Maine: University of Southern Maine, Muskie School of Public Service; 2009.

19. Geiger H. Community health centers: Health care as an instrument of social change. In: Sidel VW, Sidel R, eds. *Reforming Medicine: Lessons of the Last Quarter Century*. New York, NY: Pantheon Books; 1984:11–32.

20. Bird DC, Lambert D, Hartley D, Coburn AF, Beeson PG. Integrating primary care and mental health in rural America: a policy review. *Adm Policy Ment Health*. 1998;25(3):287–308.

21. Lambert D, Gale JA. *Integrating Primary Care and Mental Health: Current Practices in Rural Community Health Centers*. Kansas City, MO: National Rural Health Association; 2006.

22. Gale J, Lambert D. Mental healthcare in rural communities: the once and future role of primary care. *North Carolina Med J*. 2006;67(1):66–70.

23. California HealthCare Foundation. Chronicling an entry into telehealth: Open door community health centers. http://www.chcf.org/~/media/MEDIA%20LIBRARY%20Files/PDF/O/PDF%20OpenDoorTelehealth.pdf.

24. Duclos C, Hook J, Rodriguez M. Telehealth in community clinics: Three case studies in implementation. http://www.chcf.org/~/media/MEDIA%20LIBRARY%20Files/PDF/T/PDF%20TelehealthClinicCaseStudies.pdf.

25. Minnesota Department of Human Services. *Governor's Mental Health Initiative: Fast Facts. 2007 Legislative Session*. St. Paul, MN: Minnesota Department of Human Services. http://www/mhcsn.net/DHS.pdf. 2007.

26. Minnesota doctors will be eligible for bonuses tied to depression care. *Ment Health Weekly*. 2008;18(22).

27. Cherokee Health Systems. History of Cherokee Health Systems. http://www.cherokeehealth.com/index.php?page=About-Us-Timeline. 2010.

28. Takach M, Purington K, Osius E. *A Tale of Two Systems: A Look at State Efforts to Integrate Primary Care and Behavioral Health in Safety Net Settings*. Portland, Maine and Washington, DC: National Academy for State Health Policy; 2010.

29. Rosenberg L. Healthcare reform—Let's get down to business! *National Council Magazine*. http://www.thenationalcouncil.org/galleries/business-practice%20 files/Mauer.pdf. 2010; 2(6).

30. Pub L No 110-343, Division C, Section 511: Paul Wellstone and Pete Domenici Mental Health Parity and Addiction Equity Act of 2008. 122 Stat 3765; 2008, October 3. http://www.gpo.gov/fdsys/pkg/PLAW-110publ343/pdf/PLAW-110publ343.pdf.

31. Pub L No 111-148: Patient Protection and Affordable Care Act. 124 Stat 119; 2010, March 23. http://www.gpo.gov/fdsys/pkg/PLAW-111publ148/pdf/ PLAW-111publ148.pdf.

32. Levis D. Piloting mental health integration in the community care of North Carolina program. *North Carolina Med J*. 2006;67:68–70.

33. National Association of State Mental Health Program Directors and National Association of State Alcohol and Drug Abuse Directors. *Morbidity and Mortality in People with Serious Mental Illness*. Alexandria, VA: Author; 2006.

CHAPTER 7

Mental Health in Rural Areas

K. Bryant Smalley and Jacob C. Warren

As with other health outcomes, rural Americans face persistent disparities in rates, severity, and outcomes of mental illness that have remained relatively unchanged over the past several decades. Practitioners and researchers have long recognized the unique mental health challenges faced by rural Americans, but organized movements toward improving mental health in rural areas did not come to the forefront until the 1970s. At the time, the most pressing concerns were the lack of doctoral-level psychologists available at community mental health centers in rural areas, the lack of training of mental health professionals in the particular needs of rural residents, and the high rate of turnover in rural mental health positions.[1] Unfortunately, these concerns continue today, and federal funding for rural mental health research lags behind funding received for other disparity groups.

The federal response to rural mental health has heightened in the past quarter century, with one of the most significant advancements being the establishment of the Office of Rural Health Policy and the National Rural Health Advisory Committee in 1987.[2] Many other federal steps have been taken to improve rural mental health; however, despite nearly 30 years of intensified focus on rural mental health, rural populations continue to face increased mental health burden and distinct challenges in receiving mental health services.

While this chapter summarizes the current status of rural mental health, it only provides a broad introduction, briefly touching on many complex issues. A more comprehensive discussion of each of these issues can be found in individual chapters of our previous text, *Rural Mental Health*.[3]

Portions of this chapter previously appeared in the text *Rural Mental Health*.

MENTAL HEALTH IN RURAL AREAS

While there are many reasons for the disparate impact of mental health disorders in rural areas, the core issues have traditionally been summarized as a three-part problem of accessibility, availability, and acceptability of mental health services.[4,5] The combination of these three factors leads rural residents suffering from mental health disorders to enter mental health care later and with more serious symptoms, and as a result require more intensive treatment in an already access- and resource-restricted setting.[6,7]

When considering accessibility of mental health services in rural areas, core issues include transportation to and from services and the ability to pay for services. Because of the lack of public transportation and the overall economic climate of rural areas, many rural residents are unable to secure transportation to services that may be available. Transportation challenges are exacerbated by issues of poverty and geographic isolation, making it exceptionally challenging for many rural residents to participate in care (even if it is available).

Availability of services is impacted mainly by health professional shortages; more than 85% of Mental Health Professional Shortage Areas (MHPSAs) are in rural areas,[8] and more than half of all the counties in the United States do not have a single psychologist, psychiatrist, or social worker.[9,10] The shortage is so great that it would take an estimated 1,427 new mental health providers in rural areas to address the need. Practitioner shortages have been attributed to challenges in recruiting and retaining professionals because of lower salaries, limited social/cultural outlets, and increased risk of professional burnout.[4] As discussed in Chapter 4, rural providers in mental as well as physical health face additional ethical dilemmas that may serve as a deterrent to establishing and maintaining a practice in rural areas.

Acceptability of receiving psychological services in rural areas is negatively impacted by increased stigma and decreased anonymity in seeking psychological services.[4] The impact of stigma is well-recognized in rural areas, mainly related to traditional cultural beliefs and a lack of understanding of mental health issues,[11] and the level of stigma increases as the size of the community decreases.[12] In addition, because of the interconnected nature of rural communities, there is less anonymity when seeking mental health services.[13] For instance, by parking at a psychologist's office, residents face the possibility of word spreading of their use of services. The increased stigma and decreased anonymity may make rural residents less likely to seek care than their urban counterparts,[14] and may contribute to rural residents' perceptions that psychological services are less available and accessible to them.[15] As a result, despite the tight-knit nature of rural communities, rural residents with mental health concerns face increased burdens of isolation and loneliness because of the high levels of stigma regarding mental illness.

Rural Mental Health Disparities

Large-scale, systematic differences between rural and urban areas are difficult to identify due to several factors, including the difficulty in defining rurality itself (see Chapter 1), difficulty in defining mental health diagnoses themselves, and the already-described lack of mental health providers in rural settings (making it difficult to use traditional utilization-based measures of health care services). However, despite the lack of large-scale findings, some relatively consistent differences have emerged.

Substance use and suicide disparities are among the most robust differences that have been found between rural and urban areas. The reasons for these differences are complex and often intertwined with the physical and cultural realities of rural living (see Chapter 8). While illegal drugs have traditionally been thought of as an "urban" problem, methamphetamine use in particular is becoming an increasing problem in rural settings.[16] Rural youth have higher rates of substance use than their urban counterparts, including alcohol, tobacco, methamphetamines, prescription drugs, inhalants, marijuana, and cocaine.[17–19] Unfortunately, access to appropriate inpatient and outpatient substance use care is lower in rural areas and prevents rural populations from accessing evidence-based care for substance use.[20–23] Compounding difficulties in treatment of substance use disorders is the fact that up to 40% of mentally ill individuals in rural areas have a comorbid substance use disorder,[24] complicating receipt of appropriate services even more.

Rural areas also have higher rates of suicide, consistently demonstrating more suicide deaths and a higher rate of suicide completion than urban areas.[25–28] These effects can be highly impactful: In some areas, rural–urban differences are as much as 300%.[29] Differences in suicide attempts between rural and urban areas are even more striking among adolescents, sometimes demonstrated to be 15 times higher among rural adolescents when compared to urban.[30] Many factors have been identified as driving these disparities in suicide rates, including access to lethal means, geographic and social isolation, and mental health stigma.

Beyond overall rural–urban disparities, different subgroups of rural populations face varying mental health stressors and experience different mental health burdens. Rural minority groups face a disproportionate burden of poverty and an underutilization of mental health services that lead them to have an increased utilization of mental health emergency services.[31] These differences are not simply attributable to demographic differences— even when controlling for age, gender, and insurance status, rural minorities (including African Americans and Hispanics) still have been shown to receive less mental health treatment.[32–35] As with all rural populations, rural minorities face challenges in accessibility, availability, and acceptability of services. However, rural minorities are even more impacted by reduced acceptability of services: Rural African Americans have been shown to be less likely to seek mental health care services (even when needed and available) due to distrust of medical professionals and even higher levels of mental health stigma within the African American community.[36–40]

Rural lesbian, gay, bisexual, and questioning (LGBQ) residents also face unique mental health challenges due to increased prevalence of risk factors such as victimization and discrimination, internalized heterosexism, minimal social opportunities with other LGBQ individuals, lack of family and social support, and decreased comfort in disclosing their sexual identity to others.[41–45] These risk factors lead to increased concerns regarding substance abuse and suicidality,[45,46] in a setting where mental health providers often have little or no experience or training in the mental health needs of rural LGBQ clients.[47]

Rural mental health gender disparities also emerge. Rural men report poorer levels of overall mental health and higher rates of suicide.[48–50] Because of gender-based norms of stoicism and self-reliance that are particularly strong in rural areas,[51] rural men are more likely to avoid treatment and present at later stages in the course of their mental health diagnosis.[52,53] Rural women face mental health concerns in a context with limited mental health services specific for them.[54] They face increased risk of hospitalization for depression,[55] and as with their urban counterparts, frequently struggle with eating disorders and loneliness.[56] Rural women's mental health is impacted by a number of sociocultural factors including increased risk for abuse, increased isolation, economic instability, and a lack of childcare support that have each been linked with mood disorders.[57–60]

Other groups that require special consideration in provision of mental health services in rural areas include the elderly, as well as children/adolescents and their families. While the overall U.S. population is increasingly older, rural populations have higher numbers of older adults than nonrural areas,[61,62] leading to unique mental health needs in a context with typically poorer mental health status among the elderly.[63] Older adults in rural areas face many challenges (see Chapter 16), including depression, higher burden of medical care, and lack of specialized elderly mental health expertise.[64,65] Rural children and adolescents also face significant barriers to maintaining mental health, including higher rates of poverty, obesity, physical abuse, and substance use; unfortunately, these increased burdens are often paired with lower access to basic needs such as educational opportunities, transportation services, and health care.[66,67] Rural children have been shown to be at increased risk for many mental and behavioral health issues including substance use, depression, and anxiety,[68–70] but a low proportion of rural children actually receive care for diagnosed conditions.[71]

An additional group within rural settings with particular mental health needs is rural veterans. With rural recruits overrepresented in the military[72] and the increased likelihood of rural veterans experiencing combat casualties in recent armed conflicts,[73] there will be an increased demand for mental health services for veterans in rural areas in the coming years. Unfortunately, this increased need occurs in a context that is already recognized as having broad shortages in mental health care. With high rates of posttraumatic stress disorder (PTSD), other anxiety disorders, depression, substance use, and traumatic brain injuries,[74–78] rural veterans have very specific psychological needs that frequently cannot be addressed in rural settings. Unfortunately, the Veterans Affairs (VA) system—the safety net for physical and mental health care of veterans—often does not operate in rural areas, and rural veterans frequently find themselves having difficulty securing transportation to distant VA service locations.[77]

ADDRESSING CORE PROBLEMS IN RURAL MENTAL HEALTH

A number of strategies have been developed to address the problems faced by rural populations in achieving a healthy mental status. Many of these approaches directly counteract some of the barriers to maintaining mental health or receiving mental health services that rural residents face. Two of the most promising approaches are integrated care services and telehealth technologies.

Integrated care (or the provision of physical and mental health services within the same context) addresses several concerns, including increasing access to services and decreasing stigma in receipt of services. It also addresses the high degree of comorbidity between physical and mental health conditions; an estimated 34% to 41% of patients in primary care in rural areas have a diagnosable mental health disorder,[79] and more than 40% of individuals with mental health needs originally seek treatment in a primary care setting.[80] This high overlap led the President's New Freedom Commission on Mental Health to highlight the need of increasing access to and quality of mental health care in rural areas through integrated care, specifically stating there is a need to "screen for mental disorders in primary health care, across the life span, and connect to treatment and supports." [81 (p.11)] Integration can take several models, ranging from co-location of services to "reverse" integration of primary care services into mental health care contexts. Additional details on integrated care, including best practices and evidence base, can be found in Chapter 6.

Telehealth (the provision of clinical care or consultation via technology-enhanced means) also holds tremendous promise in addressing the core problems rural residents face in receiving mental health services. Such approaches improve accessibility because they can be deployed in almost any setting, improve availability because they increase the reach of providers into rural settings without requiring providers to actually be within the rural area, and improve acceptability because of their ability to be deployed within trusted settings, including doctors' offices and the home. Currently, licensure restrictions limit the ability of telehealth to fully meet the demand for such services, and policy advocacy to expand scope of practice to allow for more widespread use of tele-mental health services would help directly address the provider shortages seen in rural settings.

CONCLUSION

While there are many challenges in providing for the mental health needs of rural populations, there are also many emerging opportunities for addressing the needs of this highly underserved population. By becoming familiar with the unique needs, mental health burdens, and cultural influences of rural populations and combining that knowledge with the latest information on evidence-based approaches to address barriers to care in rural areas, mental health professionals can begin to make a difference in the lives of rural populations and address the disproportionate mental health burden they face.

REFERENCES

1. Hollingsworth R, Hendrix EM. Community mental health in rural settings. *Prof Psychol*. 1977;8:232–238.
2. DeLeon PH, Wakefield M, Schultz AJ, Williams J, VandenBos GR. Rural America: Unique opportunities for health care delivery and health services research. *Am Psychol*. 1989;44(10):1298–1306.
3. Smalley KB, Warren JC, Rainer J, eds. *Rural mental health*. New York, NY: Springer Publishing Company; 2012.
4. Health Resources and Services Administration. *Mental Health and Rural America: 1994–2005*. Rockville, MD: Author; 2005.
5. Human J, Wasem C. Rural mental health in America. *Am Psychol*.1991;46(3):232–239.
6. Rost KJ, Fortney J, Fischer E, Smith J. Use, quality, and outcomes of care for mental health: the rural perspective. *Med Care Rev*. 2002;59(3):231–265.
7. Wagenfeld MO, Murray JD, Mohatt JD, DeBruyn, JC. *Mental Health and Rural America 1980–1993: An Overview and Annotated Bibliography*. Rockville, MD: Department of Health and Human Services; 1994.
8. Bird DC, Dempsey P, Hartley D. *Addressing Mental Health Workforce Needs in Underserved Rural Areas: Accomplishments and Challenges*. Portland, ME: Maine Rural Health Research Center; 2001.
9. American Psychological Association. Caring for the rural community: 2000–2001 report. http://www.apa.org/rural/APAforWeb72.pdf. 2001.
10. National Advisory Committee on Rural Health. *Sixth annual report on rural health*. Rockville, MD: Office of Rural Health Policy, Health Resources and Services Administration; 1993.
11. Letvak S. The importance of social support for rural mental health. *Issues Ment Health Nurs*. 2002;23:249–261.
12. Hoyt DR, Conger RD, Valde JG, Weihs K. Psychological distress and help seeking in rural America. *Am J Community Psychol*. 1997;25(4):449–470.
13. Helbok CM. The practice of psychology in rural communities: Potential ethical dilemmas. *Ethics Behav*. 2003;13:367–384.
14. Wagenfeld MO, Buffum WE. Problems in, and prospects for, rural mental health services in the United States. *Int J Rural Health*. 1983;12:89–107.
15. Rost KJ, Fortney M, Zhang M, Smith J, Smith GR. Treatment of depression in rural Arkansas: Policy implications for improving care. *J Rural Health*. 1999;15(3):308–315.
16. Gfroerer JC, Larson SL, Colliver JD. Drug use patterns and trends in rural communities. *J Rural Health*. 2008;23(s1):10–15.
17. National Center on Addiction and Substance Abuse. *No Place to Hide: Substance Abuse in Mid-size Cities and Rural America*. New York: Author; 2000.
18. Substance Abuse and Mental Health Services Administration. *Summary of Findings from the 2001 National Household Survey on Drug Abuse*. Rockville, MD: Office of Applied Studies; 2001.

19. Lambert D, Gale JA, Hartley D. Substance abuse by youth and young adults in rural America. *J Rural Health*. 2008;24(3):221–228.
20. American Society of Addiction Medicine. Preface. In: Mee-Lee D, ed. *ASAM Patient Placement Criteria for the Treatment of Substance-related Disorders*. 2nd ed. Chevy Chase, MD: American Society of Addiction Medicine, Inc; 2001.
21. American Society of Addiction Medicine. *Public Policy Statement on Treatment for Alcoholism and Other Drug Dependencies*. Chevy Chase, MD: Author; 2005.
22. Sowers WE, Rohland B. American Association of Community Psychiatrists' principles for managing transitions in behavioral health systems. *Psychiatr Serv*. 2004;55(11):1271–1275.
23. Center for Substance Abuse Treatment. *Changing the Conversation: Improving Substance Abuse Treatment* (SMA Publication No. 00–3480). Rockville, MD: US Department of Health and Human Services, The National Treatment Plan Initiative; 2000.
24. Gogek LB. Letters to the editor. *Am J Psychiatr*. 1992;149:1286.
25. Goldsmith S, Pellmar T, Kleinman A, Bunney W, eds. *Reducing Suicide: A National Imperative*. Washington, DC: The National Academies Press; 2002.
26. Centers for Disease Control and Prevention. Preventing suicide. http://www.cdc.gov/violenceprevention/pdf/PreventingSuicide-a.pdf. 2007.
27. New Freedom Commission Subcommittee on Rural Issues. http://govinfo.library.unt.edu/mentalhealthcommission/subcommittee/Sub_Chairs.htm. 2003.
28. Institute of Medicine. Reducing suicide: a national imperative. http://www.nimh.nih.gov/health/topics/suicide-prevention/reducing-suicide-a-national-imperative.shtml. 2002.
29. Mulder PL, Kenken MB, Shellenberger S, et al. The behavioral health care needs of rural women. http://www.apa.org /rural/ruralwomen.pdf. 2001.
30. Forrest S. Suicide and the rural adolescent. *Adolescence*. 1988;23(90):341–346.
31. Snowden LR, Masland MC, Libby AM, Wallace N, Fawley K. Racial/ethnic minority children's use of psychiatric emergency care in California's public mental health system. *Am J Public Health*. 2008;98(1):118–124.
32. Goodwin R, Koenen KC, Hellman F, Guardino M, Struening E. Helpseeking and access to mental health treatment for obsessive-compulsive disorder. *Acta Psychiatrica Scandinavica*. 2002;106(2):143–149.
33. Padgett DK, Patrick C, Burns BJ, Schlesinger HJ. Ethnicity and use of outpatient mental health services in a national insured population. *Am J Public Health*. 1994;84(2):222–226.
34. Han E, Lui GG. Racial disparities in prescription drug use for mental illness among population in US. *J Ment Health Policy Econ*. 2005;8(3):131–143.
35. Zito JM, Safer DJ, Zuckerman IH, Gardner JF, Soeken K. Effect of Medicaid eligibility category on racial disparities in the use of psychotropic medications among youths. *Psychiatr Serv*. 2005;56(2):157–163.
36. Corbie-Smith G, Thomas SB, St. George M. Distrust, race, and research. *Arch Intern Med*. 2002;162(21):2458–2463.
37. Fox J, Merwin E, Blank M. DeFacto mental health services in the rural south. *J Health Care Poor Underserved*. 1995;6(4):434–468.
38. Fox JC, Blank M, Rovnyak VG, Barnett RY. Barriers to help seeking for mental disorders in a rural impoverished population. *Community Ment Health J*. 2001;37(5):421–436.
39. Menke R, Flynn H. Relationships between stigma, depression, and treatment in white and African American primary care patients. *J Nerv Ment Dis*. 2009;197(6):407–411.

40. Ward EC, Clark LO, Hendrich S. African American women's beliefs, coping behaviors, and barriers to seeking mental health services. *Qual Health Res.* 2009;19(11):1589–1601.

41. Kennedy M. Rural men, sexual identity and community. *J Homosex.* 2010;57(8): 1051–1091.

42. Leedy G, Connolly C. Out of the cowboy state: a look at lesbian and gay lives in Wyoming. *J Gay Lesbian Soc Serv.* 2007;19(1):17–34.

43. McCarthy L. Poppies in a wheat field: exploring the lives of rural lesbians. *J Homosex.* 2000;39(1):75–94.

44. Preston D, D'Augelli AR, Kassab CD, Starks MT. The relationship of stigma to the sexual risk behavior of rural men who have sex with men. *AIDS Educ Prev.* 2007;19(3): 218–230.

45. Willging CE, Salvador M, Kano M. Pragmatic help seeking: how sexual and gender minority groups access mental health care in a rural state. *Psychiatr Serv.* 2006;57(6):871–874.

46. Waldo CR, Hesson-McInnis MS, D'Augelli AR. Antecedents and consequences of victimization of lesbian, gay, and bisexual young people: a structural model comparing rural university and urban samples. *Am J Community Psychol.* 1998;26(2):307–334.

47. Willging CE, Salvador M, Kano M. Unequal treatment: Mental health care for sexual and gender minority groups in a rural state. *Psychiatr Serv.* 2006;57(6):867–870.

48. Hauenstein EJ, Petterson S, Merwin E, et al. Rurality, gender, and mental health treatment. *Community Health.* 2006; 29(3), 169–185.

49. Alston M. Rural male suicide in Australia. *Soc Sci Med.* 2012;74(4):515–522.

50. Dresang L. Gun deaths in rural and urban settings: recommendations for prevention. *Guns Violence Prev.* 2001;14(2):107–115.

51. Kosberg JI, Sun F. Meeting the mental health needs of rural men. *Rural Ment Health.* 2010;34(1):5–22.

52. Francis K, Boyd CP, Aisbett DL, Newnham K. Rural adolescents' perceptions of barriers to seeking help for mental health problems. *Youth Studies Australia.* 2006;25(4):42–49.

53. Murray G, Judd F, Jackson H, et al. Big boys don't cry: an investigation of stoicism and its mental health outcomes. *Pers Individ Dif.* 2008;44(6):1369–1381.

54. Thorndyke LE. Rural women's health: a research agenda for the future. *Women's Health Issues.* 2005;15;200–203.

55. Badger L, Robinson H, Farley T. Management of mental disorders in rural primary care. *J Fam Pract.* 1999;2(2):15–22.

56. Birmingham CL, Su J, Hlynsky J, Goldner EM, Gao M. The mortality rate from anorexia nervosa. *Int J Eat Disord.* 2005;38(2):143–146.

57. Boyd MR, Mackey MC. Running away to nowhere: rural women's experiences of becoming alcohol dependent. *Arch Psychiatr Nurs.* 2000;14(3):142–149.

58. Bushy A. Rural women: lifestyles and health status. *Nurs Clinics North America.* 1993;28(1):187–197.

59. Dimmitt J, Davila Y. Group psychotherapy for abused women: a survivor group prototype. *Appl Nurs Res.* 1995;8:3–8.

60. Hauenstein EJ, Boyd MR. Depressive symptoms in young women of the Piedmont: prevalence in rural women. *Women Health.* 1994;21:105–123.

61. National Advisory Committee on Rural Health and Human Services. The 2004 report to the secretary. *Rural Health Hum Serv Issues.* 2004:35–43.

62. US Census Bureau. Projections of the total resident population by 5-year age groups, race, and Hispanic origin with special age categories: Middle series,

1999–2000 and 2050–2070. http://www.census.gov/population/projections/nation/summary/np-t4.a-g.txt. 2000.

63. Guralnick S, Kemele K, Stamm BH, Greving AM. (2003). Rural geriatrics and gerontology. In Stamm BH (Ed.), *Rural Behavioral Health Care: An Interdisciplinary Guide.* Washington, DC: American Psychological Association. 2003:193–202.

64. Unutzer J, Patrick DL, Simon G, et al. Depressive symptoms and the cost of health services in HMO patients aged 65 years and older: a 4-year prospective study. *J Am Med Assoc.* 1997;277:1618–1623.

65. Buckwalter KC, Smith M, Zevenbergen P, Russell D. Mental health services of the rural elderly outreach program. *Gerontologist.* 1991;31(3):408–412.

66. Slovak K, Singer MI. Children and violence: findings and implications from a rural community. *Child Adolescent Soc Work J.* 2002;19:35–56.

67. Welsh J, Domitrovich CE, Bierman K, Lang J. Promoting safe schools and healthy students in rural Pennsylvania. *Psychol Schools.* 2003;40:457–472.

68. Peden AR, Reed DB, Rayes MK. Depressive symptoms in adolescents living in rural America. *J Rural Health.* 2005;21(4):310–316.

69. Sears HA. Adolescents in rural communities seeking help: who reports problems and who sees professionals? *J Child Psychol Psychiatry.* 2004;45(2):396–404.

70. Spoth R, Goldberg C, Neppl T, Trudeau L, Ramisetty-Mikler S. Rural-urban differences in the distribution of parent-reported risk factors for substance use among young adolescents. *J Subst Abuse.* 2001;13:609–623.

71. Angold A, Erklani A, Farmer EMZ, et al. Psychiatric disorder, impairment, and service use in rural African American and White youth. *Arch Gen Psychiatry.* 2002;59:893–901.

72. Richardson C, Waldrop J. Veterans: 2000 (Report No. C2KBR-22). United States Census Bureau website: http://www.census.gov/prod/2003pubs/c2kbr-22.pdf. 2003.

73. O'Hare W, Bishop B. U.S. rural soldiers account for a disproportionately high share of casualties in Iraq and Afghanistan. http://www.carseyinstitute.unh.edu/publications/FS_ruralsoldiers_06.pdf. 2006.

74. Hoge CW, McGurk D, Thomas JL, Cox AL, Engel CC, Castro CA. Mild traumatic brain injury in U.S. soldiers returning from Iraq. *N Engl J Med.* 2008;358:453–463.

75. Fontana A, Rosenheck R. Treatment-seeking Veterans of Iraq and Afghanistan: comparison with veterans of previous wars. *J Nerv Ment Dis.* 2008;196:513–521.

76. Petrakis IL, Rosenheck R, Desai R. Substance use comorbidity among veterans with posttraumatic stress disorder and other psychiatric illness. *Am J Addictions.* 2011;20:185–189.

77. Wallace AE, Weeks WB, Wang S, Lee AF, Kazis LE. Rural and urban disparities in health-related quality of life among veterans with psychiatric disorders. *Psychiatr Serv.* 2006;57:851–856.

78. Zatzick DF, Marmar CR, Weiss DS, et al. Posttraumatic stress disorder and functioning and quality of life in a nationally representative sample of Vietnam veterans. *Am J Psychiatry.*1997; 154:1690–1695.

79. Sears SF, Evans GD, Kuper BD. Rural social services systems as behavioral health delivery systems. In: Stamm BH, ed. *Rural Behavioral Health Care: An Interdisciplinary Guide.* Washington, DC: American Psychological Association; 2003:109–120.

80. Chapa T. *Mental Health Services in Primary Care Settings for Racial and Ethnic Minority Populations.* Rockville, MD: Office of Minority Health; 2004.

81. President's New Freedom Commission on Mental Health. *Achieving the Promise: Transforming Mental Health Care in America* (DHHS Publication No. SMA-03-3832). Rockville, MD: US Department of Health and Human Services; 2003.

CHAPTER 8

Substance Use and Abuse in Rural America

Jennifer D. Lenardson, David Hartley,
John A. Gale, and Karen B. Pearson

Rural America may seem an unlikely setting for new trends in substance abuse. Over the past 10 years, however, the research community and mainstream media have described a remarkable rise and recognition of substance abuse far from urban centers. These rural areas, often characterized by limited economic opportunity and lengthy distances to the next town, continue to be plagued by abuse of alcohol, marijuana, and inhalants, and have been infiltrated by methamphetamine and prescription drug abuse among vulnerable rural populations including adolescents, young adults, and Native Americans. Historically, rates of substance abuse between rural and urban areas are comparable; however, recent studies have found greater use of alcohol, OxyContin/oxycodone, and methamphetamine among rural youth than urban youth in the past year.[1] Rural areas have long been characterized by limited health care resources especially for specialty services such as substance abuse treatment,[2] emphasizing the need for substance abuse prevention and providing an uncertain context for treatment and recovery.

The fragility of the rural health system generally has implications for substance abuse recognition, treatment, and recovery, and the barriers to overall rural health contribute to difficulties in implementing substance abuse prevention and treatment programs in rural areas (e.g., provider shortages, long travel distances, lack of public transportation). This chapter compares rural and urban areas and the rural continuum (where available) for prevalence of substance use and abuse, efforts to prevent substance abuse, treatment availability and accessibility, and continuing care and long-term support for abstinence. It also presents models of service delivery that address resource limitations common to rural areas.

PREVALENCE OF RURAL SUBSTANCE USE AND ABUSE

Understanding patterns of substance use prevalence as well as variations in those patterns across rural and urban areas is necessary to effectively target resources as well as prevention and treatment interventions to existing and emerging problems. While national studies reveal little difference in the prevalence of substance use across the broad categories of rural and urban,[3–5] these studies may obscure patterns of substance use across smaller geographic areas and their subpopulations. Risk factors for substance use may be similar across the broad conceptualization of rural and urban, but vary by the demographic and socioeconomic characteristics of small towns.[6–8] In this discussion, examination of rural adjacency to urban areas, in addition to general rural status, allows for a continuum of rurality to be considered (urban, rural adjacent, rural nonadjacent). The distinction is important because rural residency near centralized and highly populated urban areas may improve rural residents' access to economic opportunities and health care services, thus minimizing the impact that rural living has upon substance abuse risk factors in these areas.

Patterns of Substance Use

N.B. For the following sections, the rural continuum is classified as follows by consolidating the 2003 Rural Urban Continuum Codes. We classified metropolitan counties as urban; nonmetropolitan counties with any urban population of any size adjacent to a metropolitan area as rural-adjacent; nonmetropolitan counties with an urban population of 20,000 or more that is not adjacent to a metropolitan area as rural large; and nonmetropolitan counties with an urban population of 2,500 to 19,999 and nonmetropolitan counties that are completely rural or have an urban population less than 2,500 that are not adjacent to a metropolitan area as rural small–medium.

Regardless of location, alcohol is the most commonly used and abused substance. Looking specifically at problem use, data from the 2002–2004 National Survey on Drug Use and Health indicate that prevalence of binge drinking (i.e., five or more alcoholic beverages on one occasion within the past 30 days) ranges from 14.2% in rural adjacent counties to a high of 16.6% in large rural counties, while rates for heavy drinking (i.e., binge drinking on five or more occasions within the past 30 days) range from 5.8% in medium-small rural counties to a high of 8.1% in large rural counties (Figure 8.1[9]; see definitions of rurality below). The dangers of binge and heavy drinking include long-term physical risks (including dependency as well as metabolic, circulatory, digestive, and cardiovascular problems) and short-term risks due to impaired judgment (including driving under the influence and risky social behaviors).

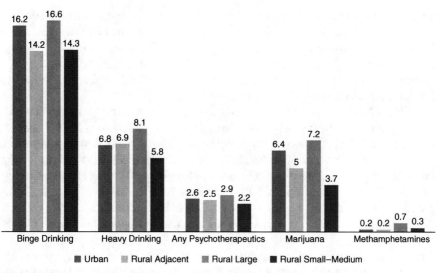

Figure 8.1 Past month substance use by location: annual average percent, 2002–2004.[9]

Marijuana is the most commonly used illicit substance, with past month rates-of-use that range from 3.7% in small or medium rural counties to 7.2% in large rural counties. The nonmedical use of any psychotherapeutic (i.e., pain reliever, tranquilizer, stimulant, and/or sedative) is the next highest category of illicit drug use, with rates that range from 2.2% in small or medium rural counties to 2.9% in large rural counties. Use rates are much lower for the nonmedical use of individual psychotherapeutics (data not shown).

As mentioned earlier, national comparisons of substance, abuse prevalence rates across all urban and rural areas tend to obscure patterns of use across smaller geographic areas and their subpopulations. A national study of the rates of substance use by youth and young adults confirms this observation. Although further study is needed to identify the specific reasons for these variations in the rates of substance use across the urban–rural continuum, past studies suggest that differences in racial and ethnic composition of these areas as well as differences in cultural, demographic, and economic factors known to influence substance use may help to explain these differences in prevalence rates.[10]

Patterns of Substance Abuse by Demographic and Socioeconomic Characteristics

In her 2006 study of rural substance abuse, Van Gundy found that substance abuse in rural areas varies by social and economic characteristics.[8] While educational attainment has not been shown to be related to alcohol use among rural young adults (ages 18–25) and older adults (ages 26 and over), fewer years of education are related to illicit drug use for young adults. According to Van Gundy, youth (ages 12–17) from low-income rural families are more likely to abuse illicit drugs than youth from high-income families.[8] Unemployment is also positively related to high rates of illicit drug use. While gender is not related to substance abuse among youth, substance abuse is higher among adult men than adult women.

Van Gundy also found that substance abuse rates vary across racial and ethnic groups, though rates differ when socioeconomic status and other factors are considered. Among rural young adults, African Americans report the lowest rates of alcohol abuse (10%). Native Americans and Asian/Pacific Islanders report the highest rates (20%), followed by Whites (18%) and Hispanics (15%). For rural youth, 14% of Native Americans abuse alcohol compared to 11% of Asian/Pacific Islanders, 9% of Hispanics, 7% of Whites, and 2% of African Americans. Among adults 26 and older, alcohol abuse ranges from a high of 14% for Native Americans to a low of approximately 3% for African Americans. Illicit drug abuse also varies by race for youth, but not for young or older adults. Among youth, Native Americans have the highest rate of illicit drug use at 13%, followed by Whites and Hispanics at roughly 5% each, and African Americans and Asian/Pacific Islanders at 2% each.[8]

Specific Substance Use Issues in Rural Communities

Nonmedical use of prescription drugs is a growing national problem and one that heavily impacts rural areas. While the rate of prescription drug use grew by 212% between 1992 and 2003 nationally, rural youth are 26% more likely than urban youth to have used prescription drugs nonmedically, adjusting for race, health, and other drug and alcohol use.[11] Factors associated with prescription drug abuse among rural youth include poor health status, presence of a major depressive episode, and other drug (marijuana, cocaine, hallucinogens, and inhalants) and alcohol use.[12]

Some, though not all, rural young adults have higher use rates of methamphetamine, prescription drugs, and alcohol compared to their urban peers. Young adults in small rural areas use methamphetamine (meth) and Oxy-Contin at rates nearly twice those of their peers in urban areas (Figure 8.2).[1,13] At least part of the greater use of meth in rural areas can be attributed to the fact that the drug is relatively easily manufactured using inexpensive chemicals readily available in rural agricultural industries, as well as the fact that rural areas, with their lower population densities, greater isolation, and supply of little-used barns and farmhouses on remote roads, provide the privacy necessary to produce the drug without detection.

In addition to the severe physiological (e.g., poor physical health and acute and long-term psychological and behavioral problems) and personal (e.g., family and child neglect, irregular work performance, and criminal behavior) effects suffered by meth addicts, meth abuse exerts a devastating toll on rural families and children, economies, law enforcement, social services, and the environment.[14–16] The family effects of meth abuse include

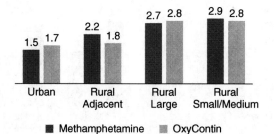

Figure 8.2 Percent of young adults (ages 18–25) using methamphetamine and OxyContin by location.[13]

child abuse, neglect, endangerment, removal of children from the family, and exposure to toxic chemicals or contaminated foods from meth production.[14–17] Societal effects include the strain and economic costs absorbed by rural schools, hospitals, emergency rooms, treatment agencies, social service agencies, and the legal and criminal justice systems in coping with the consequences of meth abuse. Environmentally, 1 pound of meth produces up to 5 or 6 pounds of toxic waste that contaminates local water systems, soil, property, and buildings as well as provides serious risk of fire, explosion, and exposure to hazardous chemicals.[14,15] Small rural communities frequently do not have the resources to address these problems.[18]

Alcohol abuse is also substantially higher among youth and young adults in specific rural communities. Youth from the smallest rural areas are more likely than their urban peers to have used alcohol and to have engaged in binge drinking, heavy drinking, and driving under the influence (Figure 8.3).[1,13] In large rural areas, nearly half of young adults report binge drinking during the last month and 20% report heavy drinking, compared to 41% and 15% of urban young adults.

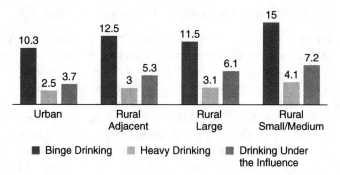

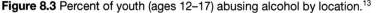

Figure 8.3 Percent of youth (ages 12–17) abusing alcohol by location.[13]

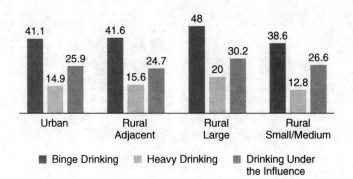

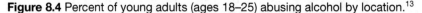

Figure 8.4 Percent of young adults (ages 18–25) abusing alcohol by location.[13]

Driving under the influence of either alcohol or drugs is a significant risk behavior and is more common among young adults and within rural communities (Figures 8.3 and 8.4). In large rural communities, 33% of young adults have driven under the influence compared to 28% of young adults in rural adjacent and 29% in urban communities. Driving under the influence is lower overall among youth; however, prevalence rates are higher in both small and large rural communities compared to urban communities. These patterns can be explained, in part, by the lack of public transportation in rural communities.

PREVENTION

At the national, state, and local levels, efforts to reduce the need for intervention and treatment of substance abuse have focused variously on early intervention, responsible use, and increasingly on primary prevention.[19] Since evidence suggests that those who become addicted to substances typically start using such substances in their adolescent years, primary prevention has focused largely on youth.

Review of Prevention Theory and Practice

As with all health promotion efforts, preference is given to promotion interventions that have been proven effective; that is, those that are "evidence-based." As a result, prevention of substance abuse has focused largely on youth, toward the goal of developing healthy behaviors early in life. For over 20 years, schools have attempted to address substance abuse in youth through programs such as Drug Abuse Resistance Education (DARE), an early effort that teaches students decision-making skills to avoid high-risk behavior. Prevention specialists have distinguished between programs that seek to help adolescents resist social influences to smoke, drink, or use drugs, and programs that seek to develop an array of cognitive-behavioral personal and social skills.[20] Both types of prevention programs have the advantage of potentially addressing multiple risk behaviors. Substantial evidence demonstrates that adolescents who take risks by using alcohol are the same adolescents who smoke, experiment with drugs, have unprotected sex, and underperform in school. Correspondingly, a majority of interventions addressing youth substance abuse embrace the "gateway hypothesis," which assumes that substance abuse often begins with the illegal use of legal substances, that is, tobacco and alcohol.[21] Discussions of prevention often feature smoking and drinking prevention as an attempt to break the gateway process. An extensive review of the inventory of prevention programs that target youth, either through social influence or personal skills approaches, found 70 such programs.[22] The evidence base for these programs varies, and unfortunately many do not focus upon the specific context of rural youth.

The probability that a young person will become involved with illegal substances is determined, in part, by both risk factors and protective factors. The two approaches described above are loosely aligned with these two determinants. Attempts to help adolescents resist social influences are focused on risk factors, while those that build social skills are focused on protective factors. Prevention strategies often involve reducing risk factors and enhancing protective factors. This is sometimes accomplished at the community or state level rather than the individual level.

The *Life Skills Training* model is an example of a school-based program that teaches students the skills needed to resist social pressure to use substances, including tobacco, marijuana, and alcohol.[23] Because it is implemented primarily in the school, it can be as effective with rural children as with urban children, as demonstrated in rigorous evaluations.[24] Because local culture affects social pressure in both positive and negative ways, some programs use the positive aspects of the community culture to build resistance to social pressure and to strengthen each child's confidence. One such program is *Project Venture*, a year-round program designed to develop skills, self-confidence, teamwork, cooperation, and trust among at-risk Native American youth. *Project Venture* includes a summer camp, 9-month school curriculum, and extensive community service.[25]

While programs targeting individual risk behaviors have shown some success,[23] community-level approaches suggest that environmental influences on youth often do not support the acquisition of good decision-making skills. Environmental or ecological models of prevention target whole communities, rather than individual children, and seek to change the standards of acceptable behavior in a neighborhood, town, or state. National surveys that gather data on substance use and abuse, such as the National Survey on Drug Use and Health, have begun to ask questions about perceptions of the acceptability of certain risky behaviors such as "To what extent do you agree with the following statement: 'My parents think it is not wrong or a little wrong for me to drink.'" Some other examples indicate the direction in which environmental prevention has gone in recent years: "To what extent do you agree: 'A kid in my neighborhood who drinks won't be caught by police,' or, 'It would be easy to get alcohol if I wanted to.'" As these questions suggest, environmental prevention efforts target the home and community environment. As one prevention specialist stated: "Holding youth solely responsible for underage drinking is like blaming fish for dying in a polluted stream" (attributed to Laurie Leiber, Center on Alcohol Awareness, Berkeley, CA).

Applying Theory and Practice to Rural Populations

Interventions that derive from perceived acceptability of risky behaviors include parent education and zero-tolerance police enforcement policies regarding youth drinking and retail sales to minors. An example of such an evidence-based environmental program is *Community Trials Intervention to Reduce High-Risk Drinking*, which employs the following strategies:

1. Using zoning and municipal regulations to restrict alcohol access through alcohol outlet density control
2. Enhancing responsible beverage service by training, testing, and assisting beverage servers and retailers in the development of policies and procedures to reduce intoxication and driving after drinking
3. Increasing law enforcement and sobriety checkpoints to raise actual and perceived risk of arrest for driving after drinking
4. Reducing youth access to alcohol by training alcohol retailers to avoid selling to minors and those who provide alcohol to minors
5. Forming coalitions to implement and support interventions that address each of these prevention components [26,27]

Environmental strategies are thought to be easier to implement because they do not target specific individuals and have the potential to impact whole populations. Such "campaigns" often involve multiple interventions, including various media (signs, radio and television spots, press conferences, etc.) as well as stepped-up law enforcement, school-based health promotion, and the participation of community leaders.[28] Rural communities may have an advantage in implementing such interventions, since they tend to be small, with relatively easily identified opinion leaders, fewer retail outlets for the sale of alcoholic beverages, and an enhanced potential to engage the whole community delivering a message to the population efficiently. Rural communities have some disadvantages as well. They often have few resources to invest in a campaign, and the effects of interventions may be harder to measure due to the small population and lack of statistical power for outcome studies. This unfortunately impacts the ability of new programs to build an "evidence base," thus making it difficult for rural-tailored programs to be developed and tested. Also, many rural communities have their own culture, values, and standards of behavior, which may include tolerance of teen drinking and of excessive adult drinking, even to the point of inconsistent enforcement of state laws. Often, interventions that involve youth not only as the "target population" but also as the designers and communicators of a program can have an impact beyond their own generation.

The *Rural Murals* project in Mendocino County, California, is an example of a low-cost environmental intervention in which youth are the designers of the medium and the message. Teams of youth design and produce murals to be posted in the community with a message designed to change social norms by dispelling "everybody does it" myths, and by presenting a positive drug and alcohol-free life style. After 9 years of experience with this program, an evaluation has found some evidence of success, citing drops in tobacco and alcohol use for some age groups, and marginal evidence of changes in perceptions.[29]

Mural design has also been a component of one of the most successful rural prevention interventions, the *Montana Meth Project*. Since 2005, this multifaceted statewide campaign has combined professionally produced media spots on television and radio with posters, press releases, billboards, and roadside murals developed by youth. Two years after launching the *Montana Meth Project*, adult meth use declined by 72% and meth-related crime decreased 62%.[30] The most recent television spots were directed by Academy Award nominee Wally Pfister. The project has been funded largely by private donations, and was recently cited as one of the most effective philanthropic endeavors in the world by *Barron's* magazine. In one of the first years of this statewide intervention, students designed and painted public service messages on the sides of barns in rural Montana. In 2010, the project included a Paint-the-State campaign described as follows:

> ... [Paint-the-State is] a statewide public art contest that leverages the creativity of Montana's youth to communicate the risks of methamphetamine use. To compete in the contest, teens throughout the state poured hundreds of hours into creating large-scale murals, massive sculptures, mixed media installations, and even live performances. Nearly half of the entries were created by grassroots organizations and community groups including Boy Scout troops, 4-H and Future Farmers of America chapters, and local Boys and Girls clubs, with groups ranging in size from 50 to 100 participants. Everything from bulldozers and jagged pieces of mirror to demolished cars and papier-mâché were used to create art that depicted lives shattered by meth. (For more information, see www.paintthestatemontana.org)

Based on a review of prevention programs in rural areas, including those mentioned previously, the following are suggested as key elements of successful rural prevention initiatives:

- Target youth, both in the schools and in the community
- Combine individual-focused strategies with environmental strategies
- Involve youth in design and communication strategies

- Engage communities, including retail outlets and law enforcement
- When possible, coordinate local interventions with statewide (or multi-tribal) campaigns

SUBSTANCE ABUSE TREATMENT

Prevention alone cannot fully address the substance abuse challenges faced in rural areas. Treatment programs must also be available for those engaged in abuse or dependence. However, substance abuse treatment overall and intensive services in particular are limited in rural areas, especially among counties not adjacent to urban areas. Since the use of specialty and intensive substance abuse services has been shown to positively affect use of continuing treatment[31] and posttreatment abstinence,[32,33] the limited availability of these services in rural areas negatively impacts long-term success. Additionally, the small range of services available in rural areas frequently precludes the individualized treatment approach and long-term follow-up recommended by professional organizations and other experts.[34-37] Providing substance abuse services in rural areas is challenged by the distribution and characteristics of providers (e.g., limited availability of specialty services and programs and travel distances to treatment). This section concludes with examples of treatment models with relevance to rural areas.

Distribution and Characteristics of Rural Providers

Overall, treatment services are relatively scarce in rural areas, with the most isolated rural areas least likely to host services. In 2006, only 9% of all 13,600 treatment facilities in the United States were located in a rural county not adjacent to an urban county, with nearly 80% of facilities located in an urban county. Though few treatment facilities are located in rural nonadjacent areas, comparing facilities to population reveals a greater supply of treatment facilities in rural areas, with 5.8 inpatient and outpatient facilities per 100,000 population in rural and 4.6 facilities in urban areas. However, limited service availability remains apparent for rural residents. Fewer inpatient and residential beds are located in rural areas (29.7 beds per 100,000 population) compared to urban areas (45.8 beds per 100,000 population).[38]

Detoxification ("detox") services, one of the most basic substance use treatment programs, are a gateway to longer-term treatment and include interventions designed to manage acute intoxication and withdrawal while minimizing the medical complications and/or physical harm caused by withdrawals from substance abuse. Unfortunately, the vast majority (82%) of rural residents live in a county without a detox provider.[39] Most rural detox providers are located in large rural towns ($n = 149$), with a lesser concentration in small rural towns ($n = 67$) and a few in isolated rural areas ($n = 19$). Most detox providers serve patients from at least 50 miles away and often greater than 100 miles away. In isolated rural areas, nearly all providers (95%) serve patients who live 51 or more miles from the facility. For alcohol abuse treatment, less than half of adults with alcohol dependence in the most rural counties have a choice between two or more facilities within 15 miles.[18] Lack of patient choice may exacerbate any disconnect between available services and local norms and beliefs, resulting in treatment avoidance.[40]

Isolated rural areas more heavily rely on less intensive community resources for treatment services following detox. Across all rural areas, patients discharged from detox programs are commonly referred to outpatient programs. However, facilities in isolated rural areas make most of their postdischarge referrals to counseling and self-help groups and less frequently to residential treatment programs and partial hospital/intensive outpatient programs.[39]

Lack of Intensive Services and Special Programs

The continuum of substance abuse treatment services needed to effectively treat a range of patients at different stages of illness are limited in rural areas (including detox, inpatient, partial hospital, intensive outpatient, outpatient, and residential care), and specialized, intensive services are often not available. Nearly all facilities across rural and urban areas provide intake, assessment, referral, and treatment.[38] However, far fewer rural facilities provide detoxification, day treatment, and long-term residential treatment, especially among facilities located in rural, not adjacent places. For example, nearly all opioid treatment programs (OTPs; programs that use methadone and other medications to treat heroin and other opiate addictions) were located in urban areas in 2006. The extremely limited supply of OTPs in rural areas could be related to the need for an adequate supply of patients to fund this type of program as well as perceived lack of privacy for specialty substance abuse treatment in rural areas.[41] Additionally, rural areas may have difficulty recruiting specialty providers to staff these programs. The urban location of OTPs may deter treatment for rural patients since opioid treatments are typically dispensed on a daily basis, requiring prohibitive travel.[42]

Special substance abuse patient populations have been shown to need key services for successful treatment outcomes, such as family therapy for adolescents or co-occurring mental health treatment for those with dual diagnoses. Nationally, less than half of treatment facilities with special programs provide these key services,[43] and it is unclear the extent to which rural treatment providers offer these programs or services. Detox providers located in isolated rural areas are less likely than providers in small and large rural towns to offer programs or groups for adolescents, co-occurring disorders, pregnant women, and criminal justice clients (see Figure 8.5). In contrast, providers in isolated rural areas are more likely to offer special programs or groups for DUI/DWI offenders.[39] The Office of National Drug Control Policy has revamped its National Youth Anti-Drug Media Campaign to concentrate on substances most often abused by adolescents and is focusing the anti-meth portion of its activities on rural and small suburban communities as well as American Indian and Native Alaskan communities.[44,45]

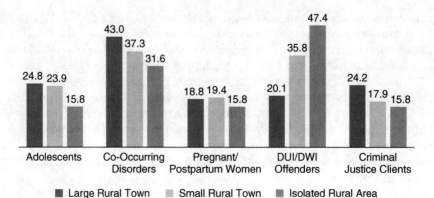

Figure 8.5 Percent of detox programs offering programs for special populations by location.[38]

Challenges to Treatment Accessibility

In addition to the geographic barriers created by long travel distances to services, access to substance abuse treatment services in rural areas may be challenged by detox treatment capacity and confidentiality concerns. Approximately one third of rural detox providers have a formal waiting list for patients wishing to access services and one third are unable to admit one or more patients within 2 months. When providers are unable to admit, patients are referred to the hospital emergency department or a provider outside their community, indicating inadequate local capacity.[39] The desire for anonymity in small, close-knit communities during substance abuse treatment may also compromise willingness to seek treatment in local settings.[46] Patients receiving behavioral health through tribal sources or the Indian Health Service were concerned with issues of confidentiality and having to receive care at facilities where friends and relatives work.[47] In an examination of barriers to receipt of substance abuse treatment, rural outpatients identified confidentiality as a primary reason why they felt uncomfortable receiving treatment (e.g., negative reactions from family, employers) in contrast to urban outpatients.[48]

Treatment Models With Relevance for Rural Providers

Treatment models with relevance for rural providers address the shortcomings of existing services. In the case of primary care, delivering treatment during a physician office visit builds on existing service providers and may address confidentiality because of the generalized nature of a primary care practice. Telehealth (defined in the following section and discussed in Chapter 17) and residential services may help address travel distances and confidentiality concerns; telehealth additionally expands treatment options.

Role of Primary Care in Identifying and Treating Substance Abuse

Primary care may play an important role in rural substance abuse treatment given the lack of specialty providers in rural areas, the likelihood of providers' regular and long-term patient contact, and the ability of the primary care setting to remove stigma associated with specialized treatment facilities. In fact, substance abuse services were one of the first mental health programs put forth as being highly needed in integrated care models (see Chapter 6). A federal consensus panel recommends that primary care clinicians include routine substance abuse screenings during office visits, brief interventions for less severe problems, assessment and treatment, referrals to specialists, and procedures to ensure confidentiality.[49] Brief interventions within primary care and hospital settings have proven effective in reducing substance abuse and across a variety of substances including cigarettes, alcohol, marijuana, opiates, and tranquilizers.[50,51]

Buprenorphine is an alternative to methadone for treating withdrawal from heroin, prescription pain medicine, and other opioids, and was approved for office-based treatment of opioid dependence in 2002. This allows physicians with appropriate training and certification to provide detox or long-term maintenance for as many as 100 patients at a time. Since 2002, the number of physicians qualified to prescribe buprenorphine has increased continuously, primarily among addiction specialists or psychiatrists, but also among family and internal medicine specialists, which greatly expands treatment capacity. The mean number of patients treated has also increased.[52] Barriers to further expansion include medication cost, difficulty obtaining reimbursement for physician services, and lack of adequate patient counseling.[53] No studies to date have examined use of buprenorphine in rural practices, but the prescribing authority of primary care physicians and the potential flexibility in service site presents possibilities for rural providers. In-home use of buprenorphine has proven successful in urban settings and may have potential for rural areas, as at-home use greatly minimizes travel burden.[53,54]

As an example of a successful training and collaboration program specific to rural health, McCarty, Rieckmann, Green, Gallon, and Knudsen describe the Opiate Medication Initiative for Rural Oregon Residents.[55] The initiative trained primary care physicians, nurse practitioners, drug abuse counselors, and pharmacists from seven rural counties in the use of buprenorphine and supported the development of community-based service models. Training regarding buprenorphine for treatment of opiate dependence was provided over 1.5 days. County-based teams were formed among participants and each team drafted clinical protocols that included assessment, referral, and treatment. The training facilitated new relationships among different providers and improved physician confidence in working with treatment facilities and caring for patients undergoing withdrawal. Following the training, 10 of 17 physicians sought federal authorization to write buprenorphine prescriptions.[55]

Telehealth

While empirical evidence is needed to assess telehealth effectiveness for substance abuse, small studies have reported high levels of patient satisfaction with mental health services,[56,57] as well as diagnosis and treatment for specific mental health conditions.[58] In a study of partial and poor responders for opioid dependency, the addition of Internet-based video conferencing for group therapy to other types of in-person treatment was satisfactory to patients and therapists; patients were also able to achieve abstinence and return to less intensive services within several weeks.[59] Potential issues to overcome include practitioner reluctance to incorporate telehealth into existing service delivery, patient lack of required technology, data security concerns, and uncertain reimbursement.[60] Additionally, other limitations include lack of direct eye contact and the potential for poor-quality connectivity affecting sound and image.[61] Overall, the ability of telehealth services to decrease travel burden and increase access to all health services, including substance abuse treatment, indicates it is a crucial line of investigation for ongoing research into treatment modalities in rural populations.

Residential Service Options

Residential programs have the advantage of minimizing transportation barriers since patients live at the facility during treatment. The *Rural Women's Recovery Program* is located in a residential addiction and mental health treatment facility in southeastern Ohio. The program follows a gender-specific treatment model and uses individualized treatment plans. Patients receive group and individual counseling and educational programming on the biological, psychological, social, and spiritual factors of addiction. The program has been certified by the Ohio Department of Drug Addiction Services and the Commission on Accreditation of Rehabilitation Services.[62] Rural in-home service options have been used in the past to address transportation and confidentiality barriers in rural areas[63]; however, few are currently in operation and provider shortages may put this out of reach for many communities. In addition, the lower absolute numbers of individuals needing treatment in rural communities tends to push such residential facilities into more populated and urbanized areas.

CONTINUING CARE AND LONG-TERM SUPPORT

Posttreatment efforts to sustain recovery are important in maintaining continued substance use abstinence[64,65] and discharge planning that transitions patients from treatment to continuing care supports continued abstinence.[66,67] Forms of long-term support include self-help groups, individual therapy, brief check-ups, peer and group counseling, and telephone-based counseling. The research literature has little to say about the availability and role of continuing care and long-term support in rural communities. Numerous studies refer informally to the limited number of 12-step meetings per week in rural areas compared to availability in urban areas. Transportation difficulties remain a factor posttreatment and patients undergoing continuing care without access to transportation are less likely to maintain abstinence than patients with access.[66] Long-term support may be compromised if the client feels group therapy attendance may unintentionally reveal substance use to community members. Continuing care interventions that bring care to the patient, through aggressive outreach or the use of low burden delivery systems (e.g., telephone), have an advantage over traditional clinic-based approaches.[67] These approaches may be particularly useful in rural areas.

Various approaches and models from the literature may be useful for promoting long-term support in rural areas. As described by the Substance Abuse and Mental Health Services Administration's (SAMHSA) *Recovery Month Toolkit*, community coalitions can be built to promote education about addiction, treatment, and recovery.[68] Coalitions can include a diverse group of organizations such as substance abuse treatment providers as well as law enforcement, social and educational agencies, religious organizations, veterans or military groups, child welfare organizations, and mental health organizations. This model may be useful to rural communities in customizing a coalition and activities to hometown needs. Through the Drug Free Communities program, federal grant money is available to community coalitions for youth drug prevention efforts. In fiscal year 2010, 62% of awards went to rural communities.[69] Faith-based organizations may also be useful in recovery and support efforts for rural communities.[70] Faith communities provide a consistent source of social support free from associations with past substance abuse behavior, and often already provide some services such as lunch programs, spiritual counseling, and space for self-help group meetings.

At the federal level, substance abuse treatment funding is targeting providers and patients in rural communities. Begun in 2004, Access to Recovery (ATR) is a grant program awarded to competing states and tribes that provides vouchers for the provision of substance abuse treatment and recovery support services (www.atr.samhsa.gov). Vouchers are given to patients in the early stages of recovery and are to be used for support services such as facilitating return to employment, transportation to self-help meetings or follow-up medical appointments, or peer-to-peer counseling. The President's 2011 fiscal year budget included a 10% requested increase to the Access to Recovery grant program.[44] Though ATR may positively impact *financial* access to services, the program does not specifically target rural areas and may not be useful in rural areas with limited service availability or lengthy travel distances.

The FY 2012 budget saw a streamlining of budget lines in SAMHSA in order to provide more flexibility in identifying and funding innovative and emerging issues in the treatment and prevention of substance abuse.[71] The fiscal impact, however, was a decrease in funding for the Access to Recovery (ATR) grant program, which saw an additional decline of $4.5 million in FY 2013.[72] The President's FY 2014 National Drug Control Budget continues to fund SAMHSA's ability to award ATR grants on a limited basis, however, and supports linkages with state health insurance exchanges.[73]

CONCLUSION

The prevalence of substance abuse among rural youth and young adults emphasizes the importance of developing intervention programs that target rural communities, particularly communities in small and remote areas. Substance abuse prevention generally targets alcohol and tobacco as initiation substances and is attentive to youth in order to stop substance use early or ideally before it begins. Prevention efforts are intended to address social influences that put youth at risk and provide social skills to resist pressure to use substances, and target individuals as well as their environment. However, a culture of drinking tolerance in many rural communities has made community-based prevention a challenge.

Few substance abuse treatment facilities operate in rural areas, particularly among the most remote rural counties. Where facilities exist, access to intensive services and the full range of professionally recommended services is limited. Travel distances for detox services are lengthy and access to specialty programs for patients for specific needs is incomplete. Treatment models should build on existing primary care and safety net providers and community resources and consider incorporating new technology approaches that could address distance and confidentiality issues. Despite the importance of continuing care and long-term support in abstinence following treatment, little research has examined the availability and role of these services in rural communities. Like other forms of substance abuse treatment, continued recovery services are likely in short supply and, where they exist, group arrangements in small communities may exacerbate confidentiality concerns. Continued financial support and additional research on the prevention and treatment needs of rural areas is essential to decreasing substance abuse in these areas.

REFERENCES

1. Lambert D, Gale JA, Hartley D. Substance abuse by youth and young adults in rural America. *J Rural Health*. 2008;24(3):221–228.
2. Schur CL, Franco SJ. Access to health care. In: Ricketts TC, ed. *Rural Health in the United States*. New York, NY: Oxford University Press; 1999:25–37.
3. Compton WM, Thomas YF, Stinson FS, Grant, BF. Prevalence, correlates, disability, and comorbidity of DSM-IV drug abuse and dependence in the United States: results from the National Epidemiologic Survey on Alcohol and Related Conditions. *Arch Gen Psychiatry*. 2007;64(5):566–576.
4. Hasin DS, Stinson FS, Ogburn E, Grant BF. Prevalence, correlates, disability, and comorbidity of DSM-IV alcohol abuse and dependence in the United States: results from the National Epidemiologic Survey on Alcohol and Related Conditions. *Arch Gen Psychiatry*. 2007;64(7):830–842.
5. Thomas YF, Compton WM. Rural populations are not protected from drug use and abuse. *J Rural Health*. 2007;23(suppl):1–3.
6. Donnermeyer JF, Tunnell K. In our own backyard: methamphetamine manufacturing, trafficking and abuse in rural America. *Rural Realities*. 2007;2(2):1–11.

7. Oetting ER, Edwards RW, Kelly KBF. Risk and protective factors for drug use among rural American youth. In: Robertson EB, Slobda Z, Boyd GM, Beatty L, Kozel NJ, eds. *Rural Substance Abuse: State of Knowledge and Issues*. Rockville, MD: US Department of Health and Human Services, National Institutes of Health, National Institute on Drug Abuse; 1997:90–130. NIDA Research Monograph 168.

8. Van Gundy K. *Reports on Rural America: Substance Abuse in Rural and Small Town America*. Durham, NH: University of New Hampshire, Carsey Institute; 2006.

9. Gale JA. Unpublished tabulations of the 2002–2004 National Survey on Drug Use and Health.

10. Conger R. The special nature of rural America. In: Robertson EB, Slobda Z, Boyd GM, Beatty L, Kozel NJ, eds. *Rural Substance Abuse: State of Knowledge and Issues*. Rockville, MD: US Department of Health and Human Services, National Institutes of Health, National Institute on Drug Use; 1997:1–5.

11. Moon MA. Rural adolescents more likely than urban ones to abuse prescription drugs. *Internal Medicine News* Digital Network. 2010. http://www.internalmedicinenews.com/news/adolescent-medicine/single-article/rural-adolescents-more-likely-than-urban-ones-to-abuse-prescription-drugs/64587a7088.html.

12. Havens JR, Young AM, Havens CE. Nonmedical prescription drug use in a nationally representative sample of adolescents: evidence of greater use among rural adolescents. *Arch Pediatr Adolesc Med*. 2010;165(3):250–255.

13. Hartley D. *Substance Abuse among Rural Youth: A Little Meth and A Lot of Booze*. Portland, ME: University of Southern Maine, Muskie School of Public Service, Maine Rural Health Research Center; 2007. Research & Policy Brief No. 35A.

14. Donnermeyer JF. The use of alcohol, marijuana, and hard drugs by rural adolescents: a review of recent research. In: Edwards R, ed. *Drug Use in Rural American Communities*. New York, NY: Haworth Press; 1992:31–75.

15. United States Environmental Protection Agency. *RCRA Hazardous Waste Identification of Methamphetamine Production Process By-Products*. [Report to Congress]. Washington, DC: US EPA; 2008.

16. Jefferson County Meth Action Team. *Methamphetamine in Jefferson County: Understanding the Impact of Methamphetamine Abuse: Issue Paper & Recommendations*. Port Townsend, WA: Jefferson County Meth Action Team; 2008.

17. Weisheit RA. *The Impact of Methamphetamine on Illinois Communities: An Ethnography*. Normal, IL: Illinois State University, Department of Criminal Justice Sciences; 2004.

18. Johnson D. Policing a rural plague: Meth is ravaging the Midwest—why it's so hard to stop. http://www.msnbc.msn.com/id/4409266/site/newsweek. March 2004.

19. Carnevale Associates. *SAMHSA's Strategic Prevention Framework*. Darnestown, MD: Carnevale Associates, LLC; 2005.

20. Botvin GJ, Wills TA. Personal and social skills training: cognitive-behavioral approaches to substance abuse prevention. *NIDA Res Monogr*. 1985;63:8–49.

21. Pentz MA, Li C. The gateway theory applied to prevention. In: Kandel DB, ed. *Stages and Pathways of Drug Involvement: Examining the Gateway Hypothesis*. New York, NY: Cambridge University Press; 2002:139–157.

22. Winters KC, Fawkes T, Fahnhorst T, Botzet A, August G. A synthesis review of exemplary drug abuse prevention programs in the United States. *J Subst Abuse Treat*. 2007;32(4):371–380.

23. Botvin GJ, Griffin KW. Life skills training as a primary prevention approach for adolescent drug abuse and other problem behaviors. *Int J Emerg Ment Health*. 2002;4(1):41–47.

24. Spoth RL, Randall GK, Trudeau L, Shin C, Redmond C. Substance use outcomes 5-1/2 years past baseline for partnership-based, family-school preventive interventions. *Drug Alcohol Depend.* 2008;96(1-2):57–68.

25. Hall M. *Project Venture: SAMHSA Model Program.* Rockville, MD: US Department of Health and Human Services, Substance Abuse and Mental Health Administration; 2004.

26. Substance Abuse & Mental Health Services Administration, Center for Substance Abuse Prevention, NREPP database. Community trials intervention to reduce high-risk drinking. 2008. http://www.nrepp.samhsa.gov/ViewIntervention .aspx?id=9.

27. Treno AJ, Gruenewald PJ, Lee JP, Remer LG. The Sacramento Neighborhood Alcohol Prevention Project: outcomes from a community prevention trial. *J Stud Alcohol Drugs.* 2007;68(2):197–207.

28. National Institute on Drug Abuse. *Preventing Drug Abuse Among Children and Adolescents: A Research-Based Guide for Parents, Educators and Community Leaders.* Bethesda, MD: Author; 2003.

29. Rural Murals Project. Environmental prevention. 2001. http://www.ruralmurals .org/prevention.shtml. 2001.

30. McGrath M. *Methamphetamine in Montana: A Follow-Up Report on Trends and Progress.* Helena, MT: Montana Department of Justice; 2008.

31. Straussner SLA. Assessment and treatment of clients with alcohol and other drug abuse problems: An overview. In: Straussner SLA, ed. *Clinical Work with Substance-Abusing Clients.* 2nd ed. New York, NY: The Guilford Press; 2004:3–36.

32. Greenfield L, Burgdorf K, Chen X, Porowski A, Roberts T, Herrell J. Effectiveness of long-term residential substance abuse treatment for women: findings from three national studies. *Am J Drug Alcohol Abuse.* 2004;30(3):537–550.

33. Mojtabi R. Use of specialty substance abuse and mental health services in adults with substance use disorders in the community. *Drug Alcohol Depend.* 2005;78(3):345–354.

34. American Society of Addiction Medicine. Preface. In: Mee-Lee D, ed. *ASAM Patient Placement Criteria for the Treatment of Substance-Related Disorders.* 2nd ed. Chevy Chase, MD: Author; 2001.

35. American Society of Addiction Medicine. *Public Policy Statement on Treatment for Alcoholism and Other Drug Dependencies.* Chevy Chase, MD: Author; 2005.

36. Center for Substance Abuse Treatment. *Changing the Conversation: Improving Substance Abuse Treatment.* Rockville, MD: US Department of Health and Human Services, The National Treatment Plan Initiative; 2000. DHHS Publication No. SMA 00-3480.

37. Sowers WE, Rohland B. American Association of Community Psychiatrists' principles for managing transitions in behavioral health services. *Psychiatr Serv.* 2004;55(11):1271–1275.

38. Lenardson JD. *Unpublished Tabulations of the 2006 National Survey of Substance Abuse Treatment Services.* Portland, ME: University of Southern Maine, Muskie School of Public Service, Maine Rural Health Research Center; 2008.

39. Lenardson J, Race M, Gale JA. *Availability, Characteristics, and Role of Detoxification Services in Rural Areas.* Portland, ME: University of Southern Maine, Muskie School of Public Service, Maine Rural Health Research Center; 2009.

40. Drug and Alcohol Services Information System. *Distance to Substance Abuse Treatment Facilities among Those with Alcohol Dependence or Abuse* [DASIS Report]. Arlington, VA: Office of Applied Studies, Substance Abuse and Mental Health Services Administration; 2002.

41. Fortney J, Mukherjee S, Curran G, Fortney S, Han X, Booth B. Factors associated with perceived stigma for alcohol use and treatment among at-risk drinkers. *J Behav Health Serv Res*. 2004;31(4):418–429.
42. Profile: Methadone treatments for heroin addicts. [transcript]. Bob Edwards. *NPR Morning Edition*. 2004. http://www.npr.org.
43. Olmstead T, Sindelar J. To what extent are key services offered in treatment programs for special populations. *J Subst Abuse Treat*. 2004;27:9–15.
44. Office of National Drug Control Policy. National Youth Anti-Drug Media Campaign [Fact Sheet]. 2010. http://www.whitehouse.gov/sites/default/files/ondcp/Fact_Sheets/national_youth_anti_drug_page_media_campaign_fact_sheet_7-16-10.pdf.
45. Humphreys K, McLellan AT. Brief intervention, treatment, and recovery support services for Americans who have substance use disorders: an overview of policy in the Obama administration. *Psychol Serv*. 2010;7(4):275–284.
46. Calloway M, Fried B, Johnson M, Morrissey J. Characterization of rural mental health service systems. *J Rural Health*. 1999;15(3):296–307.
47. Duran B, Oetzel J, Lucero J, et al. Obstacles for rural American Indians seeking alcohol, drug, or mental health treatment. *J Consult Clin Psychol*. 2005;73(5):819–829.
48. Davis WM Jr. *Barriers to Substance Abuse Treatment Utilization in Rural Versus Urban Pennsylvania* [dissertation]. Indiana: Indiana University of Pennsylvania, 2009.
49. Center for Substance Abuse Treatment. Guide to substance abuse services for primary care clinicians. In: *Treatment Improvement Protocol (TIP) Series, No. 24*. Rockville, MD: US Department of Health and Human Services, Substance Abuse and Mental Health Services Administration; 1997. DHHS Publication No. SMA 97-3139.
50. Office of National Drug Control Policy. Screening, Brief Intervention, Referral & Treatment. http://www.whitehousedrugpolicy.gov/treat/ screen_brief_intv.html. 2010.
51. Smith JG, Eisenberg SG, Bukstein OG. *Managing Substance Abuse Disorders in Primary Care Settings*. Presented at the Blending Science and Treatment NIDA Conference, Cincinnati, OH; June 2008.
52. Arfken CL, Johanson C-E, di Menza S, Schuster CR. Expanding treatment capacity for opioid dependence with office-based treatment with buprenorphine: national surveys of physicians. *J Subst Abuse Treat*. 2010;39(2):96–104.
53. Sohler NL, Li X, Kunins HV, et al. Home- versus office-based buprenorphine inductions for opioid-dependent patients. *J Subst Abuse Treat*. 2010;38(2):153–159.
54. Lee JD, Grossman E, DiRocco D, Gourevitch MN. Home buprenorphine/naloxone induction in primary care. *J Gen Intern Med*. 2008;24(2):226–232.
55. McCarty D, Rieckmann T, Green C, Gallon S, Knudsen J. Training rural practitioners to use buprenorphine: using the change book to facilitate technology transfer. *J Subst Abuse Treat*. 2004;26(3):203–208.
56. Simpson J, Doze S, Urness D, Hailey D, Jacobs P. Evaluation of a routine telepsychiatry service. *J Telemed Telecare*. 2001;7(2):90–98.
57. Skinner AG, Latchford G. Attitudes to counseling via the Internet: a comparison between in-person counseling clients and Internet support group users. *Couns Psychotherapy Res*. 2006;6(3):158–163.
58. Hilty DM, Luo JS, Morache C, Marcelo DA, Nesbitt TS. Telepsychiatry: an overview for psychiatrists. *CNS Drugs*. 2002;16(8):527–548.
59. King VL, Stoller KB, Kidorf M, et al. Assessing the effectiveness of an Internet-based videoconferencing platform for delivering intensified substance abuse counseling. *J Subst Abuse Treat*. 2009;36(3):331–338.

60. Center for Substance Abuse Treatment. *Considerations for the Provision of e-Therapy*. Rockville, MD: US Department of Health and Human Services, Substance Abuse and Mental Health Services Administration; 2009. DHHS Publication No. SMA 09-4450.

61. McGinty K, Saeed S, Simmons S, Yildirim Y. Telepsychiatry and e-mental health services: potential for improving access to mental health care. *Psychiatr Q*. 2006;77(4): 335–342.

62. Health Recovery Services. Rural women's recovery program. 2010. http://www .hrs.org/residential.html.

63. Adams KM, Ward CC. A case management model utilizing in-home treatment services for rural AODA clients: the family and children's center model. In: *Treating Alcohol and Other Drug Abusers in Rural and Frontier Areas: TAP 17* (DHHS Publication No. SMA 95-3054). Rockville, MD: US Department of Health and Human Services, Substance Abuse and Mental Health Services Administration; 1995.

64. McKay JR, Lynch KG, Shepard DS, Pettinati HM. The effectiveness of telephone-based continuing care for alcohol and cocaine dependence: 24-month outcomes. *Arch Gen Psychiatry*. 2005;62(2):199–207.

65. McKay JR, Merikle E, Mulvaney FD, Weiss RV, Koppenhaver JM. Factors accounting for cocaine use two years following initiation of continuing care. *Addiction*. 2001;96(2):213–225.

66. Schaefer JA, Harris AH, Cronkite RC, Turrubiartes P. Treatment staff's continuity of care practices, patients' engagement in continuing care, and abstinence following outpatient substance-use disorder treatment. *J Stud Alcohol Drugs*. 2008;69(5):747–756.

67. McKay JR. Continuing care research: What we have learned and where we are going. *J Subst Abuse Treat*. 2009; 36(2):131–145.

68. Center for Substance Abuse Treatment. Join the voices for recovery: now more than ever! In: *National Alcohol and Drug Abuse Recovery Month Toolkit*. Rockville, MD: US Department of Health and Human Services, Substance Abuse and Mental Health Services Administration; 2010.

69. Office of National Drug Control Policy. White House Drug Policy Director awards $85.6 million to local communities to prevent youth drug use [Press Release]. http://www.whitehousedrugpolicy.gov/pda/083110.html. 2010.

70. Hartman JC, Arndt S, Barbaer K, Wassink T. An environmental scan of faith-based and community reentry services in Johnson County, Iowa. In: *The National Rural Alcohol and Drug Abuse Network Awards for Excellence, 2004*. Rockville, MD: US Department of Health and Human Services, Substance Abuse and Mental Health Services Administration; 2006:49–58.

71. Substance Abuse and Mental Health Services Administration. *Department of Health and Human Services Fiscal Year 2012 Justification of Estimates for Appropriations Committees*. Washington, DC: SAMHSA; 2012.

72. Substance Abuse and Mental Health Services Administration. *Department of Health and Human Services Fiscal Year 2013 Justification of Estimates for Appropriations Committees*. Washington, DC: SAMHSA; 2013.

73. Office of National Drug Control Policy. *National Drug Control Budget: FY 2014 Funding Highlights*. Washington, DC: Executive Office of the President, ONDCP; April 2013.

CHAPTER 9

Heart Disease in Rural Areas

*Marylen Rimando, Jacob C. Warren, and
K. Bryant Smalley*

More than 2,200 Americans die of cardiovascular disease (CVD) each day, an average of 1 death every 39 seconds.[1] It is the leading cause of death for men and women in the United States, including Whites, African Americans, and Hispanics.[1] Among Asians, Pacific Islanders, American Indians, and Alaska Natives, heart disease is the second leading cause of death. As such, chronic CVD itself is also extremely common in the general population, affecting the majority of adults past the age of 60 years; furthermore, an estimated 82.6 million Americans or 1 in 3 adults have one or more types of CVD.[1] By 2030, an estimated 40.5% of the U.S. population or approximately 116 million people will have some form of CVD.[1] Even beyond the sheer magnitude of CVD in the United States, deaths due to CVD also have a negative effect on the population life expectancy; for instance, in 2008, 33% of deaths due to CVD occurred before age 75 (less than the average life expectancy of 77.8 years[1]). This high prevalence is associated with significant cost to the health care system; the Centers for Disease Control and Prevention (CDC) reports CVD treatment alone accounts for nearly $1 of every $6 spent on health care in the United States.[2] In total, CVD accounts for 17% of the nation's health expenditures, approximately $149 billion. CVD costs more to treat than any other diagnosis, including cancer. This includes health expenditures (direct costs such as costs of physicians and other health professionals' services, hospital services, prescribed medications, home health care) and lost productivity resulting from illness or mortality (indirect costs, which are projected to increase from an estimated $172 billion in 2010 to $276 billion in 2030).[1] CVD is therefore a significant and very expensive public health burden. While its impact is widespread, there is evidence that particular groups are even more impacted, among them rural populations. This chapter explores the various types of CVD (e.g., hypertension, heart attack, and stroke) as well as the factors that increase risk for CVD. Particular attention is paid to how rural areas differ in both prevalence and underlying risk behaviors.

HYPERTENSION

General Description

According to the 7th Report of the Joint National Committee on the Prevention, Detection, Evaluation, and Treatment of High Blood Pressure (JNC 7), hypertension (HTN) is defined as a blood pressure reading higher than 140 mmHg systolic or higher than 90 mmHg diastolic.[3] Pre-HTN is defined as a systolic blood pressure (SBP) of 120 to 139 mmHg and/or diastolic blood pressure (DBP) of 80 to 89 mmHg. Stage 1 HTN is defined as 140 to 159 mmHg SBP and/or DBP of 90 to 99 mmHg. Stage 2 HTN is defined as SBP of 160 mm Hg or higher and/or DBP of 100 mm Hg or higher.[3]

Frequently, HTN has no symptoms and is known as the "silent killer." The prevalence of HTN is approximately 76.4 million, about half of whom have uncontrolled blood pressure.[1] According to the 2005–2008 National Health and Nutrition Examination Survey (NHANES), 33.5% of U.S. adults aged 20 years and older have HTN.[1] Among hypertensive adults, approximately 80% are aware of their condition and 71% are using blood pressure medication, but only 48% of those who are aware of their condition have controlled HTN.[1] Older adults have both the highest rates of diagnosed, uncontrolled HTN and are most likely to be unaware of their condition.[4]

Older women residing in rural areas are especially susceptible to developing HTN. A study of 225 primarily White rural midwestern women between 50 and 69 years of age found that 56% of women midlife to older had pre-HTN and 20% had stage 1 or 2 HTN.[5] The high prevalence of uncontrolled HTN in older adults may be attributed to the use of fewer preventive services, although more than 80% of the elderly are estimated to have their blood pressure checked.[6]

Mortality Rates

There has been a decline in the number of deaths among Americans with HTN, but mortality rates are still higher among hypertensive people than those with normal blood pressure.[7] Ford examined death rates for adults age 25 to 74 using NHANES data. The overall death rate from 1971–1975 for adults with HTN was 42% higher compared to adults with normal blood pressure.[7] The death rate declined from 18.8 deaths per 1,000 people from 1971–1975 to 14.3 per 1,000 in 1988–1994.[7] The death rate among African Americans with HTN was higher than among Whites with HTN. The decline in deaths among men with HTN was more than 4 times larger compared to women with HTN.[7]

Changes in Rates Over Time

Trends of prevalence, awareness, and control of HTN indicate the prevalence of HTN remained at 30% and did not significantly change from 1999–2008.[8] Among those with HTN, awareness of the disease increased from 69.6% in 1999–2000 to 80.6% in 2007–2008.[8] The overall percentage of adults with controlled HTN increased from 31.6% in 1999–2000 to 48.4% in 2007–2008.[8] From 2001 to 2005, the prevalence of HTN in the Mississippi Delta increased from 31.3% to 33.3%, while the rates for the nation remained constant at 25.6% to 25.5%. Smaller declines in death rates from HTN were found in men compared to women.[7] However, a higher percentage of women received treatment and had large reductions in their blood pressure readings.[7] Additionally, African Americans had a higher mortality rate compared to Whites.[7] The small decline in death rates among women and African Americans demonstrates the need for an increased focus on education to reduce mortality rates among women and African Americans.

HEART ATTACK AND ASSOCIATED CONDITIONS

General Description

A myocardial infarction, commonly known as a heart attack, is a disease that occurs when a section of the heart muscle dies or gets damaged because of reduced blood supply.[9] Angina is chest pain or discomfort in the chest that occurs if an area of heart muscle gets insufficient oxygenated blood. Coronary heart disease (CHD), the main cause of a heart attack, occurs when plaque builds up on the inner lining of the wall of the coronary arteries that supply blood to the heart muscle.[9] Plaque consists of cholesterol deposits, blood cells, and fibrous tissue. Over time, plaque slowly enlarges, resulting in the narrowing of the cavity and stiffening of the artery wall.[10] This narrowing process is called atherosclerosis, which is responsible for almost all cases of CHD. The actual frequency of atherosclerosis is difficult to accurately determine because it is a predominantly asymptomatic condition, but develops with increasing age through ages 50 and 60.[10]

Prevalence Rates

Recent data show a high prevalence of heart attacks and associated conditions. About every 34 seconds an American will have a heart attack. Annually, approximately 1.5 million Americans have a heart attack, and about one third of those die from it. In 2009, an estimated 785,000 Americans suffered a first heart attack, and an estimated 470,000 Americans suffered a second heart attack. An additional 195,000 "silent" heart attacks are estimated to occur annually, during which the individual is ultimately unaware of the cardiac incident. Furthermore, approximately 14 million persons experience CHD and its various complications annually. An estimated 71 million adults have high cholesterol and approximately 2 of 3 people do not have it controlled.[11] More than 15 million people in the United States experience chest pain caused by CHD and angina, occurring equally among men and women.

Mortality Rates

The National Heart, Lung, and Blood Institute (NHLBI) reported that approximately 21.6% of the deaths from CVD in 2008 can be attributed to a heart attack.[12] Approximately 138,000 died from a heart attack in 2008.[12] Regionally, the southern United States has higher deaths attributed to a heart attack, stroke, and kidney failure.[13] Poor and rural areas often have the highest rates of CVD mortality, with some rural areas having mortality rates three times higher than urban areas. As such, researchers have reported a direct correlation between rurality and CVD mortality.[14] There are also racial disparities even within the geographic disparities; for instance, African American women living in rural areas have distinctly elevated mortality rates compared to White women living in rural areas.

Changes in Rates Over Time

CHD mortality rates declined over the past few decades. According to the NHLBI, the age-adjusted death rates for CHD steadily declined from 478 per 100,000 in 1963, to 234 per 100,000 in 1988, and to 123 per 100,000 in 2008.[12] The percent decline in age-adjusted CHD death rates was 74% from 1963 to 2008 and was 48% from 1998 to 2008.[12] From 1999 to 2008, death rates for CHD declined in males and females of all racial/ethnic groups.[12] From 1995 to 2005, the death rate from CHD declined 34.3%, but the actual number of deaths declined only 19.4% due to increasing population sizes.[12] Although statistics indicate a decline in mortality rates over the past few decades, high mortality rates still appear among African Americans and those living in rural areas, indicating that advances in treatment and prevention are not adequately reaching these underserved groups.

STROKE

General Description

Stroke occurs when the brain does not receive an adequate supply of blood, most commonly due to the occlusion of blood vessels. According to the American Stroke Association (ASA), stroke is characterized by left- or right-sided extremity weakness or numbness, paralysis of one side of the face, trouble speaking or understanding speech, severe sudden headaches, difficulty walking or loss of balance, sudden loss of consciousness, or vision problems.[15] Three main types of strokes are ischemic (due to brain arterial blockage), embolic (due to blood clots going to the brain), and hemorrhagic (due to bleeding inside the brain).[15] Ischemic strokes, accounting for about

88% of all strokes, frequently occur with the underlying causes slowly developing long before the stroke and remaining undetected.[15] Stroke is the third leading cause of death in the United States, as well as a leading cause of serious, long-term disability.[1] Americans paid approximately $73.7 billion in 2010 for stroke-related medical costs and disability,[15] with an estimated lifetime cost of stroke care of $140,048.[1]

Prevalence Rates

On average, every 40 seconds someone in the United States has a stroke and, on average, every 4 minutes someone dies of a stroke.[12] This accounted for 1 in every 18 deaths in the United States in 2007.[16] About 795,000 people experience a new or recurrent stroke each year, with approximately 610,000 of these strokes being first attacks, and 185,000 recurrent attacks.[1] An estimated 7 million Americans aged 20 years or older suffered a stroke. In 2010, the Behavioral Risk Factor Surveillance System (BRFSS) reported the age-adjusted prevalence of stroke among noninstitutionalized adults aged 18 years or older by state and showed that a majority of the states have a 3.1% to 4.1% stroke prevalence rate.[17] This evidence of high stroke prevalence reveals the importance of stroke as a public health concern.

Mortality Rates

In 2008, approximately 1 in 18 Americans died from a stroke.[1] From 2007 to 2009, the age-adjusted death rate from stroke in the nation among adults aged 18 and older was 54.6 per 100,000 population, with the highest rate of 72.5 per 100,000 in Alabama.[18] Overall, mortality rates were higher in the Southeast and lower in the Northeast. The CDC's Division for Heart Disease and Stroke Prevention (DHDSP) reported adults aged 35 and older in rural areas in Mississippi, Alabama, Georgia, Tennessee, and South Carolina had an age-adjusted annual death rate of 126 to 198 per 100,000, far exceeding the national average.[18]

For more than half a century there has been excess stroke mortality in the Southeast in an area known as the "Stroke Belt." According to the NHLBI, this Stroke Belt consists of 11 states with the highest age-adjusted stroke mortality in the United States.[12] In addition to being highly racially and ethnically diverse, this region contains nearly half of the people in the nation who live in poverty. Researchers investigated the Stroke Belt in depth in an attempt to elucidate ethnic differences and rural-urban disparities in access to health care and stroke rehabilitation, but were unable to reach any definitive conclusion. Even within rural areas, further disparities emerge. African Americans have a two to three times higher risk than Whites of having a stroke and dying from it, and Appalachia is characterized by high rates of stroke and heart attack.[19] Regardless of the underlying cause, there is strong indication that stroke has a particularly heavy burden in rural areas (particularly in the rural South) that merits both further investigation and development of targeted interventions.

Changes in Rates Over Time

An analysis of stroke rates from the 2005 BRFSS showed large disparities by age and mortality rates.[20] From 1996 to 2006, the stroke death rate in the United States declined 33.5%, and the number of stroke deaths decreased by 18.4%.[20] During the past 5 years, the age-adjusted prevalence of stroke remained at 2.6% to 2.7%.

CARDIOVASCULAR DISEASE RISK FACTORS

While disparities in outcomes between rural and urban populations vary by group and are sometimes difficult to detect, there are several well-established rural/urban differences in the risk factors associated with CVD. These differences in risk factors underscore the need for rural-tailored interventions to address CVD morbidity and mortality—the differential gains seen in urban populations as compared to rural populations could reflect the fact that current intervention methods are not adequately reaching rural groups. In the following sections we explore some of the best-established risk factors for CVD, with a particular focus on any existing knowledge of differences in those risk factors between rural and urban groups.

Diet

Disparities have been demonstrated in the dietary intake and cholesterol levels of rural versus urban women. Rural African American women report significantly higher daily dietary fat intake and elevated cholesterol levels compared with urban African American women in a national sample.[21] The majority (85%) of rural African American women in the study reported no prior measurement of CVD risk compared with 52% of urban African American women. Interventions for rural women aimed at CVD prevention and education can assist in reducing dietary fat intake and lowering cholesterol.

In another study, rural and urban adults self-reported their amount of fruit and vegetable consumption (five or more daily servings).[22] Notably, 37 states had a lower number of rural adults consuming at least five daily servings of fruits and vegetables, and only 11 states had a higher number of rural adults consuming at least five daily servings of fruits and vegetables.[22] Overall, fewer than one in four rural adults in the United States consumed five or more servings of fruits and vegetables.[22] Also, a higher proportion of rural residents earning less than $35,000 did not consume at least five servings of fruits and vegetables when compared to urban residents.[22] The state percentages of fruit and vegetable consumption for rural adults ranged from a low of 13.88% in Oklahoma to a high of 28.74% in Vermont.[22] These facts illustrate the need to develop tailored interventions resulting in healthier dietary choices while addressing possible issues of availability and accessibility to healthy foods unique to rural residents.

Sedentary Lifestyle

Physical activity is important for cardiovascular health, as physical inactivity increases the risk of HTN, diabetes, heart disease, and stroke. Rural residents are more likely to be sedentary than urban residents,[23,24] and even within rural settings geographic disparities exist. For instance, a higher percentage of Mississippi adults reported having a sedentary lifestyle (20.1%) as compared to Minnesota adults (9.8%).[23] Across all racial/ethnic groups, rural residents were less likely to meet recommendations for vigorous physical activity than urban residents.[24] Moreover, among rural residents, minorities were more likely to be sedentary than Whites. Only 15% of rural African Americans and 17% of rural Hispanics reported meeting the CDC's vigorous activity recommendations.[24] Similarly, 74% of rural African Americans and 69% of rural Hispanics reported sedentary behavior.[24]

Furthermore, some authors studied differences in self-reported physical activity between rural and urban women.[25] Rural middle-aged and older adults, particularly Southern and less-educated women, reported less physical activity than urban adults.[25] In most age groups, rural women were more likely to be sedentary than urban women. Rural women in the South who were African American and less educated, as well as adults aged 70 years and older, reported 60% or higher rates of sedentary behavior.[25]

Particularly, rural women described facing more personal barriers to moderate physical activity, citing their top barriers as caregiving duties and a greater body fat.[25] Rural women also reported seeing fewer adults exercise in their neighborhood, indicating lower overall social expectations for exercise.[25] Although more rural African American women reported being active or very active at work, they reported lower amounts of moderate physical activity compared to rural White women.[25]

Overall, the stark differences in sedentary lifestyle that exist when comparing urban areas to rural indicate there is a strong need for the development of rural-specific interventions designed to increase physical activity. Given obesity's role in a number of health outcomes (including CVD, diabetes, and cancer), the need for new programs is critical and is a pressing concern in effectively addressing the public health needs of rural America.

Smoking

Given the strong role of tobacco control in rural areas (particularly agricultural rural settings), it is not surprising that smoking continues to have an impact on rural residents in particular. Cigarette smoking contributes to CVD and stroke, with nearly one fifth of all deaths from CVD attributed to smoking.[26] Previous studies uncovered smoking rates that vary among rural residents. According to the 2005 BRFSS, the prevalence of cigarette smoking (23.6%) in the Mississippi Delta, for instance, was higher than those residents in Minnesota (20.0%) and higher than the national average (20.6%).[27] On the other hand, fewer rural African American women currently smoked (30.5%), as compared to rural White women (39.7%), and more women never smoked (60.7%).[26] Multiple factors such as socioeconomic status, targeted advertising, and the ability of communities to manage effective tobacco control interventions may influence smoking among ethnic minorities. Continued examination of the reasons behind rural variations in smoking patterns could reveal unique factors that could be capitalized upon in prevention efforts.

Contextual Factors

Residing in a rural and medically underserved region greatly impacts the cardiovascular health of various groups.[28] The first problem is rural adults have limited opportunities for health promotion and disease prevention services and little access to health information. Second, their occasional interaction with the health care system is only at that point when they were already unable to carry out their activities of daily living due to advanced illness. This behavior of seeking health care at a later point of time is understandable among the uninsured and it may be associated with the poor cardiovascular health outcomes eventually faced. Third, they live in difficult conditions that may negatively influence their health status. Fourth, many rural residents may face other priorities while living on a low income. For example, low-income women who are single parents may place the needs of their children and family members above their own needs, including their own health.

Rural adults also frequently face a lack of availability of healthy foods. Although rural communities produce fruits and vegetables, they typically have fewer stores that carry a wide selection of healthy, low-cost food than urban communities.[22] Thus, rural residents are more likely to live in food deserts and rural adults are less likely to consume fruits and vegetables. Another related issue is that rural residents may have to travel greater distances to food stores where a greater availability of healthy foods might be found.[22] The community food environment is an important contributor to adopting healthy lifestyles for rural individuals, and programs designed to improve the food environment are crucial in addressing the burden of CVD in rural settings.

On the other hand, research suggests that rural residents may enjoy greater social support or social cohesion than urban residents.[29] Social cohesion is defined as the degree to which groups feel connected, share resources, and provide moral support. This may include more social networks, community engagement, and participation in religious activities.[29] These influences may help protect against the daily stressors of life associated with overall health.[29] This increase in protective factors in the midst of numerous identified risk factors may partially explain why findings are inconsistent with regard to CVD disparities between rural and urban groups; the unique mixture of highly variable risk and protective factors may in part be masking differences that exist.

CARDIOVASCULAR DISEASE DISPARITIES

Several factors, including gender, race/ethnicity, and location of residence, have been associated with CVD disparities in rural populations. Following is a brief summary of these disparities.

Gender

Hypertension

Research suggests that rural women are less likely to have their HTN under adequate control. Women classified as non-White, older, obese, and living in a rural area reported a higher prevalence of HTN, which increased their risk for heart disease.[21] Also, researchers have demonstrated a high prevalence of pre-HTN and HTN, lower fitness levels, and high triglycerides in older midwestern rural women.[30]

Heart Attack and Associated Conditions

Research has demonstrated that the risk of death from a heart attack is higher in younger women compared to men in the same age group.[31] This gender disparity in mortality diminishes with increasing age, no longer statistically significant after age 74. Younger women without chest pain had a higher hospital mortality rate from a heart attack than younger men without chest pain. These gender differences in mortality rates also decreased with increasing age, from ages 45 to 75 and older.[31]

Stroke

Overall, women have a greater burden of stroke morbidity and mortality compared to men.[16] Women have a 20% lifetime risk of stroke throughout the nation, and 25% of women who experienced a stroke in any given year were under age 65.[16] Each year 55,000 more women than men experience a stroke.[16] More women than men die of stroke annually due to the disproportionately larger number of older women. In 2007, women accounted for 60.6% of stroke deaths in the United States and there is a 67% excess of stroke deaths in women in the United States.[16]

Racial and Ethnic Minorities

Hypertension

Research shows significant disparities in HTN control between rural African Americans and rural Whites. Rural African Americans are more likely to have poorer HTN control as compared to rural Whites.[21]

According to the 1988–1994 NHANES, rural African Americans were at an increased risk for uncontrolled HTN compared to rural Whites.[32] Among patients diagnosed with HTN, 11% were rural Whites, 13% were urban Whites, 20% were urban African Americans, and 23% were rural African Americans.[32]

Furthermore, based upon an analysis of 1998 National Health Interview Survey (NHIS) data, researchers reported that providers were more likely to tell rural residents of all racial/ethnic groups they had HTN than urban residents.[24] Rural African Americans reported the highest rates of HTN among any other group, at 34%.[24] Rural Hispanics with diagnosed HTN were more likely to be younger than age 65, be female, earn an annual income less than $20,000, have not graduated from high school, report poorer health, and have a greater BMI than Whites.[33] These findings support the need for more culturally sensitive education among these rural and minority populations with particular focus on HTN risk factors.

Heart Disease

CHD mortality is markedly greater in African American versus White women at all ages and time periods.[34] From 1985 to 1995, lower declines in mortality rates for premature CHD in African Americans and Whites were found to be in the rural South than other geographic areas in the nation. This effect also appears in the general population. While CHD mortality is decreasing, there is a disparity in the rate of decrease: The 5-year average annual CHD mortality declined 2.6% for White men and women, as compared to only 1.6% and 2.2% for African American men and women, respectively.

Native Americans

Another group facing large disparities in heart disease mortality rates is Native Americans.[35] CVD is the leading cause of death among Native Americans. Contributing factors for CVD include high poverty rate, high unemployment rate, low level of education, malnutrition, obesity, diabetes, and poor living conditions. Researchers have posited that the rapid shift in lifestyles associated with acculturation to Western culture, thereby moving away from traditional patterns of high physical activity and nutrition, have dramatically heightened the risk of CVD among Native populations.

Rural Native American women are among the most severely disadvantaged in today's society and one of the most understudied groups. The incidence of CVD among Native American women aged 35 years or older residing in rural counties of 50,000 or less was 406 per 100,000.[35] Previous authors report that CVD mortality rates were 57% higher among Native American women residing in rural areas compared to urban areas. This mortality rate among rural Native American women far exceeds the national average of 259 per 100,000 for all Native American women in the nation and the national average of 401 per 100,000 for all women 35 years or older.[35]

African Americans

Additionally, high heart disease mortality rates have been reported for rural African Americans. From 1991 to 1995, researchers determined the CVD mortality rates of African American women aged 35 years or older residing in selected rural counties in selected states.[36] The average heart disease mortality rate for African American women in counties of 50,000 or less was

540 per 100,000.[36] Death rates for rural counties varied from a minimum of 350 per 100,000 to a maximum of 854 per 100,000. Overall, rural African American women had significantly higher mortality rates than the general population of women in the nation (401 per 100,000).[36]

Stroke

African Americans are impacted by stroke more than any other racial group in the United States population. According to data from the 2010 BRFSS, 2.4% of men and 2.8% of women 18 years or older had a history of stroke; 2.7% of non-Hispanic Whites, 3.7% of non-Hispanic African Americans, 1.8% of Asian/Pacific Islanders, 1.8% of Hispanics, and 3.50% of multiracial individuals had a stroke.[17] African Americans' risk of having a first stroke is almost two times higher than Whites.[37] Those experiencing stroke included 2.3% Whites, 4.0% African Americans, and 2.6% Hispanics.[37] The overall age-adjusted stroke incidence rates in Americans 45 to 84 years old were 6.6 per 100,000 in African American men, 4.9 in African American women, 3.6 in White men, and 2.3 in White women.[37] These racial disparities in stroke incidence remained constant over time, and indicate a critical need for public health intervention.

Mortality data also indicate strong disparities. In addition to being more likely to have a stroke, African American women are twice as likely to die from stroke as White women.[1] This could partially be explained by the fact that African Americans are more likely to experience strokes later in life; however, the reasons are likely multifaceted and take into account differences in risk behaviors, access to care, and distance to emergency care. These disparities vary by age, with African Americans aged 35 to 54 years and older having a four times higher risk of stroke compared to Whites.[15] Even if a stroke is survived, African American stroke survivors are more likely to become disabled and experience difficulty in daily living activities.[15]

In addition to disparities found in the African American rural community, researchers from the Brain Attack Surveillance in Corpus Christi (BASIC) project revealed that Mexican Americans suffer more strokes than non-Hispanic Whites.[21] The incidence of stroke was 193 per 10,000 in Mexican Americans and 149 per 10,000 in non-Hispanic Whites.[21] Mexican Americans between the ages of 45 and 59 had a two-times higher risk of stroke compared with non-Hispanic Whites and were less likely to receive stroke prevention interventions.[21] Influences such as acculturation, low education, limited access to health care, and English-language barriers may contribute to poor stroke outcomes in this group.

Place of Residence

While there are some conflicting studies in the overall heart disease literature, a literature review revealed numerous CVD disparities between rural versus urban adults, particularly in the Southeast and Appalachians and among older White and African American men and women.

Hypertension

As with many outcomes, the view of rural–urban HTN disparities is complicated by the lack of a comprehensive, nationally representative study examining rates. Instead, individual studies must be examined to hopefully provide proper indication of areas for future study.

According to the 1996 National Health Interview Survey (NHIS), HTN was more prevalent in rural than urban areas.[38] However, in another study, there was an overall higher prevalence of undiagnosed HTN in a smaller urban sample (52.8%) from Harlem, New York, versus a larger sample (42.3%) from Pitt County, North Carolina.[39] Older women with lower socioeconomic status (SES) and lower educational levels living in rural settings were at a higher risk for developing CHD than younger White women with higher SES and more education living in urban settings.[39] However, the urban and rural samples were unequal in size and not nationally representative of the U.S. population.

Additionally, researchers measured the prevalence of HTN control in rural versus urban areas in a sample with a diagnosis of HTN and diabetes.[32] Rural Whites reported lower blood pressure than rural African Americans.[32] Urban Whites as well as urban African Americans reported lower blood pressure when compared to rural African Americans.[32] In this study, rural African Americans were at an increased risk of poor HTN control compared to rural Whites. In another study, researchers studied the determinants of CVD risk factors among a sample of rural and urban African American and White men in Georgia.[40] Self-reported HTN status differed by race, as 51.47% of rural African American men reported a HTN diagnosis compared to only 38.30% of rural White men.[40] Also, 43.05% of rural White men and 38.10% of rural African American men reported they had high cholesterol.[40] However, cholesterol rates among urban men remained constant, at about 38%. These disparities demonstrate the need for improved CVD education among rural populations. It is also difficult to determine the potential interpretation of the difference in cholesterol rates found between rural African American men and White men; it is possible that African American men are less likely to have had their cholesterol recently screened, thereby masking potential disparities. Prospective studies are necessary to better elucidate potential differences in this area.

Heart Attack and Associated Conditions

The prevalence of hospitalizations for heart attacks were highest in the Appalachians and Southeast.[21] These rural adults possibly reported a higher burden of CVD due in part to poor management of risk factors including HTN and diabetes and limited access to health care services including specialists, lack of health insurance, and concerns of the high cost of medical care.[21]

Researchers have also utilized 2008 BRFSS data to determine the prevalence of CHD or chest pain in rural versus urban settings.[41] Approximately 4% of urban adults versus 5.5% of rural adults self-reported a diagnosis of CHD or chest pain.[41] Those living in a rural environment were also more likely to report a diagnosis of CHD than those living in an urban environment, with the chance of a CHD diagnosis increased by 9% for those living in rural locations compared to those living in urban locations.[41]

Regionally, the southern United States has higher deaths attributed to heart attack and stroke than the rest of the nation.[13] This finding is supported by county-by-county profiles of heart disease mortality. Researchers have reported a significantly higher hospital mortality rate for patients with a heart attack admitted to rural hospitals (14%) than urban hospitals (6.4%).[42] While there are many potential reasons for this disparity, patients admitted to a rural hospital tend to be older and more severely ill than patients admitted to an urban hospital.[42] In a study examining Appalachian coal workers,[43] among female coal-mining workers, Appalachians were 1.17 times more likely to die of a heart attack than non-Appalachians. Among male coal-mining workers, Appalachians were 1.22 times more likely to die of a heart attack than non-Appalachians. Air pollution, water quality, and other environmental factors in Appalachia may influence the development of CVD among coal-mining workers and should be investigated more fully to determine intervention targets.

Stroke

Over the past five decades, a 153-county region comprising the coastal plains of North Carolina, South Carolina, and Georgia has had a stroke mortality rate considerably higher than the rest of the nation. This area called the "Stroke Buckle" exists within the larger Stroke Belt, which is an 8- to 12-state area in the southeast. The Stroke Buckle exhibits a stroke mortality rate about 1.3 to 1.5 times greater than the rest of the nation and consistently has the highest stroke mortality in the nation.[44] Researchers examined U.S. death certificates from 1979 to 1988 inside and outside the Stroke Buckle and distinguished residents and nonresidents.[44] Visitors to the region were 11% more likely to die of stroke than visitors to other parts of the nation. Stroke Buckle residents who left the area reduced their chances of stroke death by 10%.[44] Researchers propose that poor quality of health care, environmental toxins, other infections, and genetics may be possible explanations.

One of the most supported reasons for increased stroke mortality is delayed treatment. Researchers specifically investigating rural strokes have described delays in time to treatment of strokes in rural hospitals in Idaho.[45] These delays have been attributed to the patient's lack of knowledge of symptoms, underestimating a stroke's severity, living alone, emergency medical crews not trained to screen strokes, failure to notify hospitals of a patient having a stroke, lack of local emergency physicians, lack of access to a neurologist, lack of treatment procedures, and lack of stroke medication.[45] Optimal management of ischemic stroke involves saving as much brain tissue as possible from infarction and is governed by the time to treatment concept. Within the first 180 minutes after the development of an ischemic stroke, blood clot dissolving therapy can be administered, but after that time risks of therapy outweigh the benefits. Emergency access to health care is crucial for providing these patients with life-saving and disability-preventing treatment before the 3-hour window of opportunity closes. The 12% increase in stroke mortality among rural adults may be attributed to factors like distance and time-determined barriers to emergency medical services and the lower density of specialty health care facilities in rural areas.[46]

KNOWLEDGE AND AWARENESS OF HEART ATTACK, HEART DISEASE, AND STROKE

This section summarizes rural adults' knowledge and awareness of symptoms of heart disease, heart attack, and stroke. There is a distinct lack of nationally representative, geographically diverse studies examining these topics in rural areas; therefore, summaries of individual studies are presented.

Heart Attack and Associated Conditions

Using BRFSS data, researchers have identified the characteristics of rural adults likely to score low on knowledge questions about heart attack and stroke signs and symptoms.[47] Researchers analyzed the percentage of correct and incorrect responses by symptom question and location (rural versus urban).[47] For 9 of the 13 questions (69.3%) on heart attack and stroke symptoms, rural adults had higher percentages of incorrect answers.[47] Rural adults were more likely to score low on heart attack and stroke symptom questions if they did not graduate from high school, were older than 65, male, Hispanic and/or multiracial, single or living with a partner, earning an income less than $50,000, uninsured, and had no provider.[47]

In a study of rural men and women who had experienced a heart attack, the most common reported sign was unusual fatigue.[48] Only 30% of women in the sample reported severe chest pain and 25% reported no chest pain at all. Also, patients expected to have shortness of breath or fatigue, which did not occur. Overall, rural residents demonstrated a poor ability to recognize symptoms of a heart attack and to know the importance of seeking treatment.[48] In summary, rural adults report a lack of knowledge and awareness of heart attack symptoms, particularly older adults and women. Individuals may understand a portion but not the entire message, resulting in possible unintended consequences.[49] This may include women not seeking help because they felt chest pain, but were educated to expect shortness of breath and fatigue.[49] Public awareness efforts only describing stroke signs and symptoms is insufficient. Future education needs to indicate that each person has different symptoms and to seek immediate medical attention for a heart attack.[49]

Heart Disease

Two qualitative studies reported rural African American women's current knowledge of CVD.[50,51] In one study, rural women reported a lack of knowledge of CVD as a risk factor for women.[50] Women reported heart disease as a man's disease and breast cancer as a woman's disease. Similarly, rural African American women reported the belief that one cannot prevent heart disease if one is destined to have it.[51] They believed that fate is linked with an individual's behavior, suggesting that illness or disease may be punishment from a higher power rather the result of an individual's health behaviors.

Researchers interviewed women to determine their perceptions of the symptoms and awareness of heart disease. When they initially sought help for heart disease from health care providers, women became angered when the providers failed to resolve it.[48] Since they did not report crushing chest pain, a symptom typical in men, female patients felt that providers did not treat them as seriously as male patients. Such perceptions can jeopardize the patient–provider relationship (and thereby receipt of follow-up care and compliance with prescribed regimens); therefore, educational interventions regarding the complexities of heart disease management may help support positive and beneficial provider interactions.

Stroke

Most strokes are preventable, yet many women are unaware of their risks for stroke and are not knowledgeable of the symptoms of a stroke.[52] Authors focused on awareness of risk factors for a stroke as fundamental for stroke awareness and prevention.[53] Groups with the highest risk of stroke showed the poorest stroke knowledge. The combination of knowledge of stroke's modifiable risk factors and the proper management of these risk factors is needed to lower stroke's high mortality, particularly in rural populations.

The general population lacks sufficient knowledge of stroke warning signs. In one study, 30% to 60% of adults failed to recognize a single warning sign.[54] Only 20% to 40% recognized five symptoms and knew to call 911 if they thought someone was having a stroke.[54] In another study, rural African American stroke survivors failed to identify signs and symptoms of a stroke and call 911 immediately due to a lack of knowledge and barriers to rural health care.[51] Disparities exist for rural residents and older women in the awareness and knowledge of stroke, signs and symptoms of stroke, and the urgency for treatment, and these factors are complicated by the severe shortage of adequate stroke care in rural settings. In 2002, 21% of counties in the United States did not have a hospital, 31% lacked a hospital with an emergency department, and 77% did not have a hospital with neurological services.[51]

When looking within specific rural regions, researchers surveyed a sample of rural Mississippi Delta adults to determine their knowledge and awareness of the signs and symptoms of a stroke.[53] Particularly, 72.3% of adults identified sudden weakness/numbness, and 60% of adults identified sudden confusion and difficulty speaking as warning signs of a stroke.[50] However, less than one fourth of adults correctly identified all main stroke symptoms. Most respondents (70.2%) agreed that stroke was preventable; however, 20.2% failed to provide an answer, while 7.4% of adults stated that stroke was not preventable.[53] This evidence suggests the need for improved stroke education efforts among rural adults.

Similarly, in a study of rural residents living in West Virginia, more than one third incorrectly reported sudden chest pain as a sign of stroke and less than 20% correctly identified all stroke signs.[52] What is alarming is that almost 40% of residents were not able to identify vision loss in one eye as a stroke sign and 39% could not identify a sudden severe headache as a stroke sign. Limited knowledge about obvious stroke signs will delay medical evaluation and treatment for rural adults in a context in which access to quick care is already complicated. Thus, it is critical for rural residents to manage their CVD risks appropriately and identify symptoms of a stroke at earlier times. An increase in stroke knowledge may not necessarily indicate that patients will accurately recognize and respond appropriately to the occurrence of stroke symptoms.[16] Nevertheless, early recognition of its warning signs is the first step in obtaining immediate medical intervention when the stroke occurs.[16] To decrease stroke mortality and morbidity, the need for stroke awareness among rural population is essential.

A wide disparity in CVD knowledge and awareness exists among rural communities in the southeastern United States and Appalachia.[16,52] Future research should focus on designing and implementing interventions to improve a woman's ability to correctly identify a stroke, to practice healthy behaviors, and to improve stroke treatment outcomes for rural women and older adults. The greater burden of stroke prevalence and mortality in rural areas suggests that tailored interventions may be required to meet their unique needs. Thus, researchers and practitioners should focus on educating those with the highest risk of stroke, such as the growing population of older adults.[16] Findings suggest that culturally tailored and gender-sensitive educational strategies may assist in the improvement of knowledge and awareness of stroke signs and symptoms.

COMMUNITY-BASED PROGRAMS AND INTERVENTIONS

Challenges Faced in Improving Cardiovascular Disease in Rural Areas

Historically, rural areas have adopted health behavior changes such as smoking cessation, nutrition, and physical activity at a slower rate compared to urban areas.[38] Similarly, once CVD risk factors are adopted in rural areas, lifestyle changes occur at a slower rate than urban areas. This delay in lifestyle changes may contribute to the CVD disparities among rural versus urban adults.

Rural elderly are independent, self-sufficient, and private, and these qualities may result in their resistance to health behavior changes and inability to manage CVD. Additionally, rural residents may adhere to the role performance model of health.[55] This emphasizes that one is healthy as long as one can be productive, work, and perform daily functions. This viewpoint may influence rural residents to delay obtaining preventive services and seek medical treatment until CVD-related problems have progressed to a severe and advanced stage.[55] Cultural issues may include mistrust of the health care system and their physician. Rural residents may also be reluctant to undergo invasive procedures and have more reliance for self-care and ignore treatment. They may also be in denial of their condition and fail to realize the importance of managing their condition. Rural individuals may avoid preventive services due to concern for privacy, and discomfort with the difference in education level between themselves and their health care provider. They may have worries and concerns with the outcomes of testing and screenings and feel disgraced if they are diagnosed by a physician.[55]

Misperceptions of CVD risk may be another challenge in rural areas. Some rural residents believe they are not at risk for heart disease or stroke, and their health behaviors illustrate this misperception. This includes a decreased rate of lifestyle change from behaviors associated with CVD such as smoking, high-fat diets, and a sedentary lifestyle, especially among older rural women. Older adult women also report a low risk perception of CVD compared to men and are less likely to participate in primary prevention efforts such as health education and screening programs. This perceived lower CVD risk is worsened by the limited health screenings in rural areas.

Researchers have demonstrated southern rural African American women as a group are less likely than White women to engage in CVD prevention strategies.[51] Lower participation rates among African American women may be attributed to cultural influences on diet and exercise, the false belief that prevention strategies are useless, and fatalism.[51] Fatalism is the idea that disease and illness are not preventable and passed down from generation to generation in a family. Culturally tailored interventions that can address CVD prevention strategies within the appropriate cultural framework are sorely needed to address racial disparities in rural CVD outcomes.

Rural adults also report the specific challenges to participation in CVD programs. These challenges included lack of time in their daily schedules; transportation issues; childcare, family, and cultural pressures; low education; and low reading levels.[51] Rural adults in these programs remark that the format of a community-based program should be presented as a choice, instead of being instructed by an authority figure on what to do.[51] Rural adults in previous studies preferred a program with a group or workshop format, instead of a class format, which they associated with a lower level of education.[51] They reported written instead of visual components as more difficult to understand. In the delivery of the program, they also wanted to see regular people with regular struggles, not celebrities providing health information.

Financial difficulties are also a challenge to improving CVD in rural areas. The high cost of medical services is one barrier. Rural residents tend to be poorer with higher unemployment and lower education.[55] Rural poor are less likely to be covered by governmental assistance than urban poor. Southern rural African American women reported that the respect they received from health care providers was dependent on their health insurance status or ability to pay for their clinic visit.[47] As a result, health care providers' attitudes toward rural patients can influence the quality of medical care for CVD.[56] Health care providers have been shown to be less likely to refer patients with reduced access to health care to a cardiologist or to receive cardiac evaluation. In another study, rural health care providers agreed it was their responsibility to teach patients lifestyle modification and medication management.[56] They reported confidence in their ability to teach patients about lifestyle modification, but fewer reported confidence in their ability to actually significantly change patients' health behaviors.

Additionally, the development of improved health care facilities has been a slow, gradual process in rural areas.[41] Advances in medical care treatments such as new medicines and procedures are expensive to disseminate and may not reach poorer, rural areas compared to affluent, urban regions.[41] Diffusion of new technologies to rural areas may be limited by low education and financial resources. Innovative health care technology and resources are often used in urban areas where large populations, tertiary hospitals, and philanthropic dollars are more abundant.

As discussed elsewhere in this book, rural residents encountered numerous challenges with access to health care and service gaps in seeking treatment and preventive services.[38] These unique challenges faced by rural residents include limited access to medical personnel, screening services, and limited access to medical treatment for heart disease and stroke. Other factors include the availability of technology specialists, and limited access to cardiac rehabilitation services. In addition to health screenings, nutrition and fitness assessments are often unavailable in rural areas. Also, nonprofit organizations disseminating CVD prevention and education strategies may have limited staff and financial resources in rural areas. These unique challenges must be faced to address the burden of CVD in rural areas, particularly for older adults and minority women. Practitioners and researchers need to understand rural culture and use the unique resources of a rural community when designing and implementing health behavior change interventions in these communities. Knowledge of this literature can assist in the improvement of participation in CVD programs and interventions in rural communities.

Specific Examples of Community-Based Programs and Interventions

Three community programs specifically aimed at CVD prevention in the rural poor and underserved populations have emerged in the literature. These are described in hopes that they can serve as models for implementation, or to spark additional research in the area of heart disease prevention and management.

The CDC's DHDSP administers WISEWOMAN (Well-Integrated Screening and Evaluation for Women Across the Nation), which operated locally in 21 states and tribal organizations.[57] The purpose was to provide low-income, underinsured, or uninsured women ages 40 to 64 years old with the knowledge, skills, and opportunities to improve their nutrition, physical activity, and other health behaviors to prevent, delay, or control CVD.[57] WISE-WOMAN offered preventive services such as blood pressure and cholesterol testing and referral services as needed.[57] Also, women participated in lifestyle programs such as healthy cooking classes, walking clubs, or lifestyle counseling. From 2008 to 2010, WISEWOMAN provided 78,000 screenings to women for CVD and other risk factors and more than 43,000 women participated in at least one lifestyle intervention.[57] Results revealed WISEWOMAN participants had these risk factors: 39% had HTN, 29% had pre-HTN, 30% had high cholesterol, 16% had type 2 diabetes, 27% were smokers, 45% were obese, and 27% were overweight.[57] Results showed that 89% of WISEWOMAN participants had one or more risk factors for heart disease and stroke.

The Coronary Artery Risk Reduction in Appalachian Communities Project (CARDIAC) was developed to reduce heart disease in the rural and poor state of West Virginia.[55] The provision of a school-based statewide cholesterol screening program for fifth-grade children eliminated environmental and financial barriers commonly faced by Appalachians.[55] The CARDIAC screening program for fifth graders is one solution to increase awareness of CVD in this poor, underserved area of West Virginia.[55] The CARDIAC project provided cholesterol screening to more than 81,000 fifth-grade students, including 18.8% who were overweight, 28.3% who were obese, and 25.7% with high cholesterol.[58]

A community health education program titled Approaches to Take Absolute Control through Knowledge (ATTACK) was developed to address the high prevalence of HTN and CVD in the Mississippi Delta.[59] ATTACK was designed to promote nutrition and physical activity and provide participants with the basic knowledge of HTN and CVD.[59] ATTACK culturally adapted the program for rural, low-income African American women in the Mississippi Delta and strengthened the knowledge and skills of everyday citizens in underserved communities. Participants practiced grocery shopping and label reading in real-life situations. Results showed an increase in participants' knowledge of target blood pressure, blood glucose, cholesterol, and BMI levels after the educational sessions.[59] ATTACK demonstrates potential success for community health education programs to improve quality of life through culturally appropriate, adult learning principles.[59]

CONCLUSION

While there is sometimes conflicting evidence regarding the magnitude of CVD disparities in rural areas, there is no doubt that rural residents face unique socioeconomic, cultural, and environmental risks for CVD that are not being adequately addressed through current public health efforts. To examine rural–urban disparities in CVD, researchers often analyzed national data sets such as the BRFSS, NHIS, and NHANES to compare the morbidity and/or mortality of CVD and/or risk factors by geographic location (rural versus urban). More primary data collection of CVD knowledge and awareness in rural areas is needed in the future, as well as mixed-methods examinations aimed at developing culturally tailored prevention interventions.

Substantial differences do exist in the morbidity and mortality of CVD among White and African Americans in particular. Researchers commonly studied these differences in rural versus urban areas, particularly in the Southeast and Appalachia. Although CVD mortality rates in the United States decreased over the past decades, many rural residents are burdened by CVD and continue to face substantial challenges compared to urban residents. In recent years, researchers have designed and implemented community programs to address these challenges in rural areas, focusing on low-income populations and older adults; however, additional work in this area, including dissemination efforts, is needed to truly impact rural CVD morbidity and mortality. Practitioners, researchers, and clinicians should understand the unique barriers and challenges faced by these vulnerable populations, particularly among older women and minorities. Culturally and gender-sensitive education programs designed at the appropriate health literacy levels are necessary to address the great burden of CVD in rural populations.

REFERENCES

1. Roger VL, Go AS, Lloyd Jones D, et al. Heart disease and stroke statistics—2012 update: A report from the American Heart Association. *Circulation*. 2012, 125(1):e2–e220.
2. Centers for Disease Control and Prevention. Heart disease and stroke prevention: addressing the nation's leading killers: at a glance 2011. http://www.cdc.gov/chronicdisease/resources/publications/AAG/dhdsp.htm. Accessed September 28, 2012.
3. Chobanian AV, Bakris GL, Black HR, et al. The Seventh Report of the Joint National Committee on Prevention, Detection, Evaluation, and Treatment of High Blood Pressure: the JNC 7 Report. *JAMA*. 2003;289(19):2560–2572.
4. Hyman DJ, Pavlik VN. Characteristics of patients with uncontrolled hypertension in the United States. *N Engl J Med*. 2001;345(7):479–486.
5. Boeckner LS, Pullen CH, Walker SN, Oberdorfer MK, Hageman PA. Eating behaviors and health history of rural midlife to older women in the Midwestern United States. *J Am Diet Assoc*. 2007;107(2):306–310.
6. Kumar V, Acanfora M, Hennessy CH, Kalache A. Health status of the rural elderly. *J Rural Health*. 2001;17(4):328–331.
7. Ford E. Trends in mortality from all causes and cardiovascular diseases among hypertensive and nonhypertensive adults in the United States. *Circulation*. 2011;123:1737–1744.
8. Yoon SS, Ostchega Y, Louis, T. *Recent Trends in the Prevalence of High Blood Pressure and its Treatment and Control, 1999–2008*. 2010; Hyattsville, MD: National Center for Health Statistics.
9. Centers for Disease Control and Prevention. Heart attack. http://www.cdc.gov/heartdisease/heart_attack.htm. Accessed September 28, 2012.
10. Boudi F. Coronary artery atherosclerosis. *Medscape Reference*. http://emedicine.medscape.com/article/153647-overview. Accessed September 28, 2012.

11. OSELS. High blood pressure and cholesterol. *CDC Vital Signs.* http://www.cdc
    .gov/vitalsigns/CardiovascularDisease. Accessed September 28, 2012.
12. National Heart, Lung, and Blood Institute. Disease statistics. In: NHLBI, ed. 2011.
13. Graham-Garcia J, Raines TL, Andrews JO, Mensha GA. Race, ethnicity, and geogra-
    phy: disparities in heart disease in women of color. *J Transcult Nurs.* 2001;12(1):56–67.
14. Pearson TA, Lewis C. Rural epidemiology: insights from a rural population labo-
    ratory. *Am J Epidemiol.* 1998;148(10):949–957.
15. American Stroke Association. Together to end stroke. http://www.strokeassociation
    .org/STROKEORG. Accessed October 1, 2012.
16. Ennen KA, Beamon ER. Women and stroke knowledge: influence of age, race,
    residence location, and marital status. *Health Care Women Int.* 2012;33(10):922–942.
17. Centers for Disease Control and Prevention. Prevalence and trends data. Behav-
    ioral risk factor surveillance system. http://apps.nccd.cdc.gov/BRFSS. Accessed
    October 11, 2012.
18. Division for Heart Disease and Stroke Prevention. Maps. http://www.cdc.gov/
    dhdsp/maps/index.htm. Accessed October 1, 2012.
19. Odoi A. Needs-based population health planning: identifying barriers to health care
    services in the Appalachian region of east Tennessee. *Veterinary Vis.* 2009;8(1):10–11.
20. Fang J, Shaw K, George M. Prevalence of stroke—United States, 2006–2010.
    MMWR. 2012;61(20):379–382.
21. Bale B. Optimizing hypertension management in underserved rural populations.
    J Natl Med Assoc. 2010;102(1):10–17.
22. Lutfiyya MN, Chang LF, Lipsky MS. A cross-sectional study of US rural adults'
    consumption of fruits and vegetables: do they consume at least five servings
    daily? *BMC Public Health.* 2012;12:280.
23. Centers for Disease Control and Prevention. Adult obesity facts. Overweight and
    obesity. http://www.cdc.gov/obesity/data/adult.html. Accessed October 2, 2012.
24. Patterson P, Moore C, Probst J, Samuels M. *Hypertension, Diabetes, Cholesterol,
    Weight, and Weight Control Activities among Non-Metro Minority Adults.* Columbia,
    SC: University of South Carolina Arnold School of Public Health; 2002.
25. Wilcox S, Castro C, King AC, Housemann R, Brownson RC. Determinants of leisure
    time physical activity in rural compared with urban older and ethnically diverse
    women in the United States. *J Epidemiol Community Health.* 2000;54(9):667–672.
26. Appel SJ, Harrell JS, Deng S. Racial and socioeconomic differences in risk factors
    for cardiovascular disease among southern rural women. *J Natl Black Nurs Assoc.*
    2005;16(2):27–34.
27. Cosby A. *An Assessment of Cardiovascular Disease in the Mississippi Delta.* Starkville,
    MS: Mississippi State University; 2000.
28. Appel SJ, Giger JN, Davidhizar RE. Opportunity cost: the impact of contextual
    risk factors on the cardiovascular health of low-income rural southern African
    American women. *J Cardiovasc Nurs.* 2005;20(5):315–324.
29. Bardach S, Tarasenko Y, Schoenberg N. The role of social support in multiple mor-
    bidity: self-management among rural residents. *J Health Care Poor Underserved.*
    2011;22(3):756–771.
30. Hageman PA, Pullen CH, Walker SN, Boeckner LS. Blood pressure, fitness, and
    lipid profiles of rural women in the Wellness for Women Project. *Cardiopulmonary
    Phys Ther J.* 2010;21(3):27.
31. Canto JG, Rogers WJ, Goldberg RJ. Association of age and sex with myo-
    cardial infarction symptom presentation and in-hospital mortality. *JAMA.*
    2012;307(8):813–822.

32. Mainous AG, King DE, Garr DR, Pearson WS. Race, rural residence, and control of diabetes and hypertension. *Ann Fam Med.* 2004;2(6):563–568.

33. Mainous A, Koopman R, Geesey M. *Diabetes and Hypertension among Rural Hispanics: Disparities in Diagnosis and Management.* Columbia, South Carolina: University of South Carolina, Arnold School of Public Health; 2004.

34. Williams JE, Massing M, Rosamond WD, Sorlie PD, Tyroler HA. Racial disparities in CHD mortality from 1968–1992 in the state economic areas surrounding the ARIC study communities. Atherosclerosis risk in communities. *Ann Epidemiol.* 1999;9(8):472–480.

35. Aiello M, Fahs P. A secondary analysis cardiovascular mortality among rural Native American women. *J Multicult Nurs Health.* 2001;7(2):42–47.

36. Cort N, Fahs P. Heart disease: the hidden killer of rural black women. *J Multicult Nurs Health.* 2001;7(2):37–41.

37. Ennen KA. *Knowledge of Stroke Warning Symptoms and Risk Factors: Variations by Rural and Urban Categories.* Chicago, IL: University of Illinois, Health Sciences Center; 2004.

38. Zuniga M, Anderson DA, Alexander K. Heart disease and stroke in rural America: A literature review. *Rural Healthy People 2010: A Companion Document to Healthy People 2010.* 1999;2:73–83.

39. Geronimus AT, Colen CG, Shochet T, Lori Barer I, James SA. Urban-rural differences in excess mortality among high-poverty populations: evidence from the Harlem Household Survey and the Pitt County, North Carolina Study of African American Health. *J Health Care Poor Underserved.* 2006;17(3):532–558.

40. Quarells RC, Liu J, Davis SK. Social determinants of cardiovascular disease risk factor presence among rural and urban Black and White men. *J Mens Health.* 2012;9(2):120–126.

41. O'Connor A, Wellenius G. Rural–urban disparities in the prevalence of diabetes and coronary heart disease. *Public Health.* 2012;126(10):813–820.

42. James PA, Pengxiang L, Ward MM. Myocardial infarction mortality in rural and urban hospitals: rethinking measures of quality of care. *Ann Fam Med.* 2007;5(2):105–111.

43. Hendryx M, Zullig KJ. Higher coronary heart disease and heart attack morbidity in Appalachian coal mining regions. *Prev Med.* 2009;49(5):355–359.

44. Shrira I, Christenfeld N, Howard G. Exposure to the US Stroke Buckle as a risk factor for cerebrovascular mortality. *Neuroepidemiol.* 2008;30(4):229–233.

45. Gebhardt JG, Norris TE. Acute stroke care at rural hospitals in Idaho: challenges in expediting stroke care. *J Rural Health.* 2006;22(1):88–91.

46. Sergeev AV. Racial and rural-urban disparities in stroke mortality outside the stroke Belt. *Ethn Dis.* 2011;21(3):307–313.

47. Ford CD, Kim MJ, Dancy BL. Perceptions of hypertension and contributing personal and environmental factors among rural Southern African American women. *Ethn Dis.* 2009;19(4):407–413.

48. Swanoski MT, Lutfiyya MN, Amaro ML, Akers MF, Huot KL. Knowledge of heart attack and stroke symptomology: a cross-sectional comparison of rural and non-rural US adults. *BMC Public Health.* 2012;12:283–283.

49. Fahs PS, Kalman M. Matters of the heart: cardiovascular disease and rural nursing. *Ann Rev Nurs Res.* 2008;26:41–84.

50. Morgan DM. Effect of incongruence of acute myocardial infarction symptoms on the decision to seek treatment in a rural population. *J Cardiovasc Nurs.* 2005;20(5):365–371.

51. Liewer L, Mains DA, Lykens K, René AA. Barriers to women's cardiovascular risk knowledge. *Health Care Women Int.* 2008;29(1):23–38.
52. Evans LK. Because we don't take better care of ourselves: rural black women's explanatory models of heart disease. *J Women Aging.* 2010;22(2):94–108.
53. Sallar AM, Williams PB, Omishakin AM, Lloyd DP. Stroke prevention: awareness of risk factors for stroke among African American residents in the Mississippi Delta region. *J Natl Med Assoc.* 2010;102(2):84–94.
54. Alkadry MG, Wilson C, Nicholson D. Stroke awareness among rural residents: the case of West Virginia. *Soc Work Health Care.* 2005;42(2):73–92.
55. Deskins S, Harris CV, Bradlyn AS, et al. Preventive care in Appalachia: use of the Theory of Planned Behavior to identify barriers to participation in cholesterol screenings among West Virginians. *J Rural Health.* 2006;22(4):367–374.
56. Cook S, Drum ML, Kirchhoff AC, et al. Providers' assessment of barriers to effective management of hypertension and hyperlipidemia in community health centers. *J Health Care Poor Underserved.* 2006;17(1):70–85.
57. Division for Heart Disease and Stroke Prevention. WISEWOMAN. http://www .cdc.gov/wisewoman. Accessed October 2, 2012.
58. CARDIAC Project. Coronary artery risk detection in Appalachian communities. http://www.cardiacwv.org/index.php. Accessed April 9, 2013.
59. Mayfield-Johnson S, Young R, Mohn R, Ebersole R. Addressing chronic diseases in the Mississippi Delta through health education prevention. *Delta J Educ.* 2012;2(1):1–13.

CHAPTER 10

Obesity in Rural America

Kimberly Greder, Michelle Ihmels, Janie Burney,
and Kimberly Doudna

For the first time in U.S. history, children may have a shorter life expectancy than their parents.[1] This is largely due to obesity rates, which have reached an all-time high. More than one third of adults (men, 35.5%; women, 35.8%) and almost 17% of children and adolescents were obese in 2009–2010.[2,3]

The obesity epidemic is even more pronounced in rural America, and is a growing concern as rural adults [4,5] and children are now more likely to be obese [6] than urban adults and children.[7,8] In a 2007 national sample of rural children, 1 in 6 (16.5%) rural children were obese compared to 1 in 7 (14.4%) urban children, and the rural South claimed the highest rate of childhood overweight (34.5%) and obesity (19.5%). Within rural areas, minority groups are even more impacted by obesity. In a recent study, 1 in 4 Black children were obese (23.6%) compared to 1 in 5 Hispanic children (19%) and 1 in 8 (12%) White children. A significantly larger proportion of Black and Hispanic (41.2% and 38%, respectively) children were overweight compared to 26.7% of White children. Furthermore, overweight and obesity (44.1% and 26.3%, respectively) were more prevalent among Black rural residents than other racial and ethnic groups, which was also the case in urban areas.[6]

COSTS OF OBESITY

People who are overweight or obese are at increased risk for chronic disease and conditions such as hypertension, type 2 diabetes, coronary heart disease, stroke, gallbladder disease, osteoarthritis, sleep apnea/respiratory problems, and some types of cancers. For women, obesity also is associated with complications of pregnancy, menstrual irregularities, hirsutism, stress incontinence, and psychological disorders such as depression.[9] In a comprehensive review of 63 studies examining health risks associated with obesity in children, it was found that obese children and adolescents aged 5 to 15 years have raised serum lipids, blood pressure, glucose, and insulin, as well as increased left ventricular mass when compared to children with a healthy weight.[10] Future health implications for these children could be that they will have more heart attacks and strokes.[10] Additionally, the dramatic increase in obesity has cost the U.S. health care system billions of dollars.[11] If obesity levels of 2010 could be maintained with no increase, the savings in medical expenditures over the next 20 years could be as much as $549.5 billion.[11]

ECOLOGICAL APPROACH TO UNDERSTANDING RURAL OBESITY

Human Ecological Theory states that individuals are nested within families and other contexts, such as the sociocultural environment (e.g., characteristics of the population, values, attitudes, lifestyle, and relationships), the human-built environment (e.g., physical structures planned by people such as cities, roads, sidewalks, food stores), and the natural physical–biological environment (e.g., trees, land, water).[12] Individuals and families and the communities in which they live are part of a system—they are interrelated and influence each other. No one factor has led to the dramatic increase in obesity. Multiple changes at various system levels have resulted in Americans consuming more calories than they expend. To fully understand and effectively address obesity, research and interventions are needed that examine how various system components (i.e., individual, family, community) and policy interrelate and influence each other, and the resulting direct and indirect relationships to obesity.

Individual Factors

The first level in the ecological approach is that of the individual. While individual characteristics are important, they do not occur in a vacuum. Each individual is a member of several immediate settings such as the family, peer group, school, and work.[13] Factors within individuals serve as indicators of risk for obesity. In rural communities, women, ethnic and racial minorities, and individuals experiencing chronic stress are at greatest risk for obesity.

Gender
Obesity increased significantly between 1999 and 2010 for men and for non-Hispanic Black women and Mexican American women.[2] For other women, increases were not significant. Rural women have a higher prevalence of

obesity than urban women,[14] while men in urban and rural settings have similar rates of obesity.[5] In contrast, gender differences in youth are small.[2] Dietary fat is thought to exert a strong effect on positive energy balance leading to obesity.[15] Hermstad et al.[16] examined dietary fat intake in rural communities and reported that food in the home directly influenced dietary fat intake for rural women, but not men. For women, consumer nutrition behavior had a direct effect on dietary fat intake and operated indirectly through the home environment. Women who grocery shopped more frequently and who frequently ate at fast-food restaurants were more likely to report high-fat foods in the home and higher levels of dietary fat intake. This was not the case for men, perhaps because men do less grocery shopping/ food preparation and may therefore be less familiar with what foods are in the home.[17]

Race and Ethnicity

National survey data reveal ethnic disparities in the prevalence of obesity between White and minority populations. Non-Hispanic Black and Mexican American women[3] and Hispanic children and adolescents[2] have higher rates of obesity than White populations. Black and Mexican American youth have higher rates than Whites, and American Indian youth have the highest rates. Disparities are also seen between rural and urban communities. Urban Whites have the lowest risk of obesity, leaving rural residents of every race/ethnicity at higher risk than urban Whites.[5] Jackson et al.[4] found obesity to be most prevalent among adult African Americans and American Indians in rural counties, while Williamson et al.[8] found overweight and obesity rates very high among youth living in rural Louisiana, but more similar than different across boys and girls and Caucasian and African American youth.

Stress and Depression

Stress has been linked to obesity in adults and in children,[18] and rural residents are continually subject to the stresses of poverty, limited access to health care, and geographical and social isolation.[19,20] Depression, a psychosocial stressor, has been linked to poorer child health and to child obesity. Stress affects eating behaviors in different ways; some individuals eat more under stress while others eat less.[21] Gibson et al.[22] and Dallman[23] reported that individuals who have experienced stress increase overall consumption of calorically dense and highly palatable foods. Consuming more calorically dense foods and limited opportunities for physical activity place rural residents at a greater risk for obesity. A qualitative study of 28 rural low-income women in upper New York[24] revealed that low-income overweight and obese rural women ate in response to stress, sadness, boredom, and loneliness. The cyclic nature of the mothers' food supply was related to their strong emotional attachments to food and binge eating. Additionally, studies have shown that individuals who are chronically overexposed to stress have blunted responses to stress, resulting in decreased cortisol levels and other neurobiological dysfunctions[25,26] that have been linked to weight gain in children via direct metabolic changes and negative coping behaviors (i.e., overeating, not being physically active).[27,28]

While factors that influence overweight and obesity are ultimately controlled by an individual, available options and choices are strongly influenced by their environment, including the household and community in which they live. For children, environmental factors most commonly start with their families, child care, and educational settings. Outside of child care and school, children depend on their families for food and opportunities for physical activity. Parents play a key role in influencing a child's food consumption and physical activity.

Family and Household Factors

Poverty and Food Insecurity

Lower household incomes and higher poverty rates are more prevalent in rural communities than urban communities. In 2009, the median nonmetro household income was $40,135 compared to $51,522 for metro households.[29] In 2010, the poverty rate among nonmetro adults was 14.8%, and 24.4 among nonmetro children, compared to 13.5% among metro adults and 21.6% among metro children.[30] Low household income and poverty are associated with greater levels of adult[31] and child obesity.[32,33] In 2007, the prevalence of childhood obesity was approximately 27.2% in households below 100% of the federal poverty level (FPL) compared to 20.9% in households between 100% and 199% of the FPL, and 9.8% in households at or above 400% of the FPL.[34] Lower income, much more prevalent in rural settings, is therefore a direct risk factor for obesity in rural residents.

Additionally, studies have shown a relationship between overweight and obesity to food insecurity, which is defined as "whenever the availability of nutritionally adequate and safe food or the ability to acquire acceptable foods in socially acceptable ways is limited or uncertain."[35] Women living in food-insecure households have a higher prevalence of obesity than women living in food-secure households.[36,37] In 2010, the rates of food insecurity were higher for families with incomes near or below the FPL,[38] and was more common in rural areas and large cities than in suburban areas.

Financial Constraints and Eating Patterns

Researchers seeking to explain the associations between food insecurity and obesity have suggested that there are management strategies people adopt under economic constraints. Mothers may do without food or substitute unhealthy foods in order to make food available for their children.[24,37,39] Skipping meals and eating smaller portions[40] may lead to a cyclic pattern of under- and overeating associated with obesity.[41] Sharkey, Johns, and Dean[39] reported greater consumption of sugar-sweetened beverages and other unhealthy eating behaviors such as low fruit and vegetable intake and less frequent breakfast consumption in rural adults than in urban adults. Bove and Olson[24] reported rural low-income women in food-insecure households drank sugar-sweetened beverages as a means of coping with eating little solid food on some days, thus, illustrating maladaptive eating patterns and coping strategies that contribute to the "hunger–obesity" paradox in poor rural women.[42]

Social Home Environment

Behavioral risk factors associated with child eating and physical activity practices, sedentary behavior, and coping habits are developed within the family system[43]; thus, the family is influential in shaping child health practices.[44,45] Parents play a key role in creating home environments that either facilitate or inhibit healthy eating and physical activity by children.[46,47] Parental role modeling of physical activity, dietary and media behaviors, as well as parenting strategies and feeding practices, influence children's health behaviors and weight status.[48-51] Increased rates of obesity among rural women, who typically serve as primary caregivers of children and shape the home environment, place rural children at risk of adopting unhealthy eating and physical activity habits.

To further examine the social home environment and its relationship to rural child obesity, as well as the role of individual and family level factors and how they shape the social home environment, the authors of this chapter analyzed preliminary data from 382 rural mothers who had low incomes, had young children, and who participated in the multi-state study, *Rural Families Speak about Health*[52]. Mothers responded to various individual and family level measures such as the Family Nutrition and Physical Activity Screening Tool (FNPA)[53] that assessed the social home environment including parental attitudes, behaviors and policies regarding children's food and beverages consumption, physical activity, media usage, sleep and shared family meals and physical activity, the CES-D 10[54] which assessed maternal depressive symptomology, a modified version of the Financial Distress/Financial Well-Being Scale[55] which assessed family financial stress, a modified version of the Family Routines Inventory[56] to assess family rituals and daily routines, and the Six-Item Short Form of the Food Security Survey Module[57] to measure household food security. Additionally, children's height and weight were measured and age was identified in order to calculate body mass index.

Findings revealed that families who were characterized as having health-enhancing home environments (as measured by high FNPA scores) were more likely to have daily family routines and practice religious- or cultural-based rituals, have lower maternal depressive symptomology and perceived financial stress compared to families with a less health-enhancing home environment (low FNPA scores). Additionally, Hispanic and White mothers who had higher FNPA scores had children with lower body mass index. While the results of this study affirm previous findings, the results also suggest that additional individual (e.g., maternal depression) and family (e.g., financial stress) level factors warrant further examination.

Community Factors

In addition to lower household incomes and educational levels, rural residents are more geographically and socially isolated.[19,20] They commonly face restricted educational and vocational training opportunities, reduced flexibility in child-care options, and an absence of public transportation.[58] Rural residents experience issues related to accessing needed goods and services, lack of public health clinics, specialized health care services and state-funded mental health centers, inadequate medical insurance, and limited social support services that are also common impediments to achieving and maintaining a healthy lifestyle in rural areas.[59] These characteristics and lifestyle behaviors have been examined to identify reasons why a growing percentage of rural adults, children, and youth are overweight and obese; particular characteristics are highlighted below.

Food Access

Ironically, in rural areas where food commonly is grown to feed the rest of the country, residents may have limited access to healthy food choices such as fresh fruits and vegetables.[60] Stores in rural communities tend to skew their inventories toward inexpensive, less nutrient-dense foods while stores in nonrural communities offered a wider variety of foods that include fresh produce and low-fat products.[61] Fruit and vegetable consumption is inversely associated with risk for hypertension, cardiovascular disease, stroke, and cancer, and may prevent body weight gain.[62] Rural residents who seek a wider selection of foods and better prices commonly have to travel great distances to larger supermarkets in urban areas. However, for low-income rural residents, transportation is a problem that prevents them from accessing a wide variety of foods at affordable food prices for good health.[63] The associated concept of "food deserts" is an emerging area of inquiry in rural health, and the impact of living in an area without access to fresh produce and other healthy foods plays a critical role in sustaining obesity in rural areas.

Opportunities for Physical Activity

While lack of healthy, affordable, and accessible foods is an issue related to one side of the energy balance equation, the other side concerns barriers to physical activity in rural settings. Rural people are more likely to be inactive than people who live in urban communities during their daily living activities[4] and during their leisure time.[5,64] This holds true even when factors such as education, income, and health status are held constant.[5] Rural residents depend heavily on automobile travel to get to work, to purchase groceries, and to carry out other daily activities (e.g., doctor appointments, participation in community events), which are commonly several miles from their home. In rural West Virginia and North Carolina, commuting time to work was positively and significantly related to the risk of obesity.[65,66] More commuting means more time is spent in sedentary activity. Even rural residents who do not commute find that less human labor is required in their jobs. For example, farming used to require much more human labor than it does today. Many family farms have been replaced with corporate farms that utilize machinery and automation to perform most tasks.[19] Additionally, some rural residents perceive they have few places available for exercise[64] due to distances to recreational facilities, unpaved roads, and lack of sidewalks and streetlights,[42] all of which has been associated with obesity.[67] Lack of transportation confines some rural families to their homes and leads to sedentary lifestyles associated with obesity.[24] In a study of rural low-income women[24] transportation difficulties were twice as common among women who were overweight or obese (53%) compared to women who were normal weight or underweight (27%).

School Environment

For many families, when children are not at home, they depend on the school system to provide children with healthy food choices and to structure physical activity as part of the school day. Due to the increase in child obesity, growing concern regarding the nutritional quality of foods available at school,[68] as well as children's level of physical activity, the 2004 Child Nutrition and WIC Reauthorization Act[69] was passed making it mandatory for all schools participating in the Federal School Meal Programs to create wellness policies by 2006–2007 that would include goals for nutrition education, physical activity, and nutrition guidelines for foods served at school. Evaluation studies of school wellness policies are mixed. Some studies show positive results[70] and others indicate that some schools struggled with meeting the minimum requirements of the Act[71] and assistance from university researchers and nutrition educators would be helpful in assisting schools to implement and attain their goals.[71]

A further step to improve the nutritional quality of foods served at school and reduce child overweight and obesity was the recent Healthy Hunger-Free Kids Act of 2010.[72] This act allows for the U.S. Department of Agriculture to set nutritional standards for all foods sold in schools, including in vending machines, the "à la carte" lunch lines, and school stores. Medicaid data will be used to certify children who meet income requirements and census data will be used to determine school-wide income eligibility for school meal programs resulting in less paperwork, as well as a predicted increase in the number of eligible children enrolled in school meal programs. Furthermore, emphasis is placed on improving the nutritional quality of commodity foods used in schools.

While government and schools play a critical role in shaping eating behaviors and physical activity that affect weight, so do other community entities such as after-school programs, youth organizations, health care providers, faith-based institutions, businesses, and the media. All of these sectors and families are needed to reduce child obesity, particularly in rural areas where such agencies may be the only access point for intervention.

STRATEGIES

Studies continue to reveal relationships between broader social and economic context (i.e., household income, home ownership, mothers' educational level, family structure, race/ethnicity) and child obesity risk.[32] Therefore, strategies for reducing the prevalence of obesity in rural settings should address the spheres of influence (i.e., individual, family, community, policy) in a rural community using Human Ecological Theory (described previously).

Individual and Family Levels

Ideally, intervention through families occurs before an unhealthy weight gain trajectory is established.[73] However, despite emerging evidence for the role of parents or other adult caregivers in preventing child obesity, few interventions have been developed and proven effective that address parenting[74,75] or the family as a whole in the prevention of childhood obesity. However, for families that have low incomes, federally funded nutrition education and assistance programs such as the Expanded Food and Nutrition Education Program (EFNEP), Supplemental Nutrition Assistance Program–Education (SNAP-Ed), and WIC present opportunities to be further developed and tested to explicitly prevent child obesity in rural America. With the passing of the Healthy Hunger-Free Kids Act of 2010, obesity prevention is now a required component of SNAP-Ed.[72]

EFNEP, WIC, and SNAP-Ed are available across the United States, in some U.S. territories, and in rural communities. These programs incorporate information and skill building to help parents select foods that have nutrients their families need, healthfully prepare food, stretch their food dollars, and access community resources. Additionally, information regarding child growth and development to help parents develop appropriate expectations for their children's eating and physical activity is commonly shared. EFNEP and WIC have been shown to improve household food choices and food security[76-79] and reduce future health care costs.[80,81] EFNEP has been shown to save families money on their food bills, a particular concern of many rural families.[82] Cullen et al.[83] found that when EFNEP addressed the home environment and parenting skills, significant improvements in dietary behaviors occurred. Parents increased limit-setting regarding meals and snacks, appropriately encouraged children during meals, and modeled fruit and vegetable consumption. At the same time, negative emotional eating (i.e., eating in response to emotional distress) and instrumental feeding practices (i.e., bribing, rewarding) were reduced. Chang et al.[84] found that when mothers who participated in WIC learned how to manage their stress, they were able to eat more healthfully and be more physically active. Additionally, when WIC staff took time to discuss and demonstrate ways to modify the home environment (e.g., leaving fresh apples on the kitchen counter instead of chips or cookies), families made positive food behavior changes.

EFNEP, WIC, and SNAP-Ed, while federally funded, are implemented in communities, including rural communities. These programs help families create home environments that encourage healthful child eating and physical activity, and can continue to strengthen their partnerships with other local organizations (e.g., Head Start, child-care centers, schools, home visitation programs) that also focus on improving health and development outcomes for at-risk rural children. Such efforts need to keep in mind the complexity of individual, family, and community factors that influence parent and child behaviors and address those factors to lessen the risk for child obesity. While these programs most commonly focus on promoting home environments that encourage healthful child eating and physical activity, they should consider opportunities to partner with others to improve the sociocultural and human-built environments.

Community Level and Policies

At the community level, programs and policies should be particularly targeted to rural women with children, particularly single mothers who are not only at greater risk for food insecurity than married or cohabitating mothers, but also have greater risk for obesity. Programs such as SNAP-Ed and WIC can affect the availability of affordable, nutritious food for rural low-income families. More stores near low-income areas that accept WIC vouchers can improve healthy food availability.[85] Andreyeva et al.[86] reported improved access to healthy foods for WIC participants as a result of recent food package revisions. With no additional cost to taxpayers, WIC stores found ways to deliver new foods, which improved the local food environment for WIC participants and nonparticipants. By offering affordable, nutritious food locally, residents without adequate transportation increased their access to a healthy diet.

Role of Health Care Providers and Technology

In addition to public nutrition education programs, weight or activity counseling can come from primary care practitioners in routine office visits.[5] Probst et al.[87] reported that rural primary care practitioners were less likely than urban physicians to include clinical preventive services such as weight or activity counseling. Nurses and other professionals can be used to maximize the ability of primary care practitioners to screen and educate overweight and obese patients. Another way to maximize primary care practitioners is to deliver screening and counseling via telehealth, the use of electronic information and telecommunication technologies to support long-distance clinical health care (discussed in more detail in Chapter 17).[88] Telehealth technology can potentially deliver resources for obesity prevention and treatment that include access to weight management programs, dietitians, and psychologists.[89] In a telehealth intervention with overweight rural children, Irby et al.[90] found comparable attrition rates and improvement in weight status compared with patients in conventional treatment. Additionally, the Internet and text messaging can be further explored as tools for obesity prevention efforts. Atkinson et al. [91] found that over two thirds of rural women surveyed in Maryland had a computer and had used the Internet. Those that had not used the Internet intended to do so in the future. Women participating in the study indicated they needed and desired an intervention delivered online that would help them with nutrition, physical activity, and their food budgets.

CONCLUSION

Rural Americans are more likely to be obese than urban Americans. Rural women, racial/ethnic minorities, and low-income individuals are at greatest risk of obesity. To understand and effectively address obesity, research and interventions are needed that examine how individual, family, and community-level factors and policy interrelate and their resulting relationships to obesity. Programs and policies implemented in rural communities to prevent obesity should be designed to give attention to promoting access to affordable and healthful foods, creating opportunities for physical activity as a part of daily living, reducing chronic individual and family stressors such as depression, social isolation, unemployment and poverty, inadequate and unaffordable housing, and transportation difficulties, as well as assist individuals and families in gaining knowledge and developing skills that support healthful eating and physical activity. In rural communities, community organizations (e.g., schools and other educational entities, youth programs, health professionals, businesses, producers, faith organizations, government entities) and families need to come together to identify common goals related to obesity prevention and identify and mobilize human and community assets to implement strategies they believe will work for their community.

RESOURCES

Rural Assistance Center Obesity Section: www.raconline.org/topics/obesity
Robert Wood Johnson Foundation Childhood Obesity Page: www.rwjf.org/en/about-rwjf/program-areas/childhood-obesity.html
USDA Economic Research Service Obesity Overview: www.ers.usda.gov/topics/food-choices-health/obesity.aspx

REFERENCES

1. Catenacci VC, Hill JC, Wyatt HR. The obesity epidemic. *Clin Chest Med*. 2009; 30(3):415–444.
2. Ogden CL, Carroll MD, Kit BK, Flegal KM. *Prevalence of obesity in the United States, 2009-2010*. NCHS Data Brief 2012 (No. 82).
3. Flegal KM, Carroll, MD, Kit BK, Ogden CL. Prevalence of obesity and trends in the distribution of body mass index among US adults, 1999–2010. *JAMA*. 2012;307:491–497.
4. Jackson JE, Doescher MP, Jerant AF, Hart LG. A national study of obesity prevalence and trends by type of rural county. *J Rural Health*. 2005;21:140–148.

5. Patterson PD, Moore CG, Probst JC, Shinogle JA. Obesity and physical activity in rural America. *J Rural Health.* 2004; 20:151–158.
6. Liu J, Bennett KJ, Harun N, Zheng X, Probst JC, Pate RR. Overweight and physical inactivity among rural children aged 10-17: a National and State Portrait. *South Carolina Rural Health Research Center.* 2007. http://rhr.sph.sc.edu/report/SCRHRC_ObesityChartbook_Exec_Sum_10.15.07.pdf. Accessed September 30, 2012.
7. Scott AJ, Wilson RF. Upstream ecological risks for overweight and obesity among African American youth in a rural town in the Deep South, 2007. *Prev Chronic Dis.* 2011;8(1):A17. http://www.cdc.gov/pcd/issues/2011/jan/09_0244.htm. Accessed August 30, 2012.
8. Williamson DA, Champagne CM, Sothern MS, Stewart TM, Webber LS. Increased obesity in children living in rural communities of Louisiana. *Int J Pediatr Obes.* 2009;4(3):160–165.
9. National Institutes of Health, National Heart Lung and Blood Institute. Obesity Education Initiative. *Clinical Guidelines on the Identification, Evaluation, and Treatment of Overweight and Obesity in Adults: The Evidence Report.* NIH Publication No. 98-4083. September 1998. http://www.nhlbi.nih.gov/guidelines/obesity/ob_gdlns.pdf. Accessed September 26, 2012.
10. Friedemann C, Heneghan C, Mahtani K, Thompson M, Perera R, Ward AM. Cardiovascular disease risk in healthy children and its association with body mass index: systematic review and meta-analysis. *BMJ.* 2012;345:e4759.
11. Finkelstein EA, Trogdon JG, Cohen JW, Dietz W. Annual medical spending attributable to obesity: payer- and service-specific estimates. *Health Affairs.* 2009;28(5): w822–w831.
12. Bubolz MM, Sontag MS. Human ecology theory. In: Boss PG, Doherty WJ, LaRossa R, Schumm WR, Steinmetz SK, eds. *Sourcebook of Family Theories and Methods.* New York, NY: Springer; 1993, VI:419–450.
13. Bronfenbrenner U. *The Ecology of Human Development.* Cambridge, MA: Harvard University Press; 1979.
14. Ramsey PW, Glenn LL. Obesity and health status in rural, urban, and suburban Southern women. *Southern Med J.* 2001;95:666–671.
15. Lichtenstein AH, Kennedy E, Barrier P, et al. Dietary fat consumption and health. *Nutr Rev.* 1998;56(5, pt 2):S3– S19; discussion S19–S28.
16. Hermstad AK, Swan DW, Kegler MC, Barneete JK, Glanz K. Individual and environmental correlates of dietary fat intake in rural communities: a structural equation model analysis. *Social Science & Medicine.* 2010;71:93–101.
17. Watters JL, Satia JA. Psychosocial correlates of dietary fat intake in African-American adults: a cross-sectional study. *Nutr J.* 2009;8:15.
18. Gundersen C, Mahatmya D, Garasky S, Lohman B. Linking psychosocial stressors and childhood obesity. *Obesity Reviews.* 2011;12:e54–e63.
19. National Advisory Committee on Rural Health and Human Services. *The 2005 Report to the Secretary: Rural Health and Human Service Issues.* April 2005. ftp://ftp.hrsa.gov/ruralhealth/NAC2005.pdf. Accessed September 25, 2012.
20. Barnett E, Elmes G, Braham V, Halverson J, Lee J, Loftus S. Heart disease. In: *Appalachia: An Atlas of County Economic Conditions, Mortality, and Medical Care Resources.* Morgantown, WV: Prevention Research Center; 1998.
21. Oliver G, Wardle J. Perceived effects of stress on food choice. *Physiol Behav.* 1999;66:511–515.
22. Gibson EL. Emotional influences on food choice: sensory, physiological, and psychological pathways. *Physiol Behav.* 2006;89:53–61.

23. Dallmann MF. Stress-induced obesity and the emotional nervous system. *Trends Endocrinol Metab.* 2010;21:159–165.
24. Bove CF, Olson CM. Obesity in low-income rural women: qualitative insights about physical activity and eating patterns. *Women Health.* 2006;44(1).
25. Gunnar M, Quevedo K. The neurobiology and stress and development. *Annu Rev Psychol.* 2007;58:1522–1528.
26. Turner HA, Turner RJ. Understanding variations in exposure to social stress. *Health* 2005;9:209–240.
27. Marniemi J, Kronholm E, Aunola S, et al. Visceral fat and psychosocial stress in identical twins discordant for obesity. *J Intern Med.* 2002;251:35–43.
28. Siervo M, Wells JCK, Cizza G. The contribution of psychosocial stress to the obesity epidemic: an evolutionary approach. *Horm Metab Res.* 2009;41:261–270.
29. Economic Research Service, USDA. Prepared using data from the Annual Social and Economic Supplement (ASEC) to the Current Population Survey (P-60), US Census Bureau. http://www.ers.usda.gov/topics/rural-economy-population/rural-poverty-well-being/income-nonfarm-earnings.aspx. Accessed September 30, 2012.
30. Economic Research Service, USDA, Prepared using data from the US Census Bureau 2011 Current Population Survey, March supplement.
31. McLaren L. Socioeconomic status and obesity. *Epidemiol Rev.* 2007;29(1):29–48.
32. Grow HM, Cook AJ, Arterburn DE, Saelens BE, Drewnowski A, Lozano, P. Child obesity associated with social disadvantage of children's neighborhoods. *Soc Sci Med.* 2010;71(3):584–591.
33. Eagle TF, Sheetz A, Gurm R, et al. Understanding childhood obesity in America: linkages between household income, community resources, and children's behaviors. *Am Heart J.* 2012;163:836–843.
34. Child and Adolescent Health Measurement Initiative, Data Resource Center for Child and Adolescent Health. 2007 National Survey of Children's Health. Available at: http://www.mchb.hrsa.gov/chusa10/hstat/hsa/desc/219ooVpl.html. Accessed September 29, 2012.
35. Anderson SA, ed. Core indicators of nutritional status for difficult-to-sample populations. *J Nutr.* 1990;120:1559–1600.
36. Gross RS, Mendelsohn AL, Fierman AH, Racine AD, Messito MJ. Food insecurity and obesogenic maternal infant feeding styles and practices in low-income families. *Pediatrics.* 2012;130:254–261.
37. Martin MA, Lippert AM. Feeding her children, but risking her health: the intersection of gender, household food insecurity and obesity. *Soc Sci & Med.* 2012;74:1754–1764.
38. Coleman-Jensen A, Nord M, Andrews M, Carlson S. *Household Food Security in the United States in 2010.* ERR-125, US Department of Agriculture, Economic Research Service. 2011:37.
39. Sharkey JR, Johnson CM, Dean WR. Less-healthy eating behaviors have a greater association with a high level of sugar-sweetened beverage consumption among rural adults than among urban adults. *Food & Nutr Res.* 2011;55:5819.
40. Greder K, Brotherson MJ. Food security and low income families: research to inform policy and programs. *J Fam Consumer Sci.* 2002;94(2).
41. Polivy J. Psychological consequences of food restriction. *J Am Diet Assoc.* 1996;96:589–592.
42. Olson CM, Bove CF, Miller EO. Growing up poor: long-term implications for eating patterns and body weight. *Appetite.* 2007;49(1):198–207.
43. Davison KK, Birch LL. Childhood overweight: a contextual model and recommendations for future research. *Obesity Rev.* 2001;2(3):159–171.

44. Savage JS, Fisher JO, Birch LL. Parental influence on eating behavior: conception to adolescence. *J Law Med Ethics.* 2007;35(1):22–34.
45. Davison KK, Cutting TM, Birch LL. Parents' activity-related parenting practices predict girls' physical activity. *Med Sci Sports Exercise.* 2003;35(9):1589–1595.
46. Golan M, Weizman A. Familial approach to the treatment of childhood obesity: conceptual mode. *J Nutr Educ.* 2001; 33(2):102–107.
47. Rosenkranz RR, Dzewaltowski DA. Model of the home food environment pertaining to childhood obesity. *Nutr Rev.* 2008; 66(3):123–140.
48. Pugliese J, Tinsley B. Parental socialization of child and adolescent physical activity: a meta-analysis. *J Fam Psychol.* 2007; 21:331–343.
49. Hood MY, Ellison RC. Parental eating attitudes and the development of obesity in children. The Framingham Children's Study. *Int J Obes Relat Metab Disord.* 2000;24:1319–1325.
50. Browne M. A comparative study of parental behaviors and children's eating habits. *Infant Child Adolesc Nutr.* 2009;1:11–14.
51. Rhee KE, Lumeng JC, Appugliese DP, et al. Parenting styles and overweight status in first grade. *Pediatrics.* 2006;117:2047–2054.
52. Rural Families Speak about Health. http://ruralfamiliesspeak.org/About_the_project.html. Accessed September 28, 2012.
53. Ihmels MA, Welk GJ, Eisenmann JC, Nusser SM. Development and preliminary validation of a Family Nutrition and Physical Activity (FNPA) screening tool. *Int J Behav Nutr Phys Act.* 2009;6:14.
54. Andresen EM, Malmgren JA, Carter WB, Patrick DL. Screening for depression in well older adults: evaluation of a short form of the CES-D (Center for Epidemiologic Studies–Depression Scale). *Am J Prev Med.* 1994;10:77–84.
55. Prawitz AD, Garman ET, Sorhaindo B, O'Neill B, Kim J, Drentea P. InCharge Financial Distress/Financial Well-Being Scale: development, administration, and score interpretation. *Finan Couns Plann.* 2006;17(1): 34–50.
56. Jensen EW, James SA, Boyce WT, Hartnett SA. The Family Routines Inventory: development and validation. *Soc Sci Med.* 1983;17(4):201–211.
57. Bickel G, Nord M, Price C, Hamilton W, Cook J. *Guide to Measuring Household Food Security, Revised 2000.* Alexandria, VA: US Department of Agriculture, Food and Nutrition Service; 2000.
58. Beck RW, Jijon CR, Edwards JB. The relationships among gender, perceived financial barriers to care, and health status in a rural population. *J Rural Health* 1996;12(3):188–196.
59. Petterson S, Williams IC, Hauenstein EJ, Rovnyak V, Merwin E. Race and ethnicity and rural mental health treatment. *J Health Care Poor Underserved.* 2009;20(3):662–677.
60. Larson NI, Story MT, Nelson MC. Neighborhood environments: disparities in access to healthy foods in the U.S. *Am J Prev Med.* 2009;36(1):74–81.
61. Hosler AS. Retail food availability, obesity and cigarette smoking in rural communities. *Natl Rural Health Assoc.* 2009;25:203–210.
62. Boeing H, Bechthold A, Bub A, et al. Critical review: vegetables and fruit in the prevention of chronic diseases. *Eur J Nutr.* 2010; 51:637–663.
63. Yousefian A, Leighton A, Fox K, Hartley D. Understanding the rural food environment—perspectives of low-income parents. *Rural and Remote Health.* 2011;11:1631. http://www.rrh.org.au. Accessed September 28, 2012.
64. Parks SE, Housemann RA, Brownson RC. Differential correlates of physical activity in urban and rural adults of various socioeconomic backgrounds in the United States. *J Epidemiol Community Health.* 2003;57:29–35.

65. Amarasinghe A, D'Souza G, Brown C, Oh H, Borisova T. The influence of socio-economic and environmental determinants on health and obesity: a West Virginia case study. *Int J Environ Res Public Health*. 2009;6:2271–2287.
66. Jilcott SB, Haiyong L, Moore JB, Bethel JW, Wilson J, Ammerman AS. Commute times, food retail gaps, and body mass index in North Carolina counties. *Prev Chronic Dis* 2010;7(5):A107. http://wwcdc.gov/pcd/issues/2010/sep/09_0208. htm. Accessed August 31, 2012.
67. Boehmer TK, Lovegreen SL, Haire-Joshu D, Brownson RC. What constitutes an obesogenic environment in rural communities? *Am J Health Promot*. 2006;20:411–421.
68. Probart C, McDonnell E, Weirich J, Hartman T, Bailey-Davis L, Prabhakher V. Competitive foods available in Pennsylvania public high schools. *J Am Diet Assoc*. 2005;105:1243–1249.
69. Child Nutrition and WIC Reauthorization Act of 2004, Section 204 of Public Law 108-265—June 30, 2004. http://www.fns.usda.gov/tn/healthy/108-265.pdf. Accessed September 30, 2012.
70. Snelling AM, Kennard T. The impact of nutrition standards on competitive food offerings and purchasing behaviors of high school students. *J Sch Health*. 2009;79(11): 541–546.
71. Serrano E, Kowaleska A, Hosig K, Fuller C, Fellin L, Wigand V. Status and goals of local school wellness policies in Virginia: a response to the Child Nutrition and WIC Reauthorization Act of 2004. *J Nutr Educ Behav*. 2007;39:95–100.
72. Healthy Hunger-Free Kids Act of 2010. http://www.govtrack.us/congress/bills/111/s3307. Accessed September 30, 2012.
73. Monteiro PO, Victora CG. Rapid growth in infancy and childhood and obesity in later life—a systematic review. *Obesity Rev*. 2005;6(2):143–154.
74. Gerards SM, Sleddens EF, Dagnelie PC, deVries NK, Kremers SP. Interventions addressing general parenting to prevent or treat childhood obesity. *Int J Pediatr Obes*. 2011;6(2-2): e28–e45.
75. Davison KK, Lawson HA, Coatsworth JD. The Family-Centered Action Model of Intervention Layout and Implementation (FAMILI): the example of childhood obesity. *Health Promot Pract*. 2012;13(4):454–461.
76. Dollahite J, Olson C, Scott-Pierce M. The impact of nutrition education on food insecurity among low-income participants in EFNEP. *Fam Consum Sci Res J*. 2003;32:13.
77. Greer B, Polling R. *Impact of Participating in the Expanded Food and Nutrition Education Program on Food Insecurity*. Mississippi State, MS: Mississippi State University Southern Rural Development Center; 2001.
78. Metallinos-Katsaras E, Gorman KS, Wilde P, Kallio J. A longitudinal study of WIC participation on household food insecurity. *Matern Child Health J*. 2011;15:627–633.
79. Eicher-Miller HA, Mason AC, Abbott AR, McCabe GP, Broushey CJ. The effect of food stamp nutrition education on the food insecurity of low-income women participants. *J Nutr Educ Behav*. 2009;41:161–168.
80. Devaney B, Bilheimer LT, Schore J. *The Savings in Medicaid Costs for Newborns and Their Mothers from Prenatal Participation in the WIC Program*. Alexandria, VA: US Department of Agriculture; October 1980.
81. Rajgopal R, Cox RH, Lambur M, Lewis EC. Cost-benefit analysis indicates the positive economic benefits of the Expanded Food and Nutrition Education Program related to chronic disease prevention. *J Nutr Educ Behavior*. 2002;34(1): 26–27.
82. Burney J, Haughton B. EFNEP: a nutrition education program that demonstrates cost-benefit. *J Am Diet Assoc*. 2002;102:39–45.

83. Cullen KW, Smalling AL, Thompson D, Watson KB, Reed D, Konzelmann K. Creating healthful home food environments: results of a study with participants in the Expanded Food and Nutrition Education Program. *J Nutr Educ Behav.* 2009;41:380–388.

84. Chang M-W, Baumann LC, Nitzke S, Brown RL. Predictors of fat intake behavior differ between normal-weight and obese WIC mothers. *Am J Health Promotion.* 2005;19(4):269–277.

85. Tester JM, Yen IH, Pallis LC, Laraia BA. Healthy food availability and participation in WIC (Special Supplemental Nutrition Program for Women, Infants, and Children) in food stores around lower- and higher-income elementary schools. *Public Health Nutr.* 2010;14:960–964.

86. Andreyeva T, Luedicke J, Middleton AE, Long MW, Schwartz MB. Positive influence of the revised Special Supplemental Nutrition Program for Women, Infants, and Children food packages on access to healthy foods. *J Acad Nutr Diet.* 2012;112:850–858.

87. Probst JC, Moore CG, Baxley EG, Lammie JJ. Rural-urban differences in visits to primary care physicians. *Fam Med.* 2002;34:609–615. https://www.stfm.org/fmhub/fm2002/sept02/hsr.pdf. Accessed September 30, 2012.

88. US Department of Health and Human Services, Health Resources and Services Administration. Telehealth. Available at: http://www.hrsa.gov/ruralhealth/about/telehealth/Accessed September 6, 2012.

89. Shaikh U, Cole SL, Marcin JP, Nesbitt TS. Clinical management and patient outcomes among children and adolescents receiving telemedicine consultations for obesity. *Telemed J E Health.* 2008;14(5):434–440.

90. Irby MB, Boles KA, Jordan C, Skelton JA. TeleFIT: adapting a multidisciplinary, tertiary-care pediatric obesity clinic to rural populations. *Telemed J E Health.* April 2012; 18(3):247–249. doi:10.1089/tmj.2011.0117.

91. Atkinson NL, Billing AS, Desmond SM, Gold RS, Tournas-Hardt A. Assessment of the nutrition and physical activity education needs of low, rural mothers: can technology play a role? *J Community Health.* 2007;32:245–267.

CHAPTER 11

Diabetes in Rural Areas

Jacob C. Warren and K. Bryant Smalley

Diabetes is one of the most devastating diseases in the United States with regard to both morbidity burden and mortality rates, generating more than $170 billion in annual costs to the U.S. economy.[1] Type 2 diabetes (herein referred to as diabetes) is the second-most diagnosed chronic condition in the United States (falling behind only arthritis[2]), is the seventh-leading cause of death,[3] and is associated with a host of complications including blindness, kidney disease, amputations, cerebrovascular disease, and cardiovascular disease.[4,5] While the effect of diabetes is profound throughout the United States, the disease disproportionately impacts rural areas. Rural populations (particularly in the South) have been identified as being dramatically more impacted by diabetes; in fact, the rural South represents the core of the Centers for Disease Control and Prevention's (CDC) designated "diabetes belt"[6] (see Figure 11.1), underscoring the disparate diabetes burden that rural residents experience.

It is obvious that diabetes prevention and control is one of the most important health considerations facing rural areas; however, research and outreach focused on creating and implementing evidence-based practices unique to rural settings are limited. This chapter presents an overview of diabetes, its effects in rural areas, a description of diabetes programs that have been implemented in rural areas, and recommendations for addressing the diabetes epidemic in rural America.

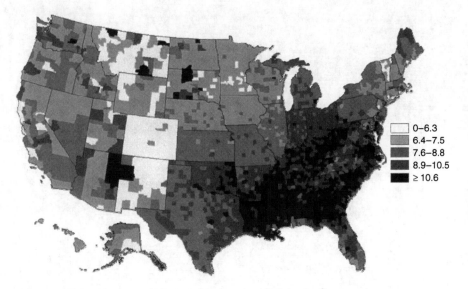

Figure 11.1 Percentage of adults with diagnosed diabetes.[6]

DIABETES IN RURAL AMERICA

As mentioned, diabetes is one of the leading health disparities faced by rural populations, and is frequently identified by rural health researchers and public health practitioners as one of the most important health issues faced by rural populations.[7] As the disparity has increased over time, so too has the perceived need to address rural diabetes. When constructing Rural Healthy People 2010, diabetes ranked as the fifth most-important health issue facing rural America, behind access to care, mental health, oral health, and educational-/community-based programs. However, in the preliminary work completed for Rural Healthy People 2020, diabetes was second in importance only to access to care, moving from an identified priority of only 26% of respondents in Rural Healthy People 2010 to a priority for over 60% of respondents for Rural Healthy People 2020.[8,9]

While the magnitude of differences between rural and urban diabetes rates varies from study to study, diabetes rates in rural areas have been shown to be higher in both self-report data (i.e., Behavioral Risk Factor Surveillance System [BRFSS]) and medical expenditure data (i.e., Medical Expenditures Panel Survey [MEPS]), even after adjusting for age, body mass index (BMI), insurance coverage, and demographic characteristics.[4] The persistence of rural–urban differences in the face of controlling for key risk factors such as weight and access to care indicates that rurality itself and not simply a combination of sociodemographic characteristics is influencing the development of diabetes. While sociodemographics certainly play a role in the maintenance of rural-based disparities, additional influences remain that must be taken into consideration when attempting to address diabetes in rural settings.

Beyond rates, prognosis of those diagnosed with diabetes is impacted in rural areas. Because they are more likely to be uninsured and more likely to have to travel greater distances to receive care, rural residents often present later in the course of the disease—a core difficulty in the management of any chronic disease. However, even after diagnosis, prevention of sequelae is impacted by rural living. Rural diabetics, although more likely to receive a quarterly hemoglobin A1c test, are less likely to receive an annual eye examination or foot check,[4] and in general receive less care than their urban counterparts.[10]

Beyond the overall health challenges faced by residents of rural areas, rural minorities face particular challenges. In the general U.S. population, African Americans are 2.1 times as likely as Whites and Hispanic populations are 1.5 times as likely as White residents to die from diabetes.[11] This disparity is magnified within rural settings, as rural African Americans have a higher prevalence of diabetes and a higher age-adjusted death rate from diabetes than rural and urban Whites and even urban African Americans.[12]

Source of Disparity

The reason for the presence of rural-based diabetes disparities is unclear, and likely represents a combination of many factors. Rural populations have shown resistance to changing high-fat diets and sedentary lifestyle,[13,14] two of the core risk factors for diabetes, indicating that current prevention efforts are not reaching this high-risk group. Rural Healthy People 2010 [8] argues that diabetes is a particular problem in rural areas because "rural life presents special cultural and structural challenges to maintaining a healthy weight."[15] While much of the risk related to diabetes has been linked to the elevated rates of overweight and obesity in rural areas,[16–17] and prevention focusing on modifiable behavioral risk factors such as diet, exercise, and weight loss has been identified as an important focus for reducing the impact of diabetes in rural areas,[18,19] control of diabetes requires more than a simple focus on weight reduction.

Many rural diabetics lack a fundamental understanding of their condition and the importance of engaging in activities to control the impact of their condition upon their health.[20] Despite this fact, current research has failed to create educational interventions focusing on diabetes that are tailored to the needs and cultural realities of rural Americans. The elevated postdiagnosis mortality rates among rural populations,[12] combined with the demonstrated lack of disease knowledge among patients, indicate that interventions focusing on health education and behavior change are sorely needed for rural patients known to have these conditions. However, rural groups have been shown to perceive diabetes as an "individual" issue more so than a "community" issue, which can complicate community-level prevention efforts in rural areas.[21] By addressing both behavioral risk factors and fundamental disease knowledge, as well as raising awareness of the community-level impact that diabetes can have, barriers such as access to care can be minimized and hopefully have a significant impact on the rural/urban diabetes disparity.

Barriers/Challenges

A core problem in addressing diabetes in rural areas is the frequent lack of diabetic education. Rural residents have been shown to be significantly less likely than their urban counterparts to receive diabetic education.[4] Because of the difficulty in accessing care, learning proper diabetes self-management techniques is critical for rural diabetics, but current efforts are not adequately reaching this group. Knowledge rates are particularly low among rural minorities. Studies have even indicated that a diagnosis of diabetes does not independently predict diabetes knowledge in rural Hispanics; that is, diagnosed Hispanic diabetics are no more knowledgeable about the disease than is the general population.[22] Addressing diabetic knowledge will be crucial in alleviating diabetes disparities.

Another barrier is the lack of available venues for physical activity. Despite the somewhat stereotypical view of rural America as full of sweeping fields ideal for physical activity, rural residents specifically identify the lack of appropriate exercise facilities as the primary barrier to becoming or remaining physically active.[23] This effect has been shown to increase with increasing rurality.[24] In their comprehensive review of the influence of the built environment upon physical activity in rural areas, Frost et al.[25] identified five key factors that could be targeted to increase physical activity in rural settings: pleasant aesthetics, availability of walking trails/paths, perceived safety and crime rate, availability of parks, and destinations that are walkable from a person's residence.

The expense of diabetes is also a difficult-to-address barrier to proper diabetic control. Because rural populations have higher rates of poverty and uninsurance, the average annual diabetes medical care cost of $13,700[26] can be exceptionally burdensome. This impacts rural residents' ability to perform even the most basic of diabetic monitoring—blood glucose monitoring—that has been shown to occur daily for less than half of rural residents.[27] In another consequence of poverty, rural residents also have very low ownership levels of diabetes-related preventive health equipment, such as specialized socks and home exercise equipment.[28] Identifying low-cost self-management strategies is even more important because of this financial burden; however, it can also be used as motivation for achieving diabetic control (highlighting to patients the financial improvement that would be associated with decreased need for diabetic care).

Promising Practices in Rural Diabetes Prevention/Control

While there is limited research to provide a full evidence base for rural-specific diabetes prevention and control programs, the Montana Diabetes Control Program is emerging as a leader in developing and evaluating promising practices that, with further study, could emerge as rural-specific evidence-based interventions for diabetes.

The first program is a countywide initiative focused on diabetes management completed by the Montana Diabetes Control Program in collaboration with the Park County Diabetes Project.[29] Together, the two groups spearheaded a health systems and coordinated diabetes education initiative designed to improve the quality of diabetes care in a frontier Montana county. The initiative involved creation of a diabetes registry that contained relevant indicators (e.g., A1c testing, blood pressure), conducting mail and telephone outreach, providing personalized patient education materials, providing continuing education workshops for health care providers in the target area, organizing 1-day foot-care clinics, establishing a lending library with patient education materials, and creating a community newsletter targeting diabetes self-management. Through this process, the county offered free classes that were not previously available, including one-on-one diabetes education and group education sessions. The initiative resulted in a higher proportion of residents receiving diabetes management education and engaging in glucose monitoring at least weekly, and a significant reduction in barriers to self-management, including difficulty making lifestyle changes, cost of glucose test strips, cost of medications, and cost of diabetes education classes.

The second program, a preventive intervention, is an adaptation of the Diabetes Prevention Program designed to be applied in rural areas.[30,31] The program, for which rural residents paid $150 to participate, involves the use of trained lifestyle coaches who deliver a 16-week core curriculum, boosted by 6 monthly postcurriculum sessions. Guest speakers at the groups covered a variety of topics including physical activity and stress management. Groups varied in size from 25 to 35 participants, which is fairly large for an intervention; however, the group size facilitates implementation in often underresourced rural settings. In addition to the educational curriculum, participants were engaged in demonstrations designed to provide specific skills (such as determining appropriate portion sizes), and the lifestyle coaches provided two supervised physical activity sessions each week, utilizing creative solutions to addressing the lack of physical activity venues in rural areas (such as having aerobics sessions in conference rooms rather than in a gym). The program had an estimated cost of $557 per participant. Retention was 83% for the 16-week component, and 64% for the 16-week plus 6-month follow-up sessions component. Participants who completed the 16-week program had a significant reduction in both weight and BMI, with 73% having a weight loss of at least 5%, and 52% having a weight loss of at least 7%. Average weight loss was 7 kg (approximately 15 pounds), and average BMI reduction was 2.5 points. For participants who also completed the 6 monthly follow-up sessions, total average weight loss was 11.1 kg (nearly 25 pounds) and average BMI reduction was 4 points.

AADE7: An Evidence-Based Model for Diabetes Prevention

The two programs discussed previously are promising practices that, with further scientific review, hold the potential to become among the first evidence-based practices for rural diabetes programming. While there are no clear evidence-based models that are specifically rural-created, there are models that with tailoring can be implemented successfully in rural settings. In a collaborative project between Georgia Southern University's Rural Health Research Institute and Mercer University's Center for Rural Health and Health Disparities, we created and implemented a telehealth-based diabetes-education program (funded by HRSA's Office of Rural Health Policy Grant D04RH23576). In selecting a model to guide our diabetes self-management education (DSME), we chose to use the evidence-based AADE7 Self-Care Behaviors model developed by and endorsed by the American Association of Diabetes Educators (AADE). According to the AADE, "the AADE7 Self-Care Behaviors framework reflects the best practice of diabetes self-management education/training by measuring, monitoring and managing outcomes."[32]

The Model

Rather than focusing simply upon the completion of certain educational processes, AADE7 focuses on measuring psychological and behavioral outcomes to ensure that the information being conveyed has been absorbed and processed by the patient. This allows a diabetes educator to return to certain information if associated behavior change has not been observed, dramatically increasing the likelihood of successful behavioral modifications. This framework has a resounding evidence base in the literature, and is endorsed by the leading association for diabetes educators in the nation. Its modular format also allows for flexibility in delivery and for easy tailoring of content to the cultural realities of rural living. Because of the significant amount of research that has gone into construction of the AADE7 framework, there are numerous existing educational materials, progress-tracking software packages, and customized evaluation tools that can assist with implementation of the model.

The AADE7 framework focuses on seven key components of diabetes education: healthy eating, being active, monitoring, taking medication, problem solving, reducing risks, and healthy coping. Each of these seven factors was included in the AADE7 model based upon a series of seven extensive literature reviews appearing in the November/December 2007 issue of *The Diabetes Educator*.[33] These reviews examined outcome-based studies focused on each of the AADE7 factors (e.g., examining all outcome studies focused on blood glucose monitoring, assessing its impact on outcomes, and, based upon that assessment, including it in the AADE7 framework). All combined, more than 400 outcome studies across these reviews formed the basis of the seven selected aspects of the AADE7 framework.

The overall AADE7 framework has been demonstrated to be effective in rural settings for both individual and group delivery when culturally tailored to the rural realities of the target population.[34] Modifications should be made to the curriculum as needed to ensure that the realities of rural living are reflected in the information provided to patients (e.g., where to find fresh vegetables, how to access low-cost care). In educational sessions, diabetes educators can address the particular AADE7 behavior that is targeted for that session using a combination of interventions, including knowledge education, behavioral contracting, situational problem solving, skill training, confidence building, goal setting, and barrier resolution.

Tailoring the AADE7 Framework

When examining the seven components of the AADE7 framework, each has tailoring opportunities to make the material and delivery more salient, relevant, and helpful to rural residents. Each component is discussed in the following paragraphs, along with an example of the rural tailoring that can help make it more impactful in rural areas.

Healthy Eating. Because of its association with not only weight control but also more fundamentally in proper control of glucose levels, healthy eating is a crucial component of diabetic self-management. In the systematic literature review that led to the inclusion of healthy eating in the AADE7 curriculum,[35] studies demonstrated an effect on weight, fat intake, saturated fat intake, and carbohydrates, but effects were not always durable—something critical to long-term change. As a result, the specific need for developing interventions focused on maintenance as well as initiation of eating behavior change was identified as a core challenge. Healthy eating aspects of diabetes self-management focus on nutrition basics, how to read a food label, how to count carbohydrates, and how to appropriately meal plan. When considering specific rural tailoring, it is important to consider the regional cuisine of the area; for instance, in Southern rural communities, the use of animal products such as ham hocks and fatback in preparation of vegetables must be addressed so that it is understood what will qualify as a "vegetable" in meal planning. Because of the sometimes increased cost of healthy eating, it is also important to work with rural patients to identify low-cost options that are readily available. In addition, because many rural areas have been identified as food deserts,[36] rural programs should also focus on teaching patients how they can access fresh produce within their area.

Being Active. As part of a larger focus on weight control, physical activity is a very important aspect of diabetes self-management. Unfortunately, given the particularly low levels of physical activity in the general population (more than half of U.S. adults do not meet physical activity guidelines[37]), this becomes particularly challenging to change. Physical inactivity is also concentrated in rural areas (see Figure 11.2), indicating that rural groups are already less physically active than their urban counterparts, making this self-management behavior all the more important. In the AADE review article on physical activity,[38] it was found that intensive exercise regimens, although effective, were not always accepted and sustained by diabetic patients. Overall, structured regimens were more effective than general exercise recommendations, although the authors identified a critical gap in the literature with regard to both effectiveness of exercise interventions in minority populations and in evaluating the economic feasibility/impact of such programs. In general, self-management strategies discussed as a part of the "being active" component of DSME should focus on addressing barriers to exercise and how to safely start an exercise routine. When considering rural-specific tailoring for encouraging activity, identifying free and safe ways to exercise is critical. As discussed, rural residents often perceive less availability of

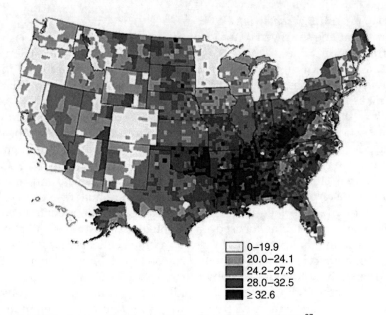

0–19.9
20.0–24.1
24.2–27.9
28.0–32.5
≥ 32.6

Figure 11.2 Physical inactivity rates in the United States, 2008.[37]

physical activity options,[25] so identifying specific locations for exercise that are accessible to patients is important in successfully encouraging an active lifestyle.

Monitoring. One of the most fundamental behaviors taught to newly diagnosed diabetics is how to monitor their blood glucose. This is often challenging, however, particularly for those with limited financial resources (test strips frequently cost $1 each, which can quickly add up for individuals struggling to pay bills or purchase food). Although inconsistently so, in general studies have shown that glucose self-monitoring leads to improved diabetic control,[39] making it an important part of diabetes self-management. Overall, glucose monitoring education should include a focus on the timing and frequency of testing, identifying target values, how to incorporate testing into a daily routine, and the importance of receiving regular medical checkups. Within rural areas, it is important to also discuss low-cost resources for obtaining testing supplies and medical care because of elevated rates of poverty, lower insurance rates, and widespread provider shortages. Rural populations have been identified as being less likely to regularly test their glucose,[27] so specifically focusing on the need for monitoring, and affordable ways in which to do it, are of particular importance.

Taking Medication. A diagnosis of diabetes is typically accompanied with prescription of a new medication to assist with control. As with many chronic conditions, adherence to prescribed medications is challenging but associated with improved outcomes. When investigating barriers to adherence, researchers have identified three main factors: regimen complexity (more than one drug to take or more than one required daily dose), comorbid depression, and difficulty remembering doses and refills.[40] Self-management focused on medication should focus on the importance of each prescribed medication, timing and dosage of medications, potential side effects to watch for, and how to travel with medicines. Within rural areas, because of increased poverty and decreased insurance, specifically developing a plan to be able to purchase medication when needed and helping patients get onto pharmaceutical company prescription assistance programs are important modifications.

Problem Solving. Because a diagnosis of diabetes frequently requires adapting to new situations and settings, problem solving (defined as "a learned behavior that includes generating a set of potential strategies for problem resolution, selecting the most appropriate strategy, applying the strategy, and evaluating the effectiveness of the strategy"[41]) is a core component of DSME. Systematic reviews[42] support that problem-solving skills are positively associated with A1c control, but are more closely related to adherence and dietary changes. Self-management skills focused on ways to adapt to blood sugar variations and what to do if glucose is too high or too low are of particular importance. Within rural settings, focusing on finding alternatives to frequently recommended practices may be of high value: Resources such as walking trails or pharmacy assistance may not be as prevalent as in urban areas, and teaching patients to be creative and persistent in finding alternatives can be of particular use.

Reducing Risks. Diabetes is associated with a host of medical sequelae, ranging from neuropathy to eye damage. In order to prevent onset of certain conditions and to prevent progression of existing ones, it is vital that diabetic patients actively engage in behaviors to reduce their risk of consequences. The AADE systematic review on reducing risks identified which risk factors need addressing and learning what is "optimal" preventive care as particularly important when addressing risks.[43] A comprehensive risk-reduction educational curriculum should address blood pressure, smoking cessation, eye exams, and foot monitoring at minimum. When considering rural areas, teaching methods to self-examine feet and individually focus on smoking cessation is important, as access to podiatric care (not to mention primary care) may be limited, as well as the availability of smoking cessation group programs. Although not measured in the same shortage designations as primary care, dental health, and mental health, decreased access to optometric services may be an important factor in rural settings (particularly given financial restrictions); therefore, recommendations for full eye dilation should be accompanied with concrete ways and sources for obtaining such services within the rural community (or as nearby as possible).

Healthy Coping. Healthy coping is the final aspect of the AADE7 framework. Issues of psychological health, emotional well-being, related risk factors, and quality of life are all key concerns of managing diabetes.[44] Because a diagnosis of diabetes doubles the risk of comorbid depression[45] (with some studies estimating a comorbidity of 20%[46]), and depression is associated with poor adherence to prescribed diabetic medical care,[47] teaching coping strategies is highly important. Self-management programs should include a focus on building motivation for change, as well as teaching relaxation and overall stress management techniques. For rural areas, information about low-cost psychological services should be provided (preferably in an integrated care setting or via telehealth in order to reduce concerns over visibility and stigma), as well as education regarding the importance of mental health and how seeking treatment is not a sign of "weakness."

Recommendations

As with many conditions, adequately addressing the needs of rural diabetes is complex and multifactorial, and will require both individual- and systems-level change. Development of rural-specific (not just rural-modified) educational interventions that address key barriers for rural populations is very important. This can include exploration of a number of novel approaches such as telehealth-based intervention strategies and church-based diabetes education programs.

Another key problem is the restrictive qualifications required to obtain the certified diabetes educator (CDE) credential. Currently, only existing licensed providers can become CDEs, and thereby eligible for special billing and compensation pathways critical to the financing of such positions. Obtaining the CDE credential requires 1,000 hours of diabetic education experience in a compensated job position, severely restricting the ability of community health centers and other rural care providers to support the credentialing of an interested provider. In addition, because the CDE credential is so difficult to obtain, anecdotal reports from rural clinics indicate that even if a CDE is able to be trained, the provider often subsequently relocates to a more urban area where compensation is much higher. The establishment of a program designed to support rural providers in obtaining their CDEs while also incentivizing them to stay in a rural practice (e.g., through a service commitment) should be explored and could hold significant impact for improving access to diabetic education.

CONCLUSION

Diabetes is a growing problem in rural areas with demonstrated disparities in both morbidity and mortality, and further demonstrated disparities among racial/ethnic groups within rural settings. The context for addressing diabetes through traditional diet and exercise-focused interventions is different from urban settings, requiring careful cultural and socioeconomic sensitivities to ensure that prevention programming meets rural residents within their own realities. By continuing to grow the rural-specific diabetes literature, researchers and practitioners can help provide evidence-based practices to rural areas that sorely need them.

REFERENCES

1. Centers for Disease Control and Prevention. *National Diabetes Fact Sheet: General Information and National Estimates on Diabetes in the United States, 2007.* Atlanta, GA: US Department of Health and Human Services, Centers for Disease Control and Prevention; 2008.
2. Xu J, Dochanek KD, Murphy SL, Tejada-Vera B. Deaths: final data for 2007. *Natl Vital Stat Rep.* 2010;58(19).
3. Hsiao C, Cherry DK, Beatty PC, Rechtsteiner EA. National Ambulatory Medical Care Survey: 2007 summary. *Natl Health Stat Rep.* 2010;27:1–32.
4. Krishna S, Gillespie KN, McBride TM. Diabetes burden and access to preventive care in the rural United States. *J Rural Health.* 2010;26(1):3–11.
5. McCollum M, Ellis SL, Morrato EH, Sullivan PW. Prevalence of multiple cardiac risk factors in US adults with diabetes. *Curr Med Res Opin.* 2006;22(6):1031–1034.
6. Centers for Disease Control and Prevention. Diabetes data and trends. http://apps.nccd.cdc.gov/DDTSTRS/default.aspx.
7. Dabney B, Gosschalk A. Diabetes in rural America. In: *Rural Healthy People 2010: A Companion Document to Healthy People 2010, Volume 1.* College Station, TX: The Texas A&M University System Health Science Center, School of Rural Public Health, Southwest Rural Health Research Center; 2003.
8. Gamm LD, Hutchison LL, Dabney BJ, Dorsey AM, eds. *Rural Healthy People 2010: A Companion Document to Healthy People 2010, Volume 1.* College Station, TX: The Texas A&M University System Health Science Center, School of Rural Public Health, Southwest Rural Health Research Center; 2003.
9. Bolin JN, Bellamy G. *Rural Healthy People 2020 Update.* College Station, TX: The Texas A&M University System Health Science Center, School of Rural Public Health, Southwest Rural Health Research Center; 2013.
10. Andrus MR, Kelley KW, Murphey LM, Herndon KC. A comparison of diabetes care in rural and urban medical clinics in Alabama. *J Community Health.* 2004;29(1):29–44.
11. Hsiao C, Cherry DK, Beatty PC, Rechtsteiner EA. National Ambulatory Medical Care Survey: 2007 summary. *Natl Health Stat Rep.* 2010;27:1–32.
12. Slifkin RT, Goldsmith LJ, Ricketts T. *Race and Place: Urban-Rural Differences in Health for Racial and Ethnic Minorities.* NC Rural Health Research and Practice Working Paper Series, No. 66; 2000.
13. Pearson TA, Lewis C. Rural epidemiology: insights from a rural population laboratory. *Am J Epidemiol.* 1998;148(10):949–957.
14. Patterson PD, Moore CG, Probst JC, et al. Obesity and physical inactivity in rural America. *J Rural Health.* 2004;20:151–159.
15. Tai-Seale T, Chandler C. Nutrition and overweight concerns in rural areas. In: Gamm LD, et al., eds. *Rural Healthy People 2010: A Companion Document to Healthy People 2010, Volume 1.* College Station, TX: The Texas A&M University System Health Science Center, School of Rural Public Health, Southwest Rural Health Research Center; 2003.
16. Noel M, Hickner J, Ettenhofer T, et al. The high prevalence of obesity in Michigan primary care practices. An UPRNet study. *J Fam Pract.* 1998;47(1):39–43.
17. Greenlund KJ, Kiefe CI, Gidding SS, et al. Differences in cardiovascular disease risk factors in black and white young adults: comparisons among five communities of the CARDIA and the Bogalusa Heart Studies. *Ann Epidemiol.* 1998;8(1):22–30.

18. Diabetes Prevention Program Research Group (DPPRG). Reduction in the incidence of type 2 diabetes with lifestyle intervention or metformin. *N Engl J Med.* 2002;346(6):393–403.

19. Tuomilehto J, Lindstrom J, Eriksson JG, et al. Prevention of type 2 diabetes mellitus by changes in lifestyle among subjects with impaired glucose tolerance. *N Engl J Med.* 1993;329(14):977–986.

20. Arcury TA, Skelly AH, Gesler WM, Dougherty MC. Diabetes beliefs among low-income, white residents of a rural North Carolina community. *J Rural Health.* 2006;21(4):337–345.

21. Della LJ. Exploring diabetes beliefs in at-risk Appalachia. *J Rural Health.* 2010;27(1):3–12.

22. Ceballos RM, Coronado GD, Thompson B. Having a diagnosis of diabetes is not associated with general diabetes knowledge in rural Hispanics. *J Rural Health.* 2010;26(4):342–351.

23. Kegler MC, Escoffery C, Alcantara I, et al. A qualitative examination of home and neighborhood environments for obesity prevention in rural adults. *Int J Behav Nutr Phys Act.* 2008;5:65–74.

24. Badland HM, Duncan MI, Mummery WK. Travel perceptions, behaviors, and environment by degree of urbanization. *Prev Med.* 2008;47:265–269.

25. Frost SS, Goins RT, Hunter RH, et al. Effects of the built environment on physical activity of adults living in rural settings. *Am J Health Prom.* 2010;24:267–283.

26. Boyle JP, Thompson TJ, Gregg EW, et al. Projection of the year 2050 burden of diabetes in the US adult population: dynamic modeling of incidence, mortality, and prediabetes prevalence. *Popul Health Metr.* 2010;8:29.

27. Skelly AH, Arcury TA, Snively BM, et al. Self-monitoring of blood glucose in a multiethnic population of rural older adults with diabetes. *Diabetes Educ.* 2005;31:84–90.

28. Bell RA, Arcury TA, Stafford JM, et al. Ethnic and sex differences in ownership of preventive health equipment among rural older adults with diabetes. *J Rural Health.* 2007;23:332–338.

29. Dettori N, Flood BN, Pessi E, et al. Improvements in care and reduced self-management barriers among rural patients with diabetes. *J Rural Health.* 2006;21:172–177.

30. Amundson HA, Butcher MK, Gohdes D, et al. Translating the Diabetes Prevention Program into practice in the general community. *Diabetes Educ.* 2009;35:209–223.

31. Vadheim LM, Brewer KA, Kassner DR, et al. Effectiveness of a lifestyle intervention program among persons at high risk for cardiovascular disease and diabetes in a rural community. *J Rural Health.* 2010;26:266–272.

32. American Association of Diabetes Education. Background. 2013. http://www.diabeteseducator.org/ProfessionalResources/AADE7/Background.html.

33. Boren SA, guest ed. AADE7 self-care behaviors: systematic reviews. *Diabetes Educ.* 2007:33(6, theme issue):931–1103.

34. Utz SW, Williams IC, Jones R, et al. Culturally tailored intervention for rural African-Americans with type 2 diabetes. *Diabetes Educ.* 2008;34(5):654–665.

35. Povey RC, Clark-Carter D. Diabetes and healthy eating: a systematic review of the literature. *Diabetes Educ.* 2007;33:931–959.

36. Morton LW, Bitto EA, Oakland MJ, Sand M. Solving the problems of Iowa food deserts: food insecurity and civic structure. *Rural Sociol.* 2009;70:94–112.

37. Centers for Disease Control and Prevention. Facts about physical activity. 2012. http://www.cdc.gov/physicalactivity/data/facts.html.

38. Kavookjian J, Elswick BM, Whetsel T. Interventions for being active among individuals with diabetes: a systematic review of the literature. *Diabetes Educ.* 2007;33:962–988.

39. McAndrew L, Schneider SH, Burns E, Leventhan H. Does patient blood glucose monitoring improve diabetes control? A systematic review of the literature. *Diabetes Educ.* 2007;33:991–1011.

40. Odegard PS, Capoccia K. Medication taking and diabetes: a systematic review of the literature. *Diabetes Educ.* 2007;33:1014–1029.

41. Mulcahy K, Maryniuk M, Peeples M, et al. Diabetes self-management education core outcomes measures. *Diabetes Educ.* 2003;29:768–784.

42. Hill-Briggs F, Gemmell L. Problem solving in diabetes self-management and control: a systematic review of the literature. *Diabetes Educ.* 2007;33:1032–1050.

43. Boren SA, Gunlock TL, Schaefer J, Albright A. Reducing risks in diabetes self-management: a systematic review of the literature. *Diabetes Educ.* 2007;33:1053–1077.

44. Fisher EB, Thorpe CT, DeVellis BM, DeVellis RF. Healthy coping, negative emotions, and diabetes management: a systematic review and appraisal. *Diabetes Educ.* 2007;33:1080–1103.

45. Lustman PJ, Clouse RE. Depression in diabetic patients: the relationship between mood and glycemic control. *J Diabetes Complications.* 2005;19:113–122.

46. Lustman PJ, Griffith LS, Clouse RE. Depression in adults with diabetes. *Semin Clin Neuropsychiatry.* 1997;2:15–23.

47. Lin EHB, Katon W, VonKorff SCD, et al. Relationship of depression and diabetes self-care, medication adherence, and preventive care. *Diabetes Care.* 2004;27:2154–2160.

HIV Prevention and Treatment Issues in Rural America: A Focus on Regional Differences

John C. Moring, Timothy F. Page,
Anne Bowen, and Julie Angiola

Since 1994, the prevalence of HIV has steadily increased, with the incidence of rural HIV cases doubling between 1994 and 2000.[1] Subsequent data indicate that this trend continues, such that nonmetropolitan statistical areas in 19 states accounted for at least 20% of newly reported AIDS cases among adults and adolescents.[2] While the incidence of HIV in rural areas at 8.9 per 100,000 is still lower than in urban areas (26.7 per 100,000[3]), there is cause for significant concern because HIV infections tend to begin in urban areas and then migrate to less-populated parts of the country.[3] Therefore, as long as the rates of HIV prevalence and incidence in metropolitan areas are maintained or increase, the prevalence of HIV in rural areas will continue to rise. This becomes a very large concern as rural-living HIV-positive individuals will have a much more difficult time managing their care given the higher presence of HIV-related stigma and decreased access to HIV specialty care in rural areas. While the overall burden of HIV is associated with decreased quality of life, increased morbidity and mortality, and increased cost of physical and mental health care,[4] individuals in rural areas face unique challenges that increase their HIV risk status, further compromising quality of life. First, due to lower prevalence rates, funding for treatment and prevention services is often limited.[5] Second, voluntary counseling and testing are challenging to promote in small communities where everyone knows everyone. Finally, rural sociocultural factors, such as poverty, discrimination, and lack of education, may increase HIV risk behaviors themselves.[6]

This chapter describes the unique issues of HIV prevention and treatment in rural areas in the United States. As for the rest of this book, it is important to keep in mind that when we discuss "rurality," it is a *culture* that varies by region and population density. The associated cultural factors can serve as barriers to accessing HIV prevention and treatment services, such as lack of insurance coverage and provider shortages in rural areas.[5]

BARRIERS TO HIV PREVENTION AND TREATMENT IN RURAL AREAS

Individuals living in rural areas face unique barriers to HIV prevention, including testing privacy, confidentiality of an HIV-positive test result, and the stigma associated with HIV in rural communities. Awareness of HIV status is a crucial step in preventing the spread of the disease. People who have been tested and are aware of their HIV status are able to take advantage of therapies, as well as protect their sexual partners or drug-use partners.[7] Individuals who are aware of their HIV-positive status are more likely to reduce risky behavior associated with HIV transmission.[8] However, people in rural areas of the United States are often reluctant to be tested. Confidentiality and privacy related to HIV testing are more difficult to maintain. Even when testing services are available, individuals distrust the health care system in terms of privacy and confidentiality.[9] There is also a greater likelihood of breaches of confidentiality or anonymity compared to metropolitan areas, and individual behaviors such as entering or exiting the HIV testing sites are more recognizable.

In addition to barriers to HIV testing, providing primary prevention interventions in rural areas is difficult. Small-group interventions are expensive to staff and to operate unless delivered to geographically concentrated at-risk groups.[10] It is doubtful that small, rural jurisdictions will ever have sufficient public health funds to provide such interventions for even the highest at-risk group; that is, rural men who have sex with men (MSM). Given the small numbers of MSM likely to reside in any rural jurisdiction (due to sheer population size and a tendency of MSM to live in more urbanized areas), it is unlikely that face-to-face, small-group interventions would ever be cost-effective. Even if small-group interventions could be inexpensively and cost-effectively provided in rural jurisdictions, fear of discovery or lack of self-identification as gay or bisexual inhibits rural MSM from attending them, especially if the interventions are identifiable or can be construed as intended for gay or bisexual men.[11] Community-level interventions are an alternative to individual or small-group interventions, but these are difficult to deliver in rural areas given the lack of identifiable MSM communities[12] and overall reduced public health infrastructure.[13]

Secondary prevention efforts involve limiting HIV transmission from people living with HIV/AIDS (PLWHA) to uninfected persons and to protect the welfare of PLWHA by lowering their risk of acquiring other strains and/or pathogens.[14,15] Strategies include teaching safer sexual practices (i.e., sexual positioning and correct condom use), safer injection behaviors, and increasing motivation and adherence to medication regimens.[14] Secondary prevention efforts also include promoting strategies within couples that decrease chances of HIV transmission. Challenges related to these strategies are similar to the challenges associated with primary prevention, and include fear of disclosure and stigma related to HIV.

Fear of disclosure in rural areas is a significant barrier to secondary prevention. At the moment of an HIV diagnosis, individuals are concerned about being stigmatized or facing discrimination.[16,17] Rural areas are associated with a greater degree of stigma than urban areas, which leads to greater isolation and concerns with anonymity.[18] Rural areas are more likely to endorse conservative values and religious beliefs, which in turn promote less tolerance of nonconventional living.[19] "Normalcy" is valued, and a stigmatized chronic condition such as HIV is not perceived as "normal." Community members in rural areas are more likely to engage in discrimination and social isolation,[20] especially since HIV is (stereotypically) associated with homosexuality, injection drug use, promiscuity, and death.[21] Increased stigma and discrimination are factors that could influence a person's decision to keep HIV status private and not seek out needed treatment and support groups that would aid in promoting secondary prevention.[22]

Treatment for PLWHA in rural areas is also challenging. Barriers to receiving health care include provider shortages and inexperience, lack of consistent primary care provider contact despite available Ryan White funds, lack of social support, and stigma.[11,23,24] Due to these barriers, rural PLWHA tend to delay seeking care, preferring to obtain care when symptoms of their illness become serious.[25] As a result, rural PLWHA are more likely to be diagnosed in later stages of illness.[26,27] Compared to urban PLWHA, those in rural areas are more likely to be uninsured,[28] have less transportation options, and travel longer distances to their health care providers.[29] These barriers to HIV treatment services result in delayed or insufficient treatment, which leads to adverse outcomes for PLWHA in rural areas.

In addition to barriers to treatment, suboptimal medication adherence is also a problem in rural areas. Highly active antiretroviral therapy medications have been an effective treatment choice and have resulted in decreased mortality and morbidity and increased the quality of life for individuals living with HIV.[30] Although the reasons for missing medications among rural populations are similar to urban populations, limited access, lack of knowledge about HIV medication regimens, and lower health literacy are even more evident among rural individuals of minority groups.[22] Barriers to adherence also include not having the medication, sleeping through dosage times, running out of the medication, and busy schedules.[31] Running out of medications is more common among rural individuals who need to travel for their health care and to receive their medications. Living farther away from downtown areas where access to treatment is more readily available has been shown to impact adherence to HIV medication regimens.[32] There is a strong link between access to health care services and engagement in medical care and adherence to antiretroviral medications, so the lack of available health care resources also presents a barrier to medication adherence.[33] Individuals in rural areas are also more likely to report skipping doses in order to decrease the possibility of disclosing their HIV status when taking the medication.[34]

The lack of social support in rural areas also contributes to low medication adherence rates. Living in a rural area, with the fear of disclosure, inhibits adequate social support systems that are important for adherence to treatment regimen. Relationships with HIV care providers, families, and children are particularly important for keeping appointments for rural women.[35] Weak social support and engaging in avoidance and denial coping strategies related to HIV management lead to lower medication adherence.[36] Heckman, Catz, Heckman, Miller, and Kalichman found that using (a) active coping strategies and (b) a good relationship with a care provider were both significantly associated with medication adherence.[37-39] Unfortunately, these support systems and substance abuse programs are not widely available in rural areas.

Regional Differences in Rural HIV/AIDS Prevention and Treatment

Barriers to HIV prevention, treatment, and medication adherence exist in rural areas nationwide, as already described. Fear of disclosure, lack of health care and support services, and limited treatment options are barriers to effective prevention and treatment in many rural areas across the country. However, each region of the United States has different geographic and cultural issues that pose problems for HIV prevention and treatment for their respective populations.

Prevalence estimates show that the rural South is especially affected, with over 31,000 reported AIDS cases through 2006, compared to the 7,400 cases in the rural Northeast, 7,400 cases in the Midwest, and 5,100 cases in the West.* Regional differences may be driven by variations in geography and the geographical distribution of high-risk groups (i.e., ethnicity, sexual

*(CDC, 2006)[40] "Southern Region" includes Alabama, Arkansas, Delaware, District of Columbia, Florida, Georgia, Kentucky, Louisiana, Maryland, Mississippi, North Carolina, Oklahoma, South Carolina, Tennessee, Texas, Virginia, and West Virginia; "Northeast Region" includes New Hampshire, New Jersey, New York, Pennsylvania, Rhode Island, and Vermont; "Midwest Region" includes Illinois, Indiana, Iowa, Kansas, Michigan, Minnesota, Missouri, Nebraska, North Dakota, Ohio, South Dakota, and Wisconsin; "Western Region" includes Alaska, Arizona, California, Colorado, Hawaii, Idaho, Montana, Nevada, New Mexico, Oregon, Utah, Washington, and Wyoming.

orientation, and drug use). For example, in the rural South, 59% of HIV-positive individuals are Black/African American, followed by 31.2% White, and 7.6% Hispanic/Latino, as compared to the other rural regions where those infected with HIV/AIDS are predominately White (e.g. Northeast, 47.9% White; Midwest, 63.7% White; and the West, 62.3% White). White, rural populations account for the highest prevalence of HIV infections in the Northeast, Midwest, and West, but incidence rates are higher for Black/African Americans and Hispanic/Latinos in all four regions.[40] Additionally, two groups are increasingly affected by HIV/AIDS in rural areas—MSM and drug users—although incidence and prevalence among these groups are difficult to assess given the hidden nature of these populations.[41] Each region has specific HIV prevention and treatment challenges related to geography and culture, and each has unique minority populations that are affected by the spread of HIV/AIDS.

Southern Region

The rural South is particularly affected by HIV/AIDS, accounting for 68% of all AIDS cases among rural populations.[42] The number of newly reported AIDS cases in the Deep South increased by 35.6% between the years 2000 and 2003, while the number of newly reported cases in other southern states increased by only 4%.[43,44] Epidemiological and demographic data concerning HIV and AIDS indicate that PLWHA in the Deep South are disproportionately African American, female, and live in rural areas.[45]

There are many factors that contribute to the above-average HIV/AIDS prevalence in the rural South. The conservative culture of the South is a possible contributor to the increased incidence of HIV and AIDS in the region.[46] For instance, most southern states adopt abstinence-based sex education, instead of teaching teens how to use condoms and prevent HIV transmission.[46] Moreover, strict laws in southern states marginalize IV drug users and sex workers, which further discourages HIV testing.[46] Additionally, individuals in the South tend to have lower income, less education, and lower literacy rates, which make prevention and treatment efforts more difficult.[47] Scott and Wilson describe a number of other determinants of health of southern rural people that may speak directly to HIV risk issues, including a lack of engagement in personal health, nonparticipation in HIV prevention activities, lack of social capital, lack of jobs and recreational venues, and the strong influence of church doctrine against condom use discussions.[48]

Access to health care and services serves as a barrier to effective prevention and treatment of HIV in the rural south, with almost half of PLWHA in the South not receiving *any* support services.[49] PLWHA in the South seek health care in different geographical areas than their homes in order to reduce the chances of being stigmatized and having their privacy compromised.[50] Basic needs, such as housing, meals, and transportation, are inadequately provided to PLWHA in the rural South. Other needs such as mental health services and alcohol and substance abuse treatment, as well as primary care providers, case managers, and social workers, are also lacking in the rural South.[39]

The cultural barriers to prevention and treatment and the lack of support services for PLWHA disproportionately affect African Americans in the rural South, who account for 50% of all rural AIDS cases. Cultural beliefs, attitudes, and misconceptions about HIV serve as barriers for African Americans to use condoms during sexual intercourse.[51] In addition, African American communities are fearful of the stigma attached to HIV and AIDS. The stigma associated with HIV affects individual behavior and prevents many African Americans in the rural South from disclosing their status.[52] HIV/AIDS is especially stigmatized for African Americans in the Deep South, making disclosure even more difficult.[6] Unfortunately, the reluctance to get tested for HIV in rural areas, combined with difficulty disclosing HIV status, increases the likelihood of HIV transmission among African Americans in the rural South.[53]

African American women are also at increased risk for HIV/AIDS in the rural South. Misconceptions about condoms, HIV prevention, and individual risk status all contribute to risky sexual behavior among African American women. Many African American women in the rural South do not use condoms because they perceive their male partner might feel discomfort or a reduction in sexual sensation.[54] Some rural African Americans also exhibit attitudes that HIV can only be transmitted among IV drug users and gay White men, which leads to the misconception that one is protected from HIV.[55] Despite engaging in high-risk behaviors, African American women endorse beliefs that they are not at risk for acquiring HIV. For example, one study found that 37% of rural African American women thought that they had no risk of acquiring the disease, even though most participants reported using multiple illicit drugs.[56]

The problems related to HIV/AIDS in the rural South are not specific to African American women. Women from all ethnic groups in the rural South are particularly vulnerable to the HIV epidemic [57] due to lower levels of education, lower levels of income, and higher poverty rates compared to their urban counterparts.[54] Lower levels of education and poverty can limit women's ability to provide financially for themselves and their families. In order to compensate for the lack of financial resources, rural women sometimes find themselves in multiple romantic relationships at the same time or in close succession to each other. Among the reasons for having multiple sex partners was "survival sex," in which women exchanged sex for money.[58] One study identified that almost 33% of a sample of rural women in the South engaged in multiple, or concurrent, sexual partnerships within a 5-year time frame.[59] Some women in this position do not perceive that they can negotiate sexual practices, such as using condoms, thereby increasing the chances for HIV transmission. A recent study found that both male and female college students residing in a rural area thought that men should be responsible for suggesting and providing condoms.[60] The power differential between rural men and women helps to explain why the primary mode for HIV transmission is through heterosexual sexual activity.[42]

Despite the problems facing PLWHA and those at risk for HIV/AIDS in the rural South, there are options for improving prevention and treatment. Media campaigns and television shows can serve to model responsible sexual behavior. Modeling can change sexual behaviors by teaching techniques and changing attitudes (i.e., attitudes regarding condom use).[61] Medina suggests that showing storylines that incorporate HIV prevention messages can serve to increase condom use among women.[62] Areas in the rural South should devote financial resources for billboards or commercials that normalize safe-sex behaviors. Increased education for women in rural communities is also needed, as well as social programs aimed to alleviate financial needs. Increased job opportunities and financial assistance could help women feel more empowered to make healthy sexual decisions, instead of relying on male assistance that can lead to the exchange of sex for money or other financial support.

Midwest

The Midwest region has the fewest reported cases of individuals living with HIV and AIDS,[63] making up 11.3% of the AIDS cases among adults and adolescents in 2006.[42] Even though this region had the fewest reported cases, there is still cause for significant concern. The Midwest experienced the second highest increase in estimated AIDS incidence in the United States, with a 10.5% increase from 1999 to 2003.[64] These statistics are particularly relevant to rural residents, who on average comprise over one quarter of the population and in some states as much as half (e.g., North and South Dakota).[65]

Rural midwestern communities are characterized by limited access to primary care, self-care education, mental health and family support services, case management, and community educational programs.[66] The limited access to these important services prevents individuals from gaining knowledge about HIV transmission, as well as HIV risk-reduction techniques. Moreover, most health care providers in the rural Midwest reported that they have no training in communication about HIV risk.[67] The same study revealed that rural and suburban health care providers were less likely to have been involved in the treatment of at least one HIV-infected patient compared to their urban counterparts. These factors produce barriers to HIV prevention and treatment for all infected or at-risk individuals in the rural Midwest.

Migrant farm workers are the minority population most at risk in the rural Midwest. Rural farmers in the midwestern region heavily utilize migrant workers from Texas, Mexico, and Latin America.[68] HIV infection among migrant Latino farm workers is estimated to be 10 times the national rate,[69] which has the potential to increase the spread of HIV within these smaller communities. Given their extreme lack of access to health care, migrant rural farm workers may be unaware of their HIV status, and return to their home communities and unknowingly transmit the disease. Latino migrant farm workers report less knowledge about condoms compared to Latino individuals in urban areas. Studies have shown over half of migrant farm workers believe that condoms were only for gay men, and less than

10% believe condoms could be used for the prevention of HIV and pregnancy.[70] Among rural heterosexual Latino immigrants, factors associated
with increased condom use included being more knowledgeable about HIV,
having higher self-efficacy of using condoms, and an adherence to more
traditional and masculine norms.[71] The positive aspects about masculinity
among this sample of heterosexual Latino men, such as personal honor and
family responsibility, were related to increased condom use.

Despite cultural beliefs about condom use and lack of knowledge about
HIV in the rural Midwest, interventions can still be effective in reducing the
spread of HIV in the region. Educational interventions have been shown to
improve knowledge of HIV risk factors among female migrant workers, but
it is important to remember that any educational and behavioral interventions in hard-to-reach rural residents should be both easily accessible and
culturally relevant. There are other potential methods for improving HIV
prevention among the migrant worker population; for example, Hispanic
female migrant workers reported that television was their main source of
information, so public announcements on Spanish television could be an
important way to deliver information regarding HIV prevention.[68] Future
research should examine whether cultural and sociodemographic characteristics of particular rural regions impact condom use to inform future prevention programming. Further, telehealth is emerging as one viable option to
deliver HIV educational services and can involve a number of technologies.
These technologies include the Internet, email, and videoconferencing; see
Chapter 17 for more details.[72]

Western Region
The rural Western region had the lowest number of AIDS diagnoses in 2009,
with 201 diagnoses per 100,000 individuals. Moreover, the rural West had
5,149 reported AIDS cases, the lowest of all four rural regions.[40] However, the
rate of AIDS cases in the West (3.4 per 100,000) was higher than the midwestern region (2.9 per 100,000),[42] suggesting that HIV still poses a threat to this
population. The West has unique characteristics that make HIV prevention
and treatment difficult, such as longer distances to travel for medical care
and high rates of substance abuse.

The rural Western region is characterized by low population densities, long distances to social activities and health services, and health care
shortages (even in comparison to other rural areas of the country). Attitudes
among residents of the rural West also provide challenges to HIV prevention
and treatment. For example, residents of the frontier West tend to endorse
beliefs about the values of independence and freedom from the status quo.[73]
The belief that each person should be self-sustaining can conflict with the
need to seek medical treatment, rely on Medicare or Medicaid, and perhaps
disclose HIV status. These problems are compounded by the high rates of
drug and alcohol abuse in the region.

One of the top priorities outlined by Healthy People 2010 was substance abuse in the Western region of the United States.[74] Men and women in

rural areas are more likely to report drinking at least five drinks in one day in the previous year compared to their metropolitan counterparts.[75] Methamphetamine (MA) is especially problematic for the rural West, and has affected the rural population since at least 1977.[76] Individuals who reside in the West are two times more likely to use MA compared to individuals who live in any other area of the country.[77] By the early 1990s, MA was considered the primary drug threat in rural western states, such as Wyoming,[78] Montana, and Colorado.[79] MA use in rural areas has continued to rise, even among adolescents.[80] The prevalence of drug and alcohol use in the Western region of the United States is problematic for HIV prevention and treatment, given the strong association between substance use and acquisition of HIV.

Individuals in rural areas are more likely to engage in IV drug use than their urban counterparts.[81] IV drug use is risky and the direct and indirect sharing of contaminated drug equipment, such as syringes, allows for the transmission of HIV. Increased chances for exposure to HIV are also present in shooting galleries (places where people can rent equipment for injection drug use) and more frequent injection drug use.[82] Given more prominent drug use in certain rural areas of the United States, it is likely that the chances for HIV transmission are also greater. In 2009, 9% of new HIV infections were injection drug users, who accounted for almost 20% of PLWHA 2008.[83] The use of drugs and alcohol prior to sexual encounters has been associated with increased risky sexual behaviors,[84] decreasing individuals' self-efficacy to use condoms.[85] A direct line of defense against HIV transmission in the West would be a focus on substance use prevention and treatment; however, treatment programs are lacking in western rural areas, and there is reluctance among drug users to seek treatment.[86] For example, there are as few as 8 residential treatment centers across Wyoming's 99,000 square miles.[87]

Prevention measures among rural individuals in the West should include a focus on substance use prevention, increased access to drug and alcohol treatment centers, and encouragement of harm reduction strategies. Increased funding for treatment centers and public health campaigns could increase the acceptability and feasibility of drug treatment in the rural West and rural America more generally.

Northeast Region

The rural Northeast region had the second highest number of AIDS diagnoses in 2009, with 221 diagnoses per 100,000 individuals. Even though the Northeast is smaller compared to other geographical regions, this area shares a substantial burden of HIV. Residents in rural areas in the Northeast experience problems similar to other regions, such as provider shortages and a lack of HIV prevention resources.

The Northeast is "small" geographically in that towns are close together, but rolling hills, winter weather, and two-lane roads separate small towns from each other and urban areas. Sixty-two percent of Vermont's[88] and 42% of Maine's population are designated as rural.[89] Challenges for Vermont residents include lack of infrastructure, distances to urban areas, low market aggregation, and other challenges to HIV prevention, such as Internet availability. In order to address these concerns, regional care clinics were established. Each clinic was staffed by part-time HIV-trained nurse practitioners and the clinics were housed in regional hospitals, which helped to ensure anonymity and confidentiality. Providing more of these clinics in remote areas of the country, even if only staffed periodically by HIV specialists, would benefit rural residents in the Northeast and other regions as well.

The dominant minority group at risk for HIV in the rural Northeast is MSM. MSM in this region face the same barriers to prevention and treatment as MSM in other parts of the country. Approximately 1.5 to 2.0 million MSM live in rural areas of the United States,[90] and almost half of diagnosed AIDS cases in the Northeast were attributed to male-to-male sexual contact in 2006.[91] MSM remain the highest HIV transmission risk group in the United States, and MSM in rural areas is the only risk group in which the incidence of HIV is increasing.[92] The prevalence of HIV/AIDS among rural MSM is two to three times greater than in cities with above-average prevalence among MSM, such as Atlanta, Philadelphia, Washington, DC, Chicago, San Francisco, or Houston.[42]

The numbers of rural MSM who are HIV infected have implications for HIV prevention strategies. Given the low population density of rural areas, if prevention programs are to be cost-effective and affordable they need to efficiently reach rural MSM across broad geographical areas. Further, rural MSM in different regions of the country have different needs related to ethnicity, religion, and geography. MSM are not a homogeneous group, as there are different group memberships and cultures that guide individual behavior.[93] Thus, there is a need for effective primary prevention programs for rural MSM that are widely available but flexible enough to be tailored to regional and individual needs.

The Future of HIV Prevention and Treatment in Rural Areas

There are several options for improving prevention and treatment for HIV/AIDS in rural areas. Given the unique risk dynamics of rural PLWHA, the Rural Center for AIDS/STD Prevention (RCAP) suggests several interventions to reduce risky HIV behaviors. These interventions include "Prevention IS Care," a social marketing campaign (www.actagainstaids.org/provider/pic) that uses educational brochures to increase knowledge about HIV. This campaign also provides broadcasts that are readily accessible via the Internet, as well as opportunities for providers to gain more knowledge about how to increase their patients' self-efficacy to make better decisions regarding their health. The one-on-one, brief, provider-initiated "The Partnership for Health"[94] and "Ask, Screen, Intervene: Incorporating HIV Prevention into Medical Care of Persons Living with HIV," are other training programs available to individual providers serving PLWHA. These programs are especially relevant to health care providers in rural areas, who might not otherwise have access to materials and information about preventing HIV and living with the disease for their rural patients. Evidence for the utility of secondary prevention initiatives among rural PLWHA is emerging.[95]

Media campaigns within small communities can lead to less stigma and increase individuals' willingness to test for HIV.[96,97] These campaigns can target communities to promote healthy sexual attitudes, including consistent condom use for nonmonogamous partners and decreased alcohol and drug use before sexual activity. Decreasing the stigma associated with HIV testing may promote healthier sexual behaviors within communities and decrease HIV transmission.

New technologies also provide a potential platform for the delivery of HIV prevention and treatment in rural areas. Some rural jurisdictions have been providing mental health and social support services to HIV-positive persons using teleconferencing technology.[98-101] Both telephone technologies and the Internet can be adapted to HIV prevention in terms of protecting the anonymity of people who might be amenable to participating[102] and providing remote access. In addition, Internet interventions have the potential to be less costly to implement due to lower reliance on trained personnel to deliver them. Although the costs of developing them are high, Internet-based interventions can be implemented and delivered at substantially lower costs than face-to-face interventions.[103] Therefore, the Internet may be an affordable and sustainable platform through which HIV-related interventions can be made available to rural populations.

Online health promotion interventions could be particularly useful for MSM living in rural areas who are at risk for HIV/AIDS.[11] Rural MSM are frequently geographically isolated and socially cut off from supportive gay communities, which tend to be in large urban areas, and in which most HIV/AIDS interventions targeting MSM are available. Rural MSM, especially those who seldom travel to urban areas, are less likely to be aware that intervention materials exist. Furthermore, materials designed to address the concerns of urban MSM are often not relevant to MSM living in rural areas. Recent studies have shown the promise of Internet-based intervention to increase HIV-related knowledge, improve condom use self-efficacy, and reduce the frequency of unprotected anal intercourse.[104,105] These interventions demonstrate the feasibility of delivering interventions to individuals who are more difficult to reach, such as rural at-risk individuals.

Technology provides a way to access rural MSM and also avoids many of the problems inherent in small-group or community-level interventions. Advertisements for HIV prevention interventions displayed on gay-oriented sites can be viewed without threatening anonymity and privacy. After seeing an Internet advertisement, interested men can go immediately to a prevention program website or access it at a time and in a place that is convenient for them. Perhaps most importantly, an Internet-based HIV prevention program does not require men to go to a public place, which might expose their sexual orientation or activities.

The Internet also provides an effective avenue for reaching a particularly high-risk group, MSM who seek sex partners online. Given their often isolation from other MSM, many rural MSM access gay-oriented sites on the Internet to socialize and look for sex partners.[106-109] MSM who seek sex partners on the Internet may be at higher risk for HIV and sexually transmitted infections (STIs) than MSM who do not seek sex partners using the Internet.[106,110,111] MSM who seek sex on the Internet tend to have greater numbers of previously diagnosed STIs, higher frequency of anal sex, greater numbers of sex partners, and higher numbers of sex partners known to be HIV-positive than non-Internet sex seekers.[112,113] MSM who met sex partners on the Internet, in addition to these other risk behaviors, also used MA more often than MSM who exclusively seek sex partners in other venues.[106]

CONCLUSION

The definition of "rural" usually involves population density within a specific geographical area. However, these methods do not capture the rural culture in terms of feelings of isolation, being limited in health care choices because of long driving distances, and lacking privacy because "everyone knows everybody." These factors are unique to rural living and may serve as barriers to HIV prevention and treatment. Once identified, steps can be made to navigate through these problems and prevent the spread of HIV in rural areas and improve the quality of life for those already infected. The treatment of HIV is also affected by the lack of resources in sparsely populated parts of the United States. Rural PLWHA need to travel longer distances for adequate health care, which impacts treatment adherence. Mental health care is also an important aspect for the treatment of PLWHA. Rural individuals who are presented with a diagnosis of HIV/AIDS are especially susceptible to depression and loneliness, but mental health and social support services in rural areas are lacking.

Incidence and prevalence rates of HIV in rural areas are slowly rising, and a thorough evaluation of the specific needs of rural individuals is needed to draw attention to the growing problem and unique challenges of HIV/AIDS in rural areas. Different rural regions face different barriers to prevention and treatment, both in terms of sociocultural characteristics and specific populations at risk; therefore, prevention programs should be targeted at specific groups of individuals. Increased testing is much needed in order for rural individuals to be aware of their HIV status and take appropriate measures to protect others. Media campaigns may be a useful strategy to decrease the stigma associated with HIV testing and communication with sexual partners, and Internet-based interventions hold much promise for expanding access to preventive care.

REFERENCES

1. Centers for Disease Control and Prevention. *HIV/AIDS surveillance report.* 2000;6:11.
2. Centers for Disease Control and Prevention. *HIV/AIDS surveillance report.* 2000;1–16.

3. Centers for Disease Control and Prevention. *HIV/AIDS surveillance in urban and nonurban areas. 2011.* www.cdc.gov/hiv/graphics/rural-urban.htm. Accessed April 1, 2012.

4. Schackman BR, Gebo KA, Walensky RP, et al. The lifetime cost of current human immunodeficiency virus care in the United States. *Med Care.* 2006;44(11):990–997.

5. Cohn SE, Berk ML, Berry SH, et al. The care of HIV-infected adults in rural areas of the United States. *J Acquir Immune Defic Syndr.* 2001;28(4):385–392.

6. Pence BW, Reif S, Whetten K, et al. Minorities, the poor, and survivors of abuse: HIV-infected patients in the US Deep South. *Southern Med J.* 2007;100(11):1114–1122.

7. Centers for Disease Control and Prevention. HIV counseling and testing at CDC-funded sites, United States, Puerto Rico, and the U.S. Virgin Islands, 2005. http://www.cdc.gov/hiv/resources/reports/pdf/2005_HIV_CT_Report.pdf. Accessed April 14, 2012.

8. Cleary, PD, Vandevanter N, Rogers TF, et al. Behavior changes after notification of HIV-infection. *Am J Public Health.* 1991;81(12):1586–1590.

9. Sutton M, Anthony MN, Vila C, et al. HIV testing and HIV/AIDS treatment services in rural counties in 10 southern states: service provider perspectives. *J Rural Health.* 2010;26(3):240–247.

10. Holtgrave D, Kelly J. The cost-effectiveness of an HIV prevention intervention for gay men. *AIDS Behav.* 1997;1:173–180.

11. Williams ML, Bowen AM, Horvath KJ. (2005). The social/sexual environment of gay men residing in a rural frontier state: implications for the development of HIV prevention programs. *J Rural Health.* 2005;21(1):48–55.

12. Kelly JD, Murphy K, Sikkema T, et al. Randomized, controlled, community-level HIV-prevention intervention for sexual-risk behavior among homosexual men in US cities. *Lancet.* 1997;350:1500–1505.

13. Hart LG, Salsberg E, Phillips DM, Lishner DM. Rural health care providers in the United States. *J Rural Health.* 2002;18(suppl):211–232.

14. Fisher JD, Smith L. Secondary prevention of HIV infection: the current state of prevention for positives. *Curr Opin HIV AIDS.* 2009;4(4):279–287.

15. Fisher JD, Smith LR, Lenz EM. Secondary prevention of HIV in the United States: past, current, and future perspectives. *J Acquir Immune Defic Syndr.* 2010;55(suppl 2): S106–S115.

16. Baumgartner LM, David KN. Accepting being poz: the incorporation of the HIV identity into the self. *Qual Health Res.* 2009;19(12):1730–1743.

17. Logie C, Gadalla TM. Meta-analysis of health and demographic correlates of stigma towards people living with HIV. *AIDS Care.* 2009;21(6):742–753.

18. Heckman TG, Somlai AM, Otto-Salaj L, Davantes BR. Health-related quality of life among people living with HIV disease in small communities and rural areas. *Psychol Health.* 1998;13:859–871.

19. Tiemann KA. Why is their picture on the wedding page? A rural community responds to a union announcement. *J Homosexuality.* 2006;51(4):119–135.

20. Gonzalez A, Miller CT, Solomon SE, Bunn JY, Cassidy DG. Size matters: community size, HIV stigma, & gender differences. *AIDS Behav.* 2009;13(6):1205–1212.

21. Swendeman D, Rotheram-Borus MJ, Comulda S, Weiss R, Ramos ME. Predictors of HIV-related stigma among young people living with HIV. *Health Psychol.* 2006;25(4):501–509.

22. Miles MS, Isler MR, Banks BB, Sengupta S, Corbie-Smith G. Silent endurance and profound loneliness: socioemotional suffering in African Americans living with HIV in the rural south. *Qual Health Res.* 2011;21(4):489–501.

23. Hall HI, Li J, McKenna MT. HIV in predominantly rural areas of the United States. *J Rural Health*. 2005;21(3):245–253.

24. McKinney MM. Variations in rural AIDS epidemiology and service delivery models in the United States. *J Rural Health*. 2002;18(3):455–466.

25. Rounds KA. AIDS in rural areas—challenges to providing care. *Soc Work*. 1988;33(3):257–261.

26. Calonge BN, Petersen LR, Miller RS, Marshall G. Human immunodeficiency virus seroprevalence in primary care practices in the United States. *West J Med*. 1993;158(2):148–152.

27. Miller RS, Green LA, Nutting PA, et al. Human immunodeficiency virus seroprevalence community based primary care practices, 1990-1992. A report from the Ambulatory Sentinel Practice Network. *Arch Fam Med*. 1995;4(12):1042–1047.

28. Hu HM. Variations in health insurance coverage for rural and urban nonelderly adult residents of Florida, Indiana, and Kansas. *J Rural Health*. 2006;22(2):147–150.

29. Schur CL, Berk ML, Dunbar JR, et al. Where to seek care: An examination of people in rural areas with HIV/AIDS. *J Rural Health*. 2002;18(2):337–347.

30. DiIorio C, McCarty F, Resnicow K, et al. Using motivational interviewing to promote adherence to antiretroviral medications: a randomized controlled study. *AIDS Care*. 2008;20(3):273–283.

31. Amico KR, Konkle-Parker DJ, Cornman DH, et al. Reasons for ART non-adherence in the Deep South: adherence needs of a sample of HIV-positive patients in Mississippi. *AIDS Care*. 2007;19(10):1210–1218.

32. Kalichman SC, Pellowski J, Kalichman MO, et al. Food insufficiency and medication adherence among people living with HIV/AIDS in urban and peri-urban settings. *Prev Sci*. 2011;12(3):324–332.

33. Messeri PA, Abramson DM, Aidala AA, Lee F. The impact of ancillary HIV services on engagement in medical care in New York City. *AIDS Care*. 2002;14:S15–S29.

34. Golin C, Isasi F, Bontempi JB, Eng E. Secret pills: HIV-positive patients' experiences taking antiretroviral therapy in North Carolina. *AIDS Educ Prev*. 2002;14(4):319–329.

35. Kempf MC, McLeod J, Boehme AK. A qualitative study of the barriers and facilitators to retention-in-care among HIV-positive women in the rural southeastern United States: implications for targeted interventions. *AIDS Patient Care STDs*. 2010;24(8):515–520.

36. Vyavaharkar M, Moneyham L, Tavakoli A, et al. Social support, coping, and medication adherence among HIV-positive women with depression living in rural areas of the southeastern United States. *AIDS Patient Care STDs*. 2007;21(9):667–680.

37. Heckman BD, Catz SL, Heckman TG, Miller JG, Kalichman SC. Adherence to antiretroviral therapy in rural persons living with HIV disease in the United States. *AIDS Care*. 2004;16(2):219–230.

38. Hoang T, Goetz MB, Yano EM, et al. The impact of integrated HIV care on patient health outcomes. *Med Care*. 2009;47(5):560–567.

39. Stewart KE, Phillips MM, Walker JF, Harvey SA, Porter A. Social services utilization and need among a community sample of persons living with HIV in the rural south. *AIDS Care*. 2011;23(3):340–347.

40. Centers for Disease Control and Prevention. Cases of HIV infection and AIDS in the United States and dependent areas. *HIV/AIDS Surveillance Report*. 2006.

41. Lieb S, Fallon SJ, Friedman SR. Statewide estimation of racial ethnic populations of men who have sex with men in the U.S. *Public Health Rep*. 2011;126:60–72.

42. Centers for Disease Control and Prevention. Estimates of new HIV infections in the United States. *CDC HIV/AIDS Facts.* August 2008.
43. Centers for Disease Control and Prevention. US HIV and AIDS cases reported through December 2001. *HIV AIDS Surveillance Rep.* 2001;13(2).
44. Centers for Disease Control and Prevention. Cases of HIV Infection and AIDS in the United States 2003. *HIV AIDS Surveillance Rep.* 2003;15.
45. Reif S, Geonnotti KL, Whetten K. HIV infection and AIDS in the Deep South. *Am J Public Health.* 2006;96:970–973.
46. Human Rights Watch. Southern exposure: human rights and HIV in the Southern United States. 2010. http://www.hrw.org/sites/default/files/related_material/BPapersouth1122_6.pdf. Accessed June 2012.
47. Peterman TA, Lindsey CA, Selik RM. This place is killing me: a comparison of counties where the incidence rates of AIDS increased the most and the least. *J Infect Dis.* 2005;191:S123–S126.
48. Scott AJ, Wilson RF. Social determinants of health among African Americans in a rural community in the Deep South: an ecological exploration. *Rural Remote Health.* 2011;11(1):1634.
49. Reif S, Whetten K, Ostermann J, Raper JL. Characteristics of HIV-infected adults in the Deep South and their utilization of mental health services: a rural vs. urban comparison. *AIDS Care.* 2006;18(S1):10–17.
50. Konkle-Parker DJ, Amico KR, Henderson MH. Barriers and facilitators to engagement in HIV clinical care in the Deep South: results from semi-structured patient interviews. *J Assoc Nurses AIDS Care.* 2011;22(2):90–99.
51. Williams PB, Sallar AM. HIV/AIDS and African American men: urban-rural differentials in sexual behavior, HIV knowledge, and attitude towards condoms use. *J Natl Med Assoc.* 2010;102(12):1139–1149.
52. Gaskins, S, Payne Foster P, Sowell R, et al. Reasons for HIV disclosure and non-disclosure: an exploratory study of rural African American men. *Issues Ment Health Nurs.* 2011;32(6):367–373.
53. Marks G, Crepaz N, Senterfitt JW, Janssen RS. Meta-analysis of high-risk sexual behavior in persons aware and unaware they are infected with HIV in the United States: implications for HIV prevention programs. *J Acquir Immune Defic Syndr.* 2005;39(4):446–453.
54. Williams PB, Ekundayo O, Udezulu IE, Omishakin AM. An ethnically sensitive and gender-specific HIV/AIDS assessment of African American women—a comparative study of urban and rural American communities. *Fam Community Health.* 2003;26(2):108–123.
55. Foster PH. Use of stigma, fear, and denial in development of a framework for prevention of HIV/AIDS in rural African American communities. *Fam Community Health.* 2007;30(4):318–327.
56. Brown EJ, Van Hook M. Risk behavior, perceptions of HIV risk, and risk-reduction behavior among a small group of rural African American women who use drugs. *J Assoc Nurses AIDS Care.* 2006;17(5):42–50.
57. Fleming PL, Lansky A, Lee LM, Nakashima AK. The epidemiology of HIV/AIDS in women in the southern United States. *Sex Transm Dis.* 2006;33(suppl 7):S32–S38.
58. Stratford D, Ellerbrock TV, Chamblee S. Social organization of sexual-economic networks and the persistence of HIV in a rural area in the USA. *Cult Health Sex.* 2007;9(2):121–135.
59. Adimora AA, Schoenbach VJ, Martinson FE, Donaldson KH, Stancil TR, Fullilove RE. Concurrent partnerships among rural African Americans with recently

reported heterosexually transmitted HIV infection. *J Acquir Immune Defic Syndr.* 2003;34(4):423–429.

60. Ross L, Moring J, Angiola J, Bowen A. The influence of sexual scripts and the "better than average" effect on condom responsibility. *J College Student Dev.* In press.

61. Bandura A. *Social Foundations of Thought and Action: A Social Cognitive Theory.* Englewood Cliffs, NJ: Prentice Hall; 1986.

62. Medina C. An alternate HIV preventive strategy: sex scripts in media for women of color. *Soc Work Public Health.* 2011;26:260–277.

63. The Henry J. Kaiser Family Foundation. State Health Facts Online. 2005. http://www.statehealthfacts.org. Accessed May 5, 2011.

64. Centers for Disease Control and Prevention. Cases of HIV Infection and AIDS in the United States 2003. *HIV AIDS Surveillance Rep.* 2003;15.

65. US Census Bureau. Census 2000 Summary File 1. 2007.

66. Baldwin KA, Marvin CL, Rodine MK. The development of a comprehensive interdisciplinary HIV/AIDS center: a community needs assessment. *J Public Health Manage Pract.* 1998;4(4):87–96.

67. Wolf MS, Linsk NL, Mitchell CG, Schechtman B. HIV prevention in practice: an assessment of the public health response of physicians and nurses in the Midwest. *J Community Health.* 2004;29(1):63–73.

68. Fitzgerald K, Chakraborty J, Shah T, Khuder S, Duggan J. HIV/AIDS knowledge among female migrant farm workers in the Midwest. *J Immigr Health.* 2003;5(1):29–36.

69. Organista KC, Organista PB, Bola JR, García de Alba JE, Castillo Morán MA. Predictors of condom use in Mexican migrant laborers. *Am J Community Psychol.* 2000;28(2):245–265.

70. Ford K, King G, Nerenberg L, Rojo C. AIDS knowledge and risk behaviors among Midwest migrant farm workers. *AIDS Educ Prev.* 2001;13(6):551–560.

71. Knipper E, Rhodes SD, Lindstrom K, Bloom FR, Leichliter JS, Montaño J. Condom use among heterosexual immigrant Latino men in the southeastern United States. *AIDS Educ Prev.* 2007;19(5):436–447.

72. Richardson LK, Frueh BC, Grubaugh AL, Egede L, Elhai JD. Current directions in videoconferencing telemental health research. *Clin Psychol.* 2009;16(3):323–338.

73. Kitayama S, Conway LG, Pietromonaco PR, Park H, Plaut VC. Ethos of independence across regions in the United States: the production-adoption model of cultural change. *Am Psychol.* 2010;65(6):559–574.

74. Gamm L, Hutchison L, Dabney B, Dorsey A, eds. *Rural Healthy People 2010: A Companion Document to Healthy People 2010.* College Station, TX: The Texas A&M University System Health Science Center, School of Rural Public Health, Southwest Rural Health Research Center. 2003;1.

75. Eberhardt M, Ingram D, Makuk D, et al. *Urban and Rural Health Chartbook. Health, United States.* Hyattsville, MD: National Center for Health Statistics; 2001.

76. Brown BS. Comparison of drug abuse clients in urban and rural settings. *Am J Drug Alcohol Abuse.* 1977;4(4):445–454.

77. United States Department of Health and Human Services. Substance Abuse and Mental Health Services Administration. Office of Applied Studies. *National Survey on Drug Use and Health,* 2007.

78. Wyoming Department of Health. *Methamphetamine Planning Study.* Cheyenne, WY: Wyoming Department of Health; 2005.

79. Executive Office of the President. *Pulse Check: Trends in Drug Abuse: January–June 2002 Reporting Period*. Washington, DC: Office of National Drug Control Policy; 2002.

80. Eaton DK, Kann L, Kinchen S, et al. Youth Risk Behavior Surveillance—United States, 2009. In: Surveillance Summaries, June 4, 2010. *MMWR*. 2009;59(SS05):1–142.

81. Young AM, Havens JR, Leukefeld CG. Route of administration for illicit prescription opioids: a comparison of rural and urban drug users. *Harm Reduct J*. 2010;7(24):1–7.

82. Himmelgreen DA, Singer M. HIV, AIDS, and other health risks: findings from a multisite study—an introduction. *Am J Drug Alcohol Abuse*. 1998;24(2):187–197.

83. Centers for Disease Control and Prevention. HIV in the United States: at a glance. 2012. http://www.cdc.gov/hiv/resources/factsheets/PDF/HIV_at_a_glance.pdf. Accessed May 20, 2012.

84. Chesney MA, Barrett DC, Stall R. Histories of substance use and risk behavior: precursors to HIV seroconversion in homosexual men. *Am J Public Health*. 1998;88(1):113–116.

85. Kalichman SC, Picciano JF, Roffman RA. Motivation to reduce HIV risk behaviors in the context of the information, motivation and behavioral skills (IMB) model of HIV prevention. *J Health Psychol*. 2008;13(5):680–689.

86. *Rural Healthy People 2010: A Companion Document to Healthy People 2010*. College Station, TX: The Texas A&M University System Health Science Center, School of Rural Public Health, Southwest Rural Health Research Center; 2010.

87. Bowen A, Moring J, Williams M, Hopper G, Daniel C. An investigation of bioecological influences associated with first use of methamphetamine in a rural state. *J Rural Health*. 2012;28(3):286–295.

88. Sawyer W. Vermont. Small. Rural. What does it mean? Center for Rural Studies, University of Vermont. 2010. http://www.uvm.edu/crs/reports/2010/vt_small_rural_2010.pdf

89. US Department of Agriculture, Economic Research Service. *State Fact Sheets*. 2012. http://www.ers.usda.gov/data-products/state-fact-sheets/state-data.aspx?StateFIPS=23&StateName=Maine. Accessed February 1, 2013.

90. Centers for Disease Control and Prevention. HIV/AIDS among men who have sex with men. *HIV/AIDS Fact Sheet*. 2007:1–9. http://www.cdc.gov/hiv/topics/msm/resources/factsheets/pdf/msm.pdf

91. Centers for Disease Control and Prevention. AIDS by region, 2006. 2009. http://www.cdc.gov/hiv/topics/surveillance/resources/slides/aids_regional. Accessed May 2, 2012.

92. Centers for Disease Control and Prevention. HIV & AIDS in the United States: a picture of today's epidemic. *CDC HIV/AIDS Media Facts*. March 2008.

93. Caceres CF, Aggleton P, Galea JT. Sexual diversity, social inclusion and HIV/AIDS. *AIDS*. 2008;22(suppl 2):S45–55.

94. Richardson JL, Milam J, McCutchan A, et al. Effect of brief safer-sex counseling by medical providers to HIV-1 seropositive patients: a multi-clinic assessment. *AIDS*. 2004;18(8):1179–1186.

95. Rose CD, Courtenay-Quirk C, Knight K, et al. HIV Intervention for Providers study: a randomized controlled trial of a clinician-delivered HIV risk-reduction intervention for HIV-positive people. *J Acquir Immune Defic Syndr*. 2010;55(5):572–581.

96. de Vroome EM, Paalman ME, Sandfort TG, Sleutjes M, de Vries KJ, Tielman RA. AIDS in the Netherlands: the effects of several years of campaigning. *Int J STD AIDS*. 1990;1(4):268–275.

97. Hausser D, Michaud PA. Does a condom-promoting strategy (the Swiss STOP-AIDS campaign) modify sexual behavior among adolescents? *Pediatrics.* 1994;93(4):580–585.
98. Heckman TG, Kalichman SC, Roffman RR, et al. A telephone-delivered coping improvement intervention for persons living with HIV/AIDS in rural areas. *Soc Work Groups.* 1999;21(4):49–61.
99. Heckman TG, Somlai AM, Kalichman SC, Franzoi SL, Kelly JA. Psychosocial differences between urban and rural people living with HIV/AIDS. *J Rural Health.* 1998;14(2):138–145.
100. Rounds KA, Galinsky MJ, Stevens SL. Linking people with AIDS in rural communities: the telephone group. *Soc Work.* 1991;36(1):13–18.
101. Rutledge SE, Mahoney C, Berghuis JP, Roffman RA, Picciano JF, Kalichman SC. Motivational enhancement counseling strategies in delivering a telephone-based brief HIV prevention intervention. *Clin Soc Work J.* 2001;29(3):291–306.
102. Hospers HJ, Harterink P, VanDen Hoek K, Veenstra J. Chatters on the Internet: a special target group for HIV prevention. *AIDS Care.* 2002;14(4):539–544.
103. Page TF, Horvath KJ, Danilenko GP, Williams M. A cost analysis of an Internet-based medication adherence intervention for people living with HIV. *J AIDS.* 2012;60(1):1–4.
104. Bowen AM, Williams ML, Daniel CM, Clayton S. Internet based HIV prevention research targeting rural MSM: feasibility, acceptibility, and preliminary efficacy. *J Behav Med.* 2008;31:463–477.
105. Rosser BR, Oakes JM, Konstan J, et al. Reducing HIV risk behavior of men who have sex with men through persuasive computing: results of the men's Internet study-II. *AIDS.* 2010;24(13):2099–2107.
106. Benotsch EG, Kalichman S, Cage M. Men who have met sex partners via the Internet: prevalence, predictors, and implications for HIV prevention. *Arch Sex Behav.* 2002;31(2):177–183.
107. Bowen A. Internet sexuality research with rural men who have sex with men: can we recruit and retain them? *J Sex Res.* 2005;42(4):317–323.
108. Elford J, Bolding G, Davis M, Sherr L, Hart G. Web-based behavioral surveillance among men who have sex with men: a comparison of online and offline samples in London, UK. *J Acquir Immune Defic Syndr.* 2004;35(4):421–426.
109. Hospers HJ, Kok G, Harterink P, de Zwart O. A new meeting place: chatting on the Internet, e-dating and sexual risk behaviour among Dutch men who have sex with men. *AIDS.* 2005;19(10):1097–2101.
110. Garofalo R, Herrick A, Mustanski BS, Donenberg GR. Tip of the iceberg: young men who have sex with men, the Internet, and HIV risk. *Am J Public Health.* 2007;97(6):1113–1117.
111. Shaw DF. Gay men and communication: a discourse of sex and identity in cyberspace. In: Jones SG, ed. *Virtual Culture: Identity and Communication in Cybersociety.* London, England: SAGE. 1997:133–145.
112. McFarlane M, Bull SS, Rietmeijer CA. The Internet as a newly emerging risk environment for sexually transmitted diseases. *JAMA.* 2000;284(4):443–446.
113. Horvath KJ, Bowen AM, Williams ML. Virtual and physical venues as contexts for HIV-risk behaviors among rural men who have sex with men. *Health Psychol.* 2006; 25(2):237–242.

Environmental and Occupational Health in Rural Areas

Simone M. Charles and
Azita K. Cuevas

There is growing evidence that environmental exposures influence several health outcomes, including, but not limited to, mental health, oncology, and respiratory illness. Environmental exposures tend to be greater in minority and low-income communities, resulting in worse health outcomes in these communities.[1,2] Rural populations, facing strong economic pressures and unique environmental exposures, are influenced by environmental exposures to a greater extent that their urban counterparts.[3] The resulting health disparities and differential burden of exposures can be viewed through the lens of environmental justice.

The National Institute of Environmental Health Sciences (NIEHS) defines environmental health broadly to include physical activity, diet, toxicant exposures, diet, and stress—an integrated view incorporating all aspects of the environment that influence exposures and exposure outcomes. While some environmental influences are shared with urban counterparts, some health status determinants are specific to rural environments.[4] For instance, compared to urban groups, rural populations face greater exposures to zoonoses,[5] reduced access to health care[6] and diagnostic and management services,[7] increased exposure to occupational hazards,[8] elevated rates of smoking,[9] lower levels of physical activity,[10] and greater psychological stress.[11] Understanding the extent to which rurality influences environmental health outcomes is important for the development of sound policy to improve rural health status.[12] Overcoming rural environmental health disadvantages requires a firm understanding of the facets that influence the health disparities—socioeconomic, demographic, discrimination, inequality, disparate resource allocation, unemployment—in tandem with environmental exposure and education.[4]

In a survey of national rural health leaders, four of the five key priority areas identified as important to rural health were "heart disease and stroke, diabetes, mental health and mental disorders, and oral health."[13] Each of these areas has roots in environmental exposures.[11,14-16] In the same survey, environmental health ranked 15th of the most important Healthy People 2010 Focus Areas among rural health professionals. Tobacco use,[9] substance abuse,[17] maternal and child health,[18] nutrition and obesity,[19] cancer,[20] infectious disease,[21] and injury and violence[22] were each ranked higher by rural professionals.[13] Interestingly, each of these health concerns has roots in the broader perspective of environmental health. Environmental health, therefore, is a highly impactful, yet often unrecognized, force in rural health.

This chapter focuses on three current environmental health issues of great importance to rural populations—environmental justice (and health inequity), gene–environment interactions, and climate change. The work is presented as a treatise on each subject but is in no way meant to be exhaustive. Rather, we touch on the critical issues facing rural populations and highlight pivotal points with case studies to guide further discussion.

ENVIRONMENTAL JUSTICE AND COMMUNITY-BASED PARTICIPATORY RESEARCH (CBPR)

CBPR: A Useful Tool for Addressing Environmental Justice Issues in Rural America

Because of the inherent population-based direct impact of many environmental exposures, community-led initiatives have particular power to address environmental health issues. CBPR is increasingly being recognized as a valuable research method for conducting research at the community level. It is defined as "a collaborative process that equitably involves all partners in the research process and recognizes the unique strengths that each brings. CBPR begins with a research topic of importance to the community with the aim of combining knowledge and action for social change to improve community health and eliminate health disparities."[23]

CBPR is an effective model used to engage communities in the research process, to increase sustainability of programs within communities, and to incorporate the true perspectives of the community when addressing complex public health issues. Research that is community based rather than community placed is more effective at translating research around complex public health issues.[24,25] Partners in the relationship contribute perspectives and share the responsibilities of formulating and conducting the research and dissemination of research findings to effect action.[26] When the community is instrumental in developing the research question, it is more likely that the community will be genuinely involved in the research and that it will lead to more meaningful action. [27]

CBPR has proven effective in several research studies, including determining the etiology of environmentally related diseases, exposure assessments, and interventions in marginalized communities. As such, it has also been effective for addressing community-level environmental justice, health equity, and for building environmental health awareness in general, but also specifically within rural communities.[28-30] Members of disenfranchised communities suffer disproportionate exposures from environmental hazards yet frequently do not receive information about the health consequences of exposure, principally in a form culturally relevant to the community. Working with rural communities in particular to develop the research strategy for addressing these issues is critical to creating sustainable change, promoting health equity and policy-related change given the unique social, cultural, and economic environment found in rural settings.

The NIEHS is committed to promoting and funding CBPR projects.[31] There are several successful CBPR studies around environmental health of rural communities, including studies focused on diabetes prevention and management,[32] lead poisoning in rural Native American children,[33] cigarette smoking among Native Americans,[34] environmental justice,[28] and malodors from hog production.[35]

Case Study: Concerned Citizens of Tillery, North Carolina, and the University of North Carolina

Hog production in North Carolina has grown over the past 20 years, to 9 million hogs in 2010.[26] Rural, African American, and low-income communities are disproportionately located near these intensive livestock operations (ILOs), resulting in adverse health effects including eye irritations and respiratory ailments,[37] cardiovascular issues,[38,39] mental health issues,[40] occupational hazards,[41] and malodor nuisances.[38,42-44] Environmental insults result from biological and chemical contaminants (including bacteria, viruses, nitrates, hydrogen sulfide, and endotoxins), particulate matter,[45,46] and noxious odors.

To help address this problem, a CBPR partnership between a local nongovernmental organization, Concerned Citizens of Tillery, and Dr. Steve Wing of University of North Carolina was created. The partnership, Community Health and Environmental Reawakening (CHER), has worked for over a decade to conduct community-based research to transform the disenfranchised communities impacted by hog industries in North Carolina. The activities of the CHER partnership, such as workshops, community presentations, and meetings, raised awareness about ILOs and built momentum for policy change.[41]

The CHER partnership is a model of successful CBPR partnerships to enact community-level change and health equity around several health outcomes. In collaboration with county government officials, CHER developed intensive livestock ordinances to impose stricter environmental controls on ILOs than state requirements. They facilitated collaborative research studies on economic, social, environmental, and health outcomes due to presence of ILOs in underrepresented, primarily minority communities.[41] The partnership has cooperated with regional universities to provide medical care (i.e., Tillery People's Clinic) and to conduct social and health equity research around environmental issues.[44] Using CBPR principles, CHER and its collaborators have advanced the health and well-being of the citizens of Tillery and surrounding communities.

Replacement of family farms with ILOs significantly impacts rural communities—family farms support local economies critical to sustaining rural communities[46]—and impedes valued traditions of rural life.[47,48] CBPR also elevates the voice of the community and all the issues concerned around a community-based issue. Dichotomous issues such as economic advancement for communities versus adverse health impacts are issues that emerge through the CBPR process not typically captured through traditional research.[49]

GENE–ENVIRONMENT INTERACTIONS: IMPORTANCE TO RURAL COMMUNITIES

As mentioned, rural and resource-poor communities experience disproportionate health outcomes that have been linked to environmental stressors. Genetic differences and susceptibilities may determine who will have worse health from short-term or protracted exposure to various environmental conditions compared to their nonexposed contemporaries. Heritable mutations from DNA damage and epigenetic modifications have the potential to affect disease development. In addition to the potential importance in the maintenance of genome stability, appropriate methylation of DNA is critical for imprinting, regulation of gene expression, and disease progression.

Genome-wide studies of adverse health impacts have shown that DNA modifications explain only a small proportion of heritability.[50] However, growing evidence indicates that interaction of environment and genotype is a potential mechanism for genetic susceptibility.[51] One specific environmental exposure that is impacting rural communities is air pollution. Air pollution is a complex, heterogeneous mixture; it varies in chemical, physical, and biological composition, and contains organic, oxidizing, gaseous, and PM components. The toxicity of the PM components is dependent upon size, surface area, concentration, and chemical composition.[52,53] Other factors that influence the toxicity of PM are geographical location and temperature.[54] As such, it remains difficult to pinpoint the exact component of air pollution reasonable for the observed health effects.

Many studies have shown the relevance of gene–environment interactions to understanding the impact of environmental toxicants specific to health outcomes. Specifically, growing evidence indicates that air pollution induces alterations in DNA methylation. Perera et al. recently showed that in-utero exposure to traffic-related pollution was associated with extensive DNA methylation changes in umbilical cord white blood cells at birth, including alterations of metabolic genes.[55] These associations have also been observed in rural communities, including the impact of organic dust on asthma atopy in children,[56] role of genetic and environmental factors on asthma morbidity in children living on rural farms,[51] gene–environment influences on adolescent substance use and negative behaviors and geographic residency (rural versus urban),[17] supportive family environments, changes in genetic characteristics, adverse physical health consequences,[57] and breast cancer.[58]

Inhalation of pesticides in the air in rural areas has been linked to gene polymorphisms that induce various negative health outcomes. One cohort study reported a statistically significant relationship between breast cancer risk and fungicides among women who had never used pesticides, but whose husbands reported exposure to a fungicide captan in farming applications in rural Iowa.[59] A more recent study was meticulously designed to explore the possible interaction between a polymorphism in CYP1A1, a cytochrome P450 enzyme that is involved in estrogen, toxin metabolism, and fungicide exposure.[60]

A recent study by Roychoudhury et al. reported the link between indoor air pollution, formed from biomass fuel burning, and the risk of airway carcinogenesis.[61] One hundred and eighty seven premenopausal women (median age 34 years) from rural eastern India were studied. All of these women exclusively cooked with biomass and were age-matched to 155 control women, who cooked with cleaner fuel. Sputum samples indicated that women using biomass fuel had a three-fold increased risk of developing metaplasia and a seven-fold higher risk of dysplasia in airway epithelial cells (AEC). Immuno-cytochemistry endpoints indicated an up-regulation, or increase, of phosphorylated proteins in AEC from women using biomass as compared with LPG users. Biomass users also had increases in various markers and precursors to DNA damage pathways, such as increases in reactive oxygen species (ROS) generation, decreased antioxidant enzymes, and superoxide dismutase (SOD) activity indicating oxidative stress via the Akt signal transduction pathway. This pathway is not only activated in response to DNA insult (DNA double-strand breaks [DSBs]) but also is responsible in DNA damage repair. As such, this study reports that cumulative exposure to biomass smoke increases the risk of cell mutagenesis leading to lung carcinogenesis. Additional research that will assist in answering these types of questions will ultimately contribute to understanding the distribution of health risk and policy implications.

IMPACT OF CLIMATE CHANGE
ON HEALTH OF RURAL COMMUNITIES

In the last century, global temperatures have increased by approximately 0.75°C, with an accelerated rate of warming of 0.18°C per decade (World Health Organization [WHO]). Greenhouse gases, such as ozone and carbon dioxide, trap heat close to the Earth's surface. While the greenhouse effect is actually an essential environmental process to sustain life on Earth, an abundance of this effect has led to environmental changes. With the range of potential atmospheric changes resulting from the warming of the atmosphere (i.e., positive radiative forcing), creating the potential for both warming and cooling events, the climate of regions around the Earth can change unpredictably. Such changes include thermal stress,[62] severe storms and weather events,[63,64] sea-level rise,[65,66] drought, increases in atmospheric ozone and particulate matter,[67] and increases in pestilence.[68] The U.N. Intergovernmental Panel of Climate Change (IPCC) uses the following definition: *"a change of climate which is attributed directly or indirectly to human activity that alters the composition of the global atmosphere and which is in addition to natural climate variability observed over comparable time periods."* Even with a lack of consensus among atmospheric scientists regarding the causes and impacts of climate change, there are a few facts on which they agree: (a) the Earth's temperature is rising, (2) at least part of that change is due to human activities, and (3) the impacts of climate change are already affecting human and ecological systems. With this warming, ecological changes are gradually occurring, which have some impact on health.

Climate Change Impacts on Rural Public Health

Effects of climate change will vary by population group and area of the globe[69] and will include impacts on public health, human rights, social equality, society, and economic well-being.[70] Public health professionals must prepare to manage and ameliorate the associated potential health burdens.[71] The poor and disenfranchised are suspected to be most affected by negative impacts of climate change; Hurricane Katrina is a pertinent example.[72] Poor nations and rural communities with limited resources and less resiliency compared to wealthier and/or urban communities have and are projected to continue to suffer even more from adverse outcomes of climate change.[73–75]

The public health response to climate change can be primary prevention (i.e., mitigation) or secondary prevention (i.e., adaptation). Adaptive capacity is defined by Eakin as "characteristics of an individual, household, or population group which enable it to alter or structurally reorganize its activities to diminish present threats to survival while enhancing its ability to address new risks."[76] To be successful at future adaptation efforts, adjustments in present-day livelihood choices and policy decisions that incorporate flexibility need to occur today.[76,77]

Scientists agree that many diseases are climate sensitive.[78] As such, climate change is suspected to contribute to the global burden of disease such as increases in diarrheal diseases, vector-borne diseases (spread and duration of breeding seasons), heat-related morbidity and mortality,[79] heart disease,[80] respiratory illness due to increased allergen counts and air pollutants,[67] low birth weight deliveries,[81] water- and food-borne disease,[82,83] and malnutrition.[78,84] Health effects are anticipated to vary by location and to be influenced by social determinants of health (e.g., poverty).[85] As a result, the health of rural, poor, underserved communities is projected to be significantly impacted by climate change in comparison to urban communities.[70] Adverse health impacts are estimated to outweigh the benefits that may accompany climate change (e.g., increased agricultural production in some areas and fewer winter depths due to increased winter temperatures), particularly for poorer areas, including rural areas.[86]

Extremes of temperature are expected with climate change, which is projected to increase respiratory and cardiovascular illness, particularly among sensitive populations (e.g., the elderly).[87] Mortality increases when temperatures are elevated primarily due to cardiovascular, cerebrovascular, and respiratory diseases.[88] High temperatures would also increase smog formation.[89] The number of weather-related natural disasters has tripled since the 1960s.[84] Flood-related deaths are often the result of rapid-rising flood waters[90] and mobilization of health hazards.[91] These disasters have destroyed homes, cost lives, created mental distress, destabilized food systems, and strained municipal and health services.[84] Climate change is also expected to alter transmission of vector- and rodent-borne infectious diseases due to increased temperatures, altered humidity, soil moisture, and sea level rise.[92]

Disease prevalence is a major climate change health concern. The WHO estimates that, by 2030, direct damage costs to health from climate change will be $2 billion to $4 billion per year.[84] Major public health concerns include increased injuries and fatalities related to increases in and severity of weather extremes; changes in vector spread and infectious diseases; contamination of food and water; increased allergies and respiratory and cardiovascular disease; and changes in food production.[71] Less obvious impacts of climate change include poor mental health and economic impacts of population dislocation.[71]

Given the uncertain balance between positive and negative outcomes on facets of human existence (e.g., social, human, institutional, natural, economic), great uncertainties exist around impacts on fragile communities. The sustainability of rural communities depends on their ability to adapt to and/or mitigate the environmental vicissitudes of climate change.[93] A study in rural Canada projected that rural communities would be hard hit by climate change[93]: reduced agricultural production, water shortages, and soil erosion. Causes included increased drought, extreme weather events, and pest infestations. Given that many rural communities rely on an agricultural economy, have a strained relationship with the health care system, and have reduced adaptation and mitigation options (in part due to a perception of no risk), they are projected to be especially hit hard by climate change.[94] A focus on risk communication and risk management is critical for rural communities in preparing them for climate change impacts and managing adverse health effects.

Point of Interest: Impact of Climate Change on Mental Health of Rural Communities

One health impact often overlooked in climate change discourses is its impact on mental health of communities. Humans obtain sustenance and psychological and emotional well-being from the environment.[95] Since research illustrates that engaging with the environment promotes mental health,[96] loss or destruction of natural assets will have adverse psychological and physical impacts.[97] For instance, climate change impacts—water shortages due to droughts, adverse economic impacts, wetland loss—compounded by other ecological issues unique to rural communities (e.g., geographical isolation, community erosion) result in emotional distress such as psychoterratic illness,*,[95,98] posttraumatic stress disorder,[99] and increased long-term psychiatric morbidity.[100] Studies in rural Australia report significant distress and adverse emotional impact from conditions such as drought and economic hardship due to drought.[100] Given the estimated increase in drought conditions with continued climate change and the dependence of many rural communities on the environment for livelihood and cultural identity, the burden of psychological illness in rural areas can be anticipated to increase.[100,101]

CONCLUSION

From the extremes of weather causing human injuries, hyper- and hypothermia, droughts resulting in famine, increases in respiratory ailments, vector- and water-borne diseases, and human displacement and death, climate is expected to continue to change with time[102] and continue to influence public health.[103,104] Preventing human health morbidity and mortality is the main justification for taking adaptive or mitigation actions on climate change.[78] Frumkin suggests implementing public health strategies for moderating impacts of climate change, including monitoring health status through surveillance, informing and educating communities, mobilizing community partnerships, and linking communities to health services.[71] These strategies are particularly important for rural communities at greater risk of adverse impacts from climate change.

Human exposure to environmental toxins is of increasing concern to communities, as evidence mounts about environmentally attributable diseases. This chapter focused on three emerging and paramount environmental health issues impacting rural populations—environmental justice, gene environment, and climate change. One must recognize, however, the vast breadth of environmental health and that, therefore, it is impossible to touch on all current issues, including aspects such as risk assessment and exposome science, built environment, occupational exposures, and industrial fracking. The fundamental message of this chapter is the critical nature of a true understanding of the facets of rurality influencing the environmental health of rural populations and that understanding environmental health

---

* Albrecht et al.[98] defines psychoterratic illness as "earth-related mental illness where people's mental wellbeing (psyche) is threatened by the severing of 'healthy' links between themselves and their home/territory."

PACKING SLIP

SPRINGER PUBLISHING COMPANY
11 W 42nd Street
New York, NY 10036-8002
t: 212 431-4370
fx: 212 941-7842
www.springerpub.com

760143

	Page	Customer ID	Invoice ID
	1	2387347	760143
PO #		Ref Date	Invoice Date
		6/21/2016	6/21/2016

Sold To:
Linda Nelms
1720 Old Newport Hwy
Sevierville, TN 37876

Ship To:
Linda Nelms
Walters State Comm Coll
1720 Old Newport Hwy
Sevierville, TN 37876 5100

Customer PO #	Rep	Warehouse	Shipped Via	Terms	Ordered By
		2 PSSC	USPS STD B SPEC		

ProdCode	Title	List Price	Ordered	Shipped	Corrected Shipped
978-0-8261-0894-4	Rural Public Health	75.00	1	1	
0-8261-0894-6					

ALL PRODUCTS MANUFACTURED IN THE U.S.A

Please send all returns to:

Publishers Storage and Shipping Corporation
46 Development Road
Fitchburg, MA 01420

All returns send to our New York address will be refused.
For any Customer Service questions, please call toll free: 1-877-687-7476

THIS IS NOT A BILL.

Total Units Ordered	Total Units Shipped This Warehouse
1	1

reight: _____

y: _____

in its broadest nature, preventive health, is imperative for making positive change in the rural environmental health.

RESOURCES

Funding Opportunities

Funding agencies of greatest relevance to environmental health are numerous. Below is a nonexhaustive list:

- National Institute of Environmental Health Sciences (http://www.niehs.nih.gov)
- United States Environmental Protection Agency (www.epa.gov)
- United States Department of Agriculture (www.usda.gov)
- National Environmental Education Foundation (http://www.neefusa.org)
- Water Environment Federation (www.wef.org)
- National Science Foundation (www.nsf.gov)
- Oak Ridge Institute for Science and Education (www.orise.orau.gov)
- Health Effects Institute (www.healtheffects.org)

Organizations/Groups/Websites

- National Institute of Environmental Health Sciences (http://www.niehs.nih.gov)
- United States Environmental Protection Agency (www.epa.gov)
- United States Department of Agriculture (www.usda.gov)
- National Center for Environmental Research (www.epa.gov/ncer)
- USDA National Resources Conservation Service (www.nrcs.usda.gov)
- Intergovernmental Panel on Climate Change (www.ipcc.ch)
- National Environmental Health Association (www.neha.org)
- World Health Organization, Public Health and Environment (www.who.int/phe/en)
- World Health Organization, Health and Environment Linkages Initiative (www.who.int/heli/en)
- Agency for Toxic Substances and Disease Registry (www.atsdr.cdc.gov)
- National Environmental Public Health Tracking Program (www.cdc.gov/nceh/tracking)

Toolkits

- World Health Organization, Health and Environment Linkages Initiative, Scientific Assessment Tools (www.who.int/heli/tools/en)
- United States National Library of Medicine TOXNET (http://www.toxnet.nlm.nih.gov)

REFERENCES

1. Bullard R, Mohai P, Saha R, Wright B. Toxic wastes and races at twenty: why race still matters after all of these years. *J Environ Law.* 2008;38:371–411.
2. Payne-Sturges D, Gee GC. National environmental health measures for minority and low-income populations: tracking social disparities in environmental health. *Environ Res.* 2006;102(2):154–171.

3. Strickland J, Strickland, DL. Barriers to preventive health services for minority households in the rural south. *J Rural Health*. 1996;12(3):206–217.
4. Smith K, Humphreys J, Wilson M. Addressing the health disadvantage of rural populations: how does epidemiological evidence inform rural health policies and research? *Aust J Rural Health*. 2008;16:56–66.
5. Gerrard CE. Farmers' occupational health: cause for concern, cause for action. *J Adv Nurs*.1998;28:155–163.
6. Dejardin O, Bouvier A, Herbert C, et al. Social and geographic disparities in access to reference care site for patients with colorectal cancer in France. *Br J Cancer*. 2005;92(10):1842–1845.
7. Robertson R, Campbell N, Smith S, et al. Factors influencing time from presentation to treatment of colorectal and breast cancer in urban and rural areas. *Br J Cancer*. 2004;90(8):1479–1485.
8. Luque JS, Reyes-Ortiz C, Marella P, et al. Mobile farm clinic outreach to address health conditions among Latino migrant farmworkers in Georgia. *J Agromedicine*. 2012;17(4):386–397.
9. Hosler A. Retail food availability, obesity, and cigarette smoking in rural communities. *J Rural Health*. 2009;25(2):203–210.
10. Brownson R, Hoehner C, Day K, Forsyth A, Sallis J. Measuring the built environment for physical activity: state of the science. *Am J Prev Med*. 2009;36(suppl 4): S99–S123.
11. Hiott A, Grzywacz J, Davis S, Quandt S, Arcury T. Migrant farmworker stress: mental health implications. *J Rural Health*. 2008;24(1):32–39.
12. Humphreys J, Hegney D, Lipscombe J, Gregory G, Chater B. Whither rural health? Reviewing a decade of progress in rural health. *Aust J Rural Health*. 2002;10:2–14.
13. Gamm L, Hutchison L. Rural health priorities in America: where you stand depends on where you sit. *J Rural Health*. 2003:19(3):209–213.
14. Ahn S, Burdine J, Smith M, Ory M, Phillips C. Residential rurality and oral health disparities: influences of contextual and individual factors. *J Prim Prev*. 2011;32(1):29–41.
15. Hermstad A, Swan D, Kegler M, Barnette J, Glanz K. Individual and environmental correlates of dietary fat intake in rural communities: a structural equation model analysis. *Soc Sci Med*. 2010;71(1):93–101.
16. Hamman R. Genetic and environmental determinants of non-insulin-dependent-diabetes mellitus (NIDDM). *Diabetes Metab Rev*. 2009;8(4):287–338.
17. Legrand L, Keyes M, McGue M, Iacono W, Krueger R. Rural environments reduce the genetic influence on adolescent substance use and rule-breaking behavior. *Psychol Med*. 2008;38(9):1341–1350.
18. Physicians for Social Responsibility. *In Harm's Way: Toxic Threats to Child Development*. Boston, MA: Author; 2000.
19. Lutfiyya M, Lipsky M, Wisdom-Behounek J, Inpanbutr-Martinkus M. Is rural residency a risk factor for overweight and obesity for U.S. children? *Obesity*. 2007:15(9):2348–2356.
20. Gomez S, Glaser S, McClure L, et al. The California neighborhoods data system: a new resource for examining the impact of neighborhood characteristics on cancer incidence and outcomes in populations. *Cancer Causes Control*. 2011;22(4):631–647.
21. Semenza J, Menne B. Climate change and infectious diseases in Europe. *Lancet Infect Dis*. 2009;9(6):365–375.

22. Johnson G, Lu X. Neighborhood-level built environment and social characteristics associated with serious childhood motor vehicle occupant injuries. *Health Place.* 2011;17(4):902–910.

23. Kellogg Foundation Community Health Scholars Program. Overview. http://www.kellogghealthscholars.org/about/community.cfm.

24. Jacquez F, Vaughn L, Wagner E. Youth as partners, participants or passive recipients: a review of children and adolescents in community-based participatory research (CBPR). *Am J Community Psychol.* 2013;51(1-2):176–189.

25. Horowitz C, Robinson M, Seifer S. Community-based participatory research from the margin to the mainstream: are researchers prepared? *Circulation.* 2009;119(19):2633–2642.

26. Israel BA, Schultz AJ, Parker EA, et al. Critical issues in developing and following community based participatory research principles. In: Minkler M, Wallerstein N, eds. *Community-Based Participatory Research for Health.* San Francisco, CA; Jossey-Bass; 2003:53–76.

27. Cook WK. Integrating research and action: a systematic review of community-based participatory research to address health disparities in environmental and occupational health in the United States. *J Epidemiol Community Health.* 2008;62(8):668–676.

28. Minkler M, Vasquez V, Tajik M, Petersen D. Promoting environmental justice through community-based participatory research: the role of community and partnership capacity. *Health Educ Behav.* 2006;35(1):119–137.

29. O'Fallon LR, Dearry A. Community-based participatory research as a tool to advance environmental health sciences. *Environ Health Perspect.* 2002;110(suppl 2):155–159.

30. O'Fallon LR, Dearry A. Commitment of the national institute of environmental health sciences to community-based participatory research for rural health. *Environ Health Perspect.* 2001;109(suppl 3):469–473.

31. O'Fallon LR, Wolfle GM, Brown D, Dearry A, Olden K. Strategies for setting a national research agenda that is responsive to community needs. *Environ Health Perspect.* 2003;111(16):1855–1860.

32. Parker EA, Eng E, Laraia B, et al. Coalition building for prevention: lessons learned from the North Carolina community-based public health initiative. *J Public Health Manag Pract.* 1998;4(2):25–36.

33. Kegler M, Malcoe L. Results from a lay-health advisor intervention to prevent lead poisoning among rural native American children. *Am J Health Promot.* 2004;94(10):1730–1735.

34. Daley CM, Greiner KA, Nazir N, et al. All nations breath of life: using community-based participatory research to address health disparities in cigarette smoking among American Indians. *Ethn Dis.* 2010;20(4):334–338.

35. Wing S. Social responsibility and research ethics in community-driven studies of industrialized hog production. *Environ Health Perspect.* 2005;110(5):437–444.

36. Agricultural Statistics. Hogs: inventory and value. http://www.ncagr.com/stats/livestock/hoginv.htm.

37. Bullers S. Environmental stressors, perceived control, and health: the case of residents near large-scale hog farms in eastern North Carolina. *Hum Ecol.* 2005;33:1–16.

38. Wing S, Horton R, Rose K. Air pollution from industrial swine operations and blood pressure of neighboring residents. *Environ Health Perspect.* 2013;121(1):92–96.

39. Nagai M, Wada M, Usui N, Tanaka A, Hasebe Y. Pleasant odors attenuate the blood pressure increase during rhythmic handgrip in humans. *Neurosci Lett.* 2000;289(3):227–229.

40. Horton R, Wing S, Marshall S, Brownley K. Malodor as a trigger of stress and negative mood in neighbors of industrial hog operations. *Am J Public Health.* 2009;99(suppl 3): S610–S615.

41. Wing S. Social responsibility and research ethics in community-driven studies of industrialized hog production. *Environ Health Perspect.* 2002;110(5):437–444.

42. O'Connor A, Auvermann B, Bickett-Weddle D, et al. The association between proximity to animal feeding operations and community health: a systematic review. *PLoS One.* 2010;5(3):e9530–e9530.

43. Farquhar S, Wing S. Methodological and ethical considerations in environmental justice research. In: Minkler M, Wallerstein N, eds. *Community-Based Participatory Research for Health.* 2nd ed. San Francisco, CA: Jossey-Bass; 2008.

44. Tajik M, Minkler M. Environmental justice research and action: a case study in political economy and community-academic collaboration. *Int Q Community Health Educ.* 2007;26(3):213–231.

45. Schinasi L, Horton R, Guidry V, Wing S, Marshall S, Morland K. Air pollution, lung function, and physical symptoms in communities near concentrated swine feeding operations. *Epidemiology.* 2011;22(2):208–215.

46. Cole D, Todd L, Wing S. Concentrated swine feeding operations and public health: a review of occupational and community health effects. *Environ Health Perspect.* 2000;108(8):685–699.

47. Tajik M, Muhammad N, Lowman A, Thu K, Wing S, Grant G. Impact of odor from industrial hog operations on daily living activities. *New Solut.* 2008;18:193–205.

48. Thu K. Industrial agriculture, democracy, and the future. In: Ervin A, Holtslander C, Qualman D, Sawa R, eds. *Beyond Factor Farming: Corporate Hog Barns and the Threat to Public Health, the Environment, and Rural Communities.* Saskatoon, Saskatchewan, Canada: Canadian Center for Policy Alternatives; 2003:9–28.

49. Snell M. Downwind in Mississippi: the struggle to keep a community from going to the hogs. *Sierra Magazine.* March/April 2001:22–26.

50. Manolio TA, Collins FS, Cox NJ, et al. Finding the missing heritability of complex diseases. *Nature.* 2009;461:747–753.

51. Ege MJ, Strachan DP, Cookson CM, et al. Gene-environment interaction for childhood asthma and exposure to farming in Central Europe. *Am Acad Allergy Asthma Immunol.* 2010;127:138–144.

52. United States Environmental Protection Agency. www.epa.gov. 2004.

53. Araujo JA, Nel AE. Particulate matter and atherosclerosis: role of particle size, composition and oxidative stress. *Part Fibre Toxicol.* 2009;6:24.

54. Araujo JA. Particulate air pollution, systemic oxidative stress, inflammation, and atherosclerosis. *Air Qual Atmos Health.* 2010;4(1):79–93.

55. Perera FP, Wang S, Vishnevetsky J, et al. Polycyclic aromatic hydrocarbons-aromatic DNA adducts in cord blood and behavior scores in New York City children. *Environ Health Perspect.* 2011;119(8):1176–1181.

56. Schwartz D. Gene-environment interactions and airway disease in children. *Pediatrics.* 2009;123:S151–S159.

57. Brody GH, Yu T, Chen Y, et al. Supportive family environments, genes that confer sensitivity, and allostatic load among rural African American emerging adults: a prospective analysis. *J Fam Psychol.* 2013;27(1):22–29.

58. Ashley-Martin J, VanLeeuwen J, Cribb A, Andreou P, Guernsey JR. Breast cancer risk, fungicide exposure and CYP1A1*2A gene-environment interactions in a province-wide case control study in Prince Edward Island, Canada. *Int J Environ Res Public Health.* 2012;9(5):1846–1858.

59. Engel LS, Hill DA, Hoppin JA. Pesticide use and breast cancer risk among farmers' wives in the Agricultural Health Study. *Am J Epidemiol.* 2005;161:121–135.

60. Cribb AE, Knight MJ, Dryer D, Guernsey J, Hender K, Tesch M, Saleh TM. Role of polymorphic human cytochrome p450 enzymes in estrone oxidation. *Cancer Epidemiol Biomarkers Prev.* 2006;15(3):551–558.

61. Roychoudhury S, Mondal NK, Mukherjee S, Dutta A, Siddique S, Ray MR. Activation of protein kinase B (PKB/Akt) and risk of lung cancer among rural women in India who cook with biomass fuel. *Toxicol Appl Pharmacol.* 2011;259(1):45–53.

62. Meehl GA, Tebaldi C. More intense, more frequent and longer lasting heat waves in the 21st century. *Science.* 2004;305(5686):994–997.

63. Piekle RA, Downton MW. Precipitation and damaging floods: trends in the United States, 1932–1997. *J Clim.* 2000;13:3625–3627.

64. Kunkel KE, Pielke RA Jr., Changnon SA. Temporal fluctuations in weather and climate extremes that cause economic and human health impacts: a review. *Bull Am Meteorol Soc.* 1999;80(6):1077–1098.

65. Rignot E, Kanagaratnam P. Changes in the velocity structure of the Greenland Ice Sheet. *Science.* 2006;311:963–964.

66. McCarthy J, et al, eds. *Climate Change 2001: Impacts, Adaptations, and Vulnerability.* Contribution of Working Group II to the Third Assessment Report of the Intergovernmental Panel on Climate Change. New York, NY: Cambridge University Press; 2001.

67. Bernard SM, Samet JM, Grambsch A, Ebi KL, Romieu I. The potential impacts of climate variability and change on air pollution-related health effects in the United States. *Environ Health Perspect.* 2001;109(suppl 2):199–209.

68. Subak S. Effects of climate on variability in Lyme disease incidence in the northeastern United States. *Am J Epidemiol.* 2003;157(6):531–538.

69. Longstreth J. Public health consequences of global climate change in the United States—some regions may suffer disproportionately. *Environ Health Perspect.* 1999;107:169–179.

70. Morello-Frosch R, Pastor M, Sadd J, Shonkoff SB. *The Climate Gap: Inequalities in How Climate Change Hurts Americans & How to Close the Gap.* The Climate Gap Report. Available at: http://college.usc.edu/geography/ESPE/perepub.html. 2010.

71. Frumkin H, Hess J, Luber G, Malilay J, McGeehin M. Climate change: the public health response. *Am J Public Health.* 2008;98(3):435–445.

72. Katrina, climate change and the poor. *CMAJ.* 2005;173:837–839.

73. Adger WN, Paavola J, Huq S, Mace MJ, eds. *Fairness in Adaptation to Climate Change.* Cambridge, MA: MIT Press; 2006.

74. Claussen E, McNeilly L. *Equity and Climate Change: The Complex Elements of Global Fairness.* Arlington, VA: Pew Center on Global Climate Change; 2001.

75. Jamieson D. Climate change and global environmental justice. In: Miller CA, Edwards PN, eds. *Changing the Atmosphere: Expert Knowledge and Environmental Governance.* Cambridge, MA: MIT Press; 2001: 287–307.

76. Eakin H. Institutional change, climate risk, and rural vulnerability: cases from Central Mexico. *World Dev.* 2005;33(11):1923–1938.

77. Ebi KL, Kovats RS, Menne B. An approach for assessing human health vulnerability and public health interventions to adapt to climate change. *Environ Health Perspect*. 2006;114:1930–1934.

78. Kovats RS, Campbell-Lendrum D, Matthies F. Climate change and human health: estimating avoidable deaths and disease. *Risk Analysis*. 2005; 25(6):1409–1418.

79. McGeehin MA, Mirabelli M. The potential impacts of climate variability and change on temperature-related morbidity and mortality in the United States. *Environ Health Perspect*. 2001;109(suppl 2):185–189.

80. Blindauer KM, Rubin C, Morse DL, McGeehin M. The 1996 New York blizzard: impact on noninjury emergency visits. *Am J Emerg Med*. 1999;17(1):23–27.

81. Chen L, Yang W, Jennison BL, Goodrich A, Omaye ST. Air pollution and birth weight in northern Nevada, 1991–1999. *Inhal Toxicol*. 2002;14(2):141–157.

82. D'Souza RM, Becker NG, Hall G, Moodie KBA. Does ambient temperature affect foodborne disease? *Epidemiology*. 2004;15(1):86–92.

83. Rose JB, Epstein PR, Lipp EK, Sherman BH, Bernard SM, Patz JA. Climate variability and change in the United States: potential impacts on water and foodborne diseases caused by microbiologic agents. *Environ Health Perspect*. 2001;109(suppl 2):211–221.

84. World Health Organization, Public Health and Environment. Available at: www .who.int/phe/en/. 2003.

85. Basu R, Samet JM. Relation between elevated ambient temperature and mortality: a review of the epidemiologic evidence. *Epidemiol Rev*. 2002;24(2):190–202.

86. McMichael AJ, Confalonieri UE, Githeko AK, et al. Human health. In: Metz B, Davidson OR, Martens WJ, van Rooijen SNM, McGrory LVW, eds. *Methodological and Technological Issues in Technology Transfer*. Cambridge: Cambridge University Press; 2001:331–347.

87. Johnson H, Kovats RS, McGregor GR, et al. The impact of the 2003 heatwave on mortality and hospital admissions in England. *Health Stat Q*. 2005;25:6–11.

88. Le Tertre A, Lefranc A, Eilstein D, et al. Impact of 2003 heat wave on all-cause mortality in 9 French cities. *Epidemiology*. 2006;17(1):75–79.

89. Peel J, Haeuber R., Garcia V, Russell A, Neas L. Impact of nitrogen and climate change interactions on ambient air pollution and human health. *Biogeochemistry*. 2012. 1–14.

90. French J, Ing R, Von Allmen S, Wood R. Mortality from flash floods: a review of National Weather Service reports, 1969–1981. *Public Health Rep*. 1983;98(6):584–588.

91. Ahern M, Kovats RS, Wilkinson P, Few R, Matthies F. Global health impacts of floods: epidemiologic evidence. *Epidemiol Rev*. 2005;27:36–46.

92. Haines A, Kovats RS, Campbell-Lendrum D, Corvalan C. Climate change and human health: impacts, vulnerability and public health. *Public Health*. 2006;120(7):585–596.

93. Wall E, Marzall K. Adaptive capacity for climate change in Canadian rural communities. *Local Environ*. 2006;11(4):373–397.

94. Davidson D, Williamson T, Parkins J. Understanding climate change risk and vulnerability in northern forest-based communities. *Canadian J Forest Res*. 2003;33:2252–2261.

95. Maller C, Townsend M, Pryor A, Brown P, St Leger L. Healthy nature healthy people: 'contact with nature' as an upstream health promotion intervention for populations. *Health Promot Int*. 2005;21(1):45–54.

96. Townsend M. Feel blue? Touch green! Participation in forest/woodland management as a treatment for depression. *Urban for Urban Greening*. 2006;5(3):111–120.

97. Scull J. Reconnecting with nature. *Encompass*. 2001;5:1–5.

98. Albrecht G, Sartore GM, Connor L, et al. Solastalgia: The distress caused by environmental change. *Australas Psychiatry.* 2007;15(suppl 1):S95–S98.
99. Hajat S, Ebi KL, Kovats S, Menne B, Edwards S, Naines A. The human health consequences of flooding in Europe and the implications for public health: a review of the evidence. *Appl Environ Sci Public Health.* 2003;1(1):13–21.
100. Sartore GM, Kelly B, Stain H, Albrecht G, Higginbotham N. Control, uncertainty, and expectations for the future: a qualitative study of the impact of drought on a rural Australian community. *Rural Remote Health.* 2008(3);8:950.
101. Campbell D, Stafford Smith M, Davies J, Kuipers P, Wakerman J, McGregor MJ. Responding to health impacts of climate change in the Australian desert. *Rural Remote Health.* 2008;8(3):1008.
102. Wigley TML. The climate change commitment. *Science.* 2005; 438:310–317.
103. Haines A, Patz JA. Health effects of climate change. *JAMA.* 2004;291(1):99–103.
104. Patz JA, Campbell-Lendrum D, Holloway T, Foley JA. Impact of regional climate change on health. *Nature.* 2005;438(7066):310–317.

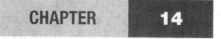

Rural Minority Health:
Race, Ethnicity, and Sexual Orientation

Jacob C. Warren, K. Bryant Smalley, Marylen Rimando,
K. Nikki Barefoot, Arthur Hatton, and Kayla LeLeux-LaBarge

Although rural populations in general face disparities in a variety of outcomes discussed throughout this book, minority groups are even more impacted by health disparities within rural areas; for instance, rural African Americans have a higher prevalence of certain chronic diseases (e.g., diabetes and heart disease) and a higher age-adjusted death rate from those diseases than rural and urban Whites, and even urban African Americans.[1] Differences in both disease prevalence and outcome occur—often with outcome-linked disparities tied back to: (a) later presentation within the course of an illness, and (b) lower access to health care services.

When considered through the lens of the multiple minority effect, minorities residing in rural settings are functionally impacted by two over-lapping disparity processes; that is, the disparities associated with being rural, which are presented throughout this book, in addition to disparities associated with being a member of the particular minority group. This dual impact results in not only additive impact, but sometimes exponential impact in health outcomes. For example, diabetes rates are higher in both rural groups and in African American groups, leading rural African Americans to have higher rates of diabetes than both the general rural population and the general African American population.[1] Such effects make rural minority health a critical issue to investigate. They also demonstrate the strong need to develop innovative public health interventions to address these effects; however, such research is unfortunately very limited.

We describe four specific minority groups within rural areas: African American; Hispanic; lesbian, gay, bisexual, and transgender (LGBT); and American Indian/Alaskan Native. As mentioned, the literature is unfortunately limited when it comes to rural subgroup health; therefore, much of the information is regional or even anecdotal, and certain other rural groups (e.g., rural Asian populations) do not even have robust enough literature to present in the current chapter. We hope that this chapter not only helps to bring together the information in a way that provides a useful resource, but also helps to highlight the stark need for additional research in this area.

RURAL AFRICAN AMERICAN HEALTH

In the United States, African Americans make up 13.6% of the population (43.9 million), and as this number continues to increase, so do the health disparities they experience.[2,3] Within the overall African American community, key disparities include hypertension, obesity, lack of physical activity, and maternal/child health.[4] These health concerns are exacerbated for African Americans living in rural areas, as unique geographic and cultural obstacles serve to further impede the ability to obtain adequate health care.

Rural African Americans comprise approximately 8.2% of all rural inhabitants,[5] with representation concentrated in the rural South. When considering overall barriers to health, rural African American adults and children are less likely to have health insurance, have lower rates of health care visits, and are less likely to have a personal physician.[5-7] African Americans living in rural areas are also more likely to be obese and are less likely to meet Centers for Disease Control and Prevention (CDC) recommendations for moderate physical activity.[8]

Cardiovascular Disease

Heart disease is the leading cause of death across the nation, and African Americans and other racial and ethnic minorities are particularly affected by heart-related disorders (e.g., heart failure, heart attack).[9] Approximately 600,000 individuals die each year from coronary heart disease,[10] and African Americans are about 30% more likely to die from this disease when compared to White men.[11] Some risk factors that are prevalent for rural African Americans in particular are diabetes, poor diet, alcohol use, lack of physical activity,[10] high blood pressure, and tobacco use.[6] Other factors such as poverty are also directly linked to rates of heart disease, indicating systematic barriers to both help-seeking behaviors as well as receipt of adequate care postdiagnosis.[9,12]

Diabetes

As discussed in Chapter 11, diabetes is a leading health concern across rural groups, and is the seventh leading cause of death in the overall U.S. population.[12] There are approximately 4.9 million African Americans with diagnosed and undiagnosed diabetes,[13] and rural African Americans are 20% more likely to be diagnosed with diabetes than are urban residents.[9] Unfortunately, rural African Americans also have poorer diabetes disease control when compared to their urban peers, leading to increased rates of complications and severe sequelae.[14–15]

Stroke

Strokes are responsible for the death of approximately 795,000 individuals each year, making it the fourth leading cause of death in the nation.[16] African Americans experience strokes 60% more frequently and with increased severity as compared to other racial and ethnic groups.[17] Some risk factors for having a stroke include high blood pressure, smoking, being overweight, and being diagnosed with diabetes,[16] most of which are elevated in rural African American populations. Rural African Americans suffer from strokes at such increased rates that the southern states, in which many rural African Americans reside, have been nicknamed "The Stroke Belt."[18] Researchers have also recently uncovered treatment approach inadequacies, namely, the underutilization of evidence-based treatments with minorities in rural areas, which is believed to exacerbate negative health outcomes for rural African Americans.[19]

Hypertension

The CDC reported hypertension as a primary cause for about 348,000 deaths in 2008,[11] and estimates that about 36 million individuals nationwide do not appropriately manage their blood pressure. African Americans are 40% more likely to have hypertension than their White counterparts,[20] and the National Institutes of Health[21] suggest genetic risk factors combine with established risks such as obesity, poor diet, and physical inactivity to sustain this disparity. African Americans living in rural communities are found to have less control of diastolic blood pressure across race and geographic location,[22] making them the group most impacted by poor hypertension control.

Research has identified barriers to adherence as playing a significant role in hypertension disparities among rural African Americans.[23] When considering health promotion efforts surrounding hypertension, adherence is influenced by much more than simple individual choice; as such, adherence improvement efforts must be viewed within the cultural context of rural African Americans (impacted by issues of poverty, access to care, availability of transportation, and general health insurance coverage). Some recommendations for decreasing blood pressure-related problems include increasing treatment sensitivity when working with rural African Americans with hypertension and using both appropriate educational approaches regarding treatment nonadherence and directly addressing specific barriers that may be influencing an individual's ability to adhere.[22]

Cancer

Cancer is the second leading cause of death in the United States.[24]African Americans have the highest prevalence of death for most cancers, as well as the shortest postdiagnosis life expectancy when compared to other racial and ethnic groups.[25] The most commonly diagnosed cancers in African Americans include prostate, colorectal, and lung for men; and breast, lung, and colorectal for women.[25] Individuals living in rural areas face barriers to preventive care (such as early-detection services and availability and access to necessary medications and treatment services) that impact all rural residents, but in particular rural African Americans.[9, 24] African American adults over the age of 50 living in rural areas are less likely to be screened for colorectal cancer,[9] and this pattern is seen for other cancers as well. Themes concerning prostate cancer prevention identified among rural African Americans include a perceived lack of importance of prevention, mistrust of the health care system, and perceived threats to manhood.[26] This suggests the need to create and implement cultural adaptations of health care provision and education to address such attitudes. Similar cancer disparities are observed in African American women living in rural areas, as they have the highest breast cancer mortality rates when compared to other racial and ethnic populations.[27] Wilson-Anderson and colleagues suggest addressing this gap in rural care by training community members to help implement and maintain positive breast cancer-related health behaviors[27]; this can be particularly effective in working within African American communities that have traditionally been viewed as having a high sense of community and interconnectedness.

Recommendations

For rural African American communities, community-based settings like churches have been found to engender higher participation and retention rates for health promotion programs.[8,28] Other studies identify general psychoeducational approaches in rural African American communities as a method to increase awareness about prevention of chronic disease and promote positive gains in overall health.[29,30] These recommendations have promise for decreasing health disparities for rural African Americans. Unfortunately, these recommendations are inappropriate for such unique health challenges as ability to access health care due to geographic restrictions, availability of health care providers, health insurance, and poverty. The development of culturally sensitive interventions should take these underlying components into account, and also view these disparities through a larger health equity and social justice lens. Continuing to expand the research and overall understanding of the complex interplay of environmental, community, and geographic influences on African American health will allow for integrative intervention approaches that address context-specific health behaviors and practices.

HEALTH DISPARITIES AMONG RURAL HISPANICS

Hispanics are the fastest growing population in rural America; since 1980 the growth of this population outpaces other major racial and ethnic groups. Between 1980 and 2000, the Hispanic population increased from 1.4 to 2.7 million in rural America.[31] Hispanics comprise 6.3% of the national rural population and about 3.2 million Hispanics live in rural America.[32] Based on projected growth rates, Hispanics will become the largest minority group in rural America by about 2025.[31]

The Hispanic population in rural America is very diverse, comprised of many nationalities from Mexico, Latin America, the Caribbean, and Spain.[32] Hispanics who recently moved to rural counties are more likely than other rural residents to be younger and male.[31] They may relocate to rural areas for employment opportunities to support their families in their home country. Rural Hispanic men have employment rates similar to rural White men; however, Hispanic women have a 10% lower employment rate than White women.[31] Rural Hispanics are more likely to work in lower skilled jobs such as agriculture, construction, and manufacturing and are less likely to have occupations requiring college degrees.[31] They also have high levels of employment without benefits, such as health insurance.[32]

Rural Hispanics have the lowest educational attainment of racial and ethnic groups.[33] Half of Hispanics did not graduate from high school and only 6.5% were college graduates in 2000.[31] Recent immigrants often originate from a poor, rural community with few available educational or career options. Limited proficiency in English-language skills may also be a disadvantage in rural areas—over 50% of immigrant Mexican Americans are poor English speakers compared with 11.6% of nonimmigrant Mexican Americans.[34] This combination of low-paying jobs, limited education, and limited English proficiency may present unique challenges for rural Hispanics with a broad-sweeping impact on health. This section describes leading health issues such as diabetes, heart disease, stroke, hypertension, and cancer among rural Hispanics, contributing factors to health disparities among rural Hispanics, and offers recommendations to improve health and eliminate disparities among rural Hispanic populations.

Diabetes

Diabetes is a leading health issue among rural Hispanics. In a national sample, rural Hispanics had a significantly greater prevalence of diagnosed diabetes (8.2%) than urban Whites (4.6%), rural Whites (6.5%), or urban Hispanics (4.5%).[35] The overall diabetes prevalence, based on self-report and glucose testing, was 21.3% in a rural Arizona sample.[36] Previous research reported the disproportionate burden of diabetes among rural Hispanics in the United States–Mexico border region[37-39]; however, similar research in other geographic areas is limited.

When considering the design of diabetes education for rural Hispanics, Hispanic women reported more general knowledge of diabetes as compared to Hispanic men in rural Washington State,[40] indicating the presence of a gender gap in health education for rural Hispanics. Rural Hispanics were *significantly* less likely to manage their diabetes with diet and exercise than rural non-Hispanic Whites (36% vs. 61.3%), indicating management behaviors are not adequately addressed within rural communities.[41] Even within rural communities, Hispanic diabetics report less engagement with diabetes education/classes (47.6% of rural Hispanics reported attending classes compared to 57.2% of rural non-Hispanic Whites).[41] Although interventions have been developed for urban Hispanics, diabetes education programs for Hispanics in rural areas remain limited.[37, 40]

Heart Disease, Stroke, and Hypertension

In addition to diabetes, there is a burden of hypertension, heart disease, and stroke among rural Hispanics. Undiagnosed hypertension is significantly higher among rural Hispanics (9.2%) compared with 5.9% in urban Hispanics, 7.3% in urban Whites, and 8.4% in rural Whites.[35] Urban Hispanics with diagnosed hypertension were significantly less likely to have uncontrolled blood pressure (34.9%) than rural Hispanics (42.9%).[35] From 1984 to 1998, the crude mortality rate for heart disease was 2.4 per 1,000 person-years in rural Hispanic men, but only 1.7 per 1,000 person-years in non-Hispanic White men in rural Colorado.[42] The crude mortality rate for stroke is also higher for rural Hispanic men (1.0 per 1,000 person-years in rural Hispanic men and 0.7 per 1,000 person-years in non-Hispanic men).[42] In 2001, the deaths per 1,000 adult hospital admissions for a heart attack were higher for Hispanics in micropolitan and nonbased statistical core areas than Hispanics in metropolitan areas.[43] Although this evidence highlights disparities among rural Hispanics, more research is needed to better understand heart disease, hypertension, and stroke disparities among rural Hispanics.

Cancer

Research shows disparities in cancer incidence and outcomes among rural Hispanics in both directions (protective for some cancers, but increasing risk of others). In a national study from 1998 to 2001, the age-adjusted colorectal cancer incidence rate for rural Hispanic men 20 years and older was lower at 74.8 per 100,000 compared to 90.6 per 100,000 for rural non-Hispanics, 76.3 per 100,000 for urban Hispanics, and 94.2 per 100,000 for urban non-Hispanics.[44] Similarly, the age-adjusted colorectal incidence rate for rural Hispanic women was lower at 51.5 per 100,000 compared to 66.7 per 100,000 for rural non-Hispanic women, 51.7 per 100,000 for urban Hispanic women, and 68.2 per 100,000 for urban non-Hispanic women.[44] From 1999 to 2007, the cervical cancer mortality rate in the nation was 3.0 per 100,000 for rural Hispanics compared to 3.3 per 100,000 for urban Hispanics.[45] In the opposite direction, however, the 5-year survival rate for Hispanic women diagnosed with cervical cancer was 19% lower in rural versus urban areas (57.8% vs. 70.9%).[45] This indicates that although underlying rates may be lower (or, alternatively, diagnosis is less likely to occur), there are still disparities in postdiagnosis outcomes. However, limited research exists on cancer diagnosis rates and cancer outcomes among rural Hispanics and the disparities between urban and rural Hispanics.

Beyond outcomes, disparities have been observed in screening practices as well. Rural Hispanic women are less likely to have a mammogram within 1 year and a Pap smear within 3 years compared to urban Hispanic women.[46] In a national sample, rural Hispanics reported lower colorectal cancer screening rates (40.8%) than urban Hispanics (43.7%), rural Whites (44.3%), and urban Whites (49.5%).[47] Given these findings, researchers have identified an important unmet need to raise cancer awareness and improve screening rates among rural Hispanics.

Factors Contributing to Disparities Among Rural Hispanics

Factors such as poverty, health insurance, and having a health care provider contribute to the health disparities among rural Hispanics. About 28% of rural Hispanics lived in poverty, which is twice the rate of Whites, but less than the rate of African Americans.[32] Lack of health insurance is also common; more than 50% of rural Hispanics under the age of 65 are estimated not to have health insurance during the past year.[43] Also, only 57.1% of rural Hispanics reported having a personal health care provider, compared to 83.4% of rural Whites and 78.4% of rural African Americans.[48]

The cost of health care, lack of bilingual staff, and transportation needs all contribute to disparities among rural Hispanics. In a national sample, 25.3% of rural Hispanics reported deferring health care due to cost, compared to 23.6% of rural African Americans and only 13.3% of rural Whites.[48] In another study, rural Hispanics reported that lack of qualified medical interpreters and bilingual medical staff were significant barriers to accessing health care.[49] In addition, one third of rural Hispanics report they do not own their own vehicle and have to rely on private transportation to reach hospitals, clinics, or physicians' offices,[49] which serves as a major barrier to receipt of not only preventive and diagnostic care, but also appropriate follow-up care and case management. When considering these needs and barriers, accessing health care is a significant concern for rural Hispanics that merits a high level of research inquiry.

Future Recommendations

To address communication barriers, more Hispanic health professionals, including physicians and nurses, should be recruited to rural areas. Also, hospitals and private physicians can train and hire qualified medical interpreters and bilingual staff to reduce language barriers and increase recruitment of Hispanic patients.[49] To increase rural Hispanics' disease awareness in their community, the education and training of health professionals, community volunteers, and health educators could occur, including cultural sensitivity training of health educators[50]—the community health worker/lay health worker model has also shown tremendous promise in improving health of rural Hispanic groups. Other suggestions could be to create or enhance existing health education materials for rural Hispanics and disseminate them to clinics.[50] These education materials can provide simple messages for symptoms, disease management, and lowering disease risk at the appropriate reading level.

RURAL LGBT HEALTH

Although there are currently no data on the exact population of sexual minorities in rural areas, geomapping research reveals there are significant populations of same-sex couples (i.e., 100 or more households) in both urban and rural parts of the United States.[51] Although there is sometimes a general assumption that LGBT individuals tend to live in more urban areas, according to recent census data approximately 19% of same-sex couples in the United States reside in rural or nonurban counties,[52] roughly mirroring the overall distribution of rural residents for the general U.S. population.

There are many social and cultural characteristics of rurality that can further stigmatize and ostracize sexual-minority groups (e.g., emphasis on conformity to social norms, conservative political climate, greater focus on traditional gender and heteronormative family structures, and fundamental religiosity).[53] Therefore, it is not surprising that stigma and discrimination of sexual minorities tend to be even more prevalent in rural areas,[54–56] and that a significant portion of rural sexual minorities report experiencing heterosexism while interacting with traditional systems within the community.[55] However, despite these apparent vulnerabilities, little is known about the specific physical health challenges that rural sexual minorities face.

The majority of what is known about rural sexual minorities is based largely on small and geographically limited qualitative studies involving rural lesbians and gay men and/or a combined examination of sexual-minority health in general. Given the documented health disparities of both sexual-minority and rural populations independently, rural gay men and lesbians have been described in the literature as a "multiply marginalized" group[57] that remains virtually unstudied.

Substance Use

An examination of previous research suggests that sexual minorities in the general population tend to have significantly higher rates of substance use and related dependence disorders compared to heterosexual adults.[58,59] More specifically, research suggests higher rates of alcohol use and cigarette smoking among sexual minorities, especially women, when compared to heterosexuals.[60] Previously noted aspects of rural living and related increases in homophobia and heterosexist beliefs can create challenges and vulnerabilities for sexual minorities that may result in higher minority stress[56] and susceptibility for maladaptive coping such as substance use. Research with rural adults in general suggests greater alcohol and substance abuse compared to urban populations[61,62]; therefore, it is likely that being a sexual minority residing in a rural context results in even more heightened risk for alcohol and substance use.

For example, although not exclusively a rural sample, a recent study by Austin and Irwin[63] that included both rural and nonrural sexual minorities living in the southern United States found that individuals in their sample reported more frequent episodes of binge drinking. Furthermore, rural sexual-minority youth have been found to endorse greater marijuana and alcohol use compared to their heterosexual peers.[64]

Risk-Taking Behaviors

Previous research has highlighted the risky health and sexual behaviors of sexual minorities in the general population and within minority LGBT groups.[65–68] For example, individuals who identify as gay or lesbian may have a tendency to engage in greater sexual risk-taking behavior such as unprotected sexual activity, while having limited access to appropriate and affirmative safe-sex education related to the prevention of sexually transmitted diseases such as HIV/AIDS that is specific for sexual minorities.[65, 69–71] More specifically, recent research suggests that sexual risk taking may actually be a maladaptive coping response by rural sexual minorities who experience distress caused by increased levels of discrimination, rejection, and victimization within the community, their families, and the health care system.[72] Of additional concern is the fact that the rate of HIV/AIDS is increasing in rural areas at three or more times the rates of more urban locations.[73–75] Unfortunately, despite the apparent vulnerabilities and potential for greater health disparities, there are limited HIV/AIDS-related research and prevention efforts focusing specifically on sexual minorities residing in rural areas.

Mental Health

Although there is a scarcity of research focusing specifically on rural LGBT mental health, research indicates sexual minorities in the general population are at higher risk for psychological distress and mental health disorders.[76–78] What little research is available suggests that, because of the homophobic climate of many rural areas,[79–81] rural LGBT-identified individuals may be more vulnerable than their urban counterparts to minority stress and psychological risk factors related to greater experiences of discrimination and enacted stigma.[56] In fact, Cohn and Leake[82] found that rural sexual minorities reported higher levels of affective distress compared to their rural heterosexual peers. Therefore, mental health concerns such as experiences of depression, anxiety, and stress may be further exacerbated by these unique vulnerabilities. Due to the increased vulnerabilities to mental health concerns that rural sexual minorities may face, access to quality, LGBT-friendly mental health care is crucial. Despite the need for LGBT-affirming mental health service providers to address the unique risk factors faced by rural sexual and gender minorities, these services may not be readily available in many rural areas.

LGBT Women's Health

Recent research has demonstrated that sexual-minority women in the general population are at greater risk for being overweight or obese (twice as likely compared to heterosexual women),[83] developing cardiovascular disease,[84] and developing the majority of female-associated cancers (i.e., breast and ovarian).[85] Underlying these disparities is a number of identified risk factors, including higher rates of smoking and alcohol use, lower levels of physical exercise, and diets with fewer fruits and vegetables.[85] In addition, sexual-minority women are more likely to be nulliparous and less likely to engage in reproductive behaviors that are protective against cancers, such as using oral contraceptives.[85, 86]

It is likely that rural sexual-minority women experience similar health risks as their urban counterparts. However, there are aspects of rurality that may make rural sexual-minority women even more susceptible to physical health problems. These include lower socioeconomic status, inaccessibility of regular quality health care, lack of adequate health care coverage, living more sedentary lifestyles, and having diets that are higher in fat.[87] In fact, previous research has established that rates of heart disease and obesity are greater for women in the rural South.[88] Although not exclusively conducted on a rural population, Austin and Irwin's survey[63] of southern lesbians found that, compared to women in the general population, these women reported greater involvement in risky health behaviors such as cigarette smoking, alcohol consumption, and unhealthy patterns of eating, all of which are related to increased risk for women's health-related problems. This is consistent with research conducted with samples of rural women in general that reveals that they too evidence greater health risks.[87] Therefore, it is reasonable that sexual-minority women residing in rural areas may present with even more health-related risk factors and outcomes. Interventions to promote rural LGBT women's health are currently limited by the complete lack of research focused on this group; future research is highly needed in this area.

Barriers to Care

Overall, lesbians and gay men have a long history of being stigmatized on a societal level as sexual minorities, which is also true on a systemic level with regard to health care (wherein homosexuality was considered a disease or mental illness until the late 1970s).[89] In fact, homophobia and heterosexism continue to be one of most common forms of discrimination in the U.S. health care system.[57,89,90] Currently, there are a variety of issues impacting sexual minorities' access to and quality of health care and subsequent health disparities. Such barriers include the limited availability of providers with adequate training to treat sexual minorities in a culturally competent manner, in addition to sexual-minority patients' previous negative experiences with the health care system, which may hinder them from even being honest about their sexuality. This can significantly impact the quality of care they receive,[67] and thus contribute to health disparities.

Rural sexual minorities are not only more likely to experience unique physical and mental health risks due to barriers to care and other previously mentioned vulnerabilities of rural living,[91, 92] but also have a tendency to be less comfortable disclosing their sexual identity to others, including medical providers, due to the conservative climate of the majority of rural areas.[63, 92–95] Rural sexual minorities are often fearful of disclosing their sexual orientation to their primary care provider because they see being known as gay or lesbian as potentially threatening or dangerous.[93, 95] Namely, they indicate concern that if their sexual orientation is disclosed to their provider and they are rejected or discriminated against, they would be unable to access safe and appropriate care given the scarcity of providers in rural areas.[95] When rural patients avoid disclosing their sexual orientation to health care providers, they may not receive adequate, LGBT-specific and affirming health care.[96] Given that previous research shows that fear of disclosure is one of the major barriers to accessing appropriate care for sexual minorities,[63,69,96] it is likely that as a result rural sexual minorities experience even greater health disparities compared to their urban counterparts.

Due to fears of disclosure and other barriers to care related to accessibility, availability, and acceptability, sexual minorities disproportionately lack adequate and ongoing physical and mental health care compared to heterosexual individuals.[67] These barriers to care contribute to the inaccessibility and/or avoidance of routine medical and preventive care, which represents the most significant medical risk factor for sexual minorities.[69] More specifically, issues related to barriers to care may be particularly challenging for rural sexual minorities. For example, with the availability of general physical and mental health care services in rural areas already scarce,[97] providers who are LGBT-friendly or affirming, let alone culturally competent in working with LGBT-related issues, may be largely unavailable.[67,98,99] Furthermore, financial concerns and related limitations on transportation options,[100] as well as lack of referrals to affirmative health care services due to limited LGBT community networks, prevent many rural sexual minorities from traveling to nearby urban areas to receive appropriate and affirming services.[101] For example, Austin and Irwin's sample of sexual minorities reported facing several barriers to receiving adequate health care, including low socioeconomic status and/or inadequate health insurance and a lack of a regular mental and physical health provider.[63]

Overall, one of the major barriers to access to care for sexual-minority patients is the significant lack of cultural competency for providers to not only be aware of, but also adequately address, the unique needs and risk factors of this population.[102] Research indicates both rural and urban providers significantly lack adequate training on LGBT issues and culturally sensitive practice.[103] In fact, recent studies have demonstrated that many rural providers continue to report negative attitudes toward sexual minorities[101,103] and rural patients report previous experiences of heterosexism, discrimination, and/or inappropriate care while accessing rural health care systems.[55] Unfortunately, there is a large information/research gap that impedes the development of such competency trainings: When the leading health issues are not well known within the scientific community due to a substantial lack of rural LGBT research, it is virtually impossible to adequately train providers in the unique needs of rural LGBT groups. In the interim, however, improving overall LGBT cultural competency can begin the process of increasing access to (and acceptability of) care for all LGBT individuals regardless of geographic background.

Specifically, there is a need for more cultural competency training with regard to facilitating safe and positive disclosure experiences and increasing the availability and accessibility of appropriate preventive care and education to sexual and gender minorities in an affirming manner. Rural providers should seek out consultation and training opportunities aimed at improving their knowledge and skills related to best practices in sexual- and gender-minority health. This type of training can improve their cultural competency to work with rural sexual minorities through increasing their understanding of gay and lesbian culture and common language, LGBT-specific health issues and barriers to care, and health issues and risk factors that are rural specific. Environmental considerations are also crucial. For example, in order to ensure that rural treatment settings are welcoming and affirming of sexual-minority patients, Hastings and Hoover-Thompson recommend having LGBT-friendly reading material in the waiting room and having some visible symbol that the agency is LGBT affirming.[104] Other environmental recommendations to take into consideration may be the type of art work and decorations used; the information on bulletin boards, posters, and brochures; and the type of television programs displayed.

Recommendations

Research into potential avenues for eliminating rural LGBT health disparities is highly limited; however, research into community-identified recommendations for improving overall LGBT health care engagement include: (a) support for legislation and public policy that advocate for equal rights for sexual and gender minorities in order to increase financial resources and access to health coverage, (b) provide public education related to the impact of homophobia related to discrimination and victimization on sexual minorities' overall health and well-being, and (c) improve efforts to increase community resources and connect local LGBT-identified individuals together in order to increase the visibility of sexual minorities within the rural community.[105]

Therefore, following are a set of integrated community and clinical recommendations for improving the experiences of rural sexual minorities in order to address health risks and barriers to care that are based on the work and recommendations outlined by Oswald and colleagues[105,106] to be more specific to public health: (a) increase the availability and visibility of mental and physical health resources and outreach programming in rural communities; (b) improve the community support for rural sexual minorities through such means as diversity education, advocacy, and public policy efforts; (c) coordinate with local and nearby urban LGBT community networks in order to collaborate on prevention efforts and to connect them with local resources; and (d) orchestrate LGBT-affirming and culturally sensitive didactic training to school professionals, law enforcement, health care workers, and other community-service providers on LGBT issues.

RURAL AMERICAN INDIAN AND ALASKA NATIVE HEALTH

Native Americans, classified in the U.S. Census under American Indian or Alaska Native (hereafter AIAN), make up a small but growing population in the United States. According to the 2010 U.S. Census, 2.9 million people, or about 0.9% of the U.S. population, reported AIAN ethnicity, and 2.3 million, or 0.7% of the population, reported AIAN race in combination with one or more other races.[107] The AIAN-only group experienced a rate of growth almost twice as fast as the general U.S. population, whereas those identifying as AIAN in combination with one or more other races grew at an even faster rate.[107]

The AIAN community has unique challenges that set it apart from others: AIANs are highly rural, experience high rates of poverty, and are younger than the general population. Those reporting AIAN race are highly concentrated in a small number of counties, particularly those designated as American Indian areas such as federal reservations, state reservations, or federal- or state-designated American Indian statistical areas.[107] The AIAN population is the most rural of any other racial group, with 40% residing in rural-designated areas.[108] There are a large proportion of young people in the AIAN community, with 31% of the AIAN population younger than 15 years old, compared to 21% for the general population.[109]

There are a number of specific health challenges faced by AIANs, and these may be attributable to genetic influences, social inequities, historical trauma, rural living, and cultural factors.[110] By 2002 to 2004, the life expectancy for AIANs had improved, but was still 5 years less than the U.S. all-races average.[109] According to a 2012 CDC report, the five leading causes of death among AIANs were cancer, heart disease, unintentional injuries, diabetes, and chronic liver disease and cirrhosis.[111] In a 2012 summary of U.S. health statistics,[112] the CDC reported that AIANs have the highest proportion of people who report being either limited in their daily activities or unable to work due to one or more chronic conditions, indicating overall health efforts are not adequately reaching AIAN populations. Major health problems experienced by AIANs include a web of interrelated conditions such as obesity, diabetes, cardiovascular disease, and psychological distress that complicate public health intervention within this group.

Unfortunately, due in part to a somewhat prevailing perception that all AIANs reside in rural settings, specific research into rural AIAN populations is scarce. We therefore present the overall research knowledge base for AIAN health in the United States (commenting on its rural specificity when appropriate). To truly advance AIAN health, it will be important for future research to specifically investigate the separate needs of rural versus urban AIAN individuals.

Diabetes and Cardiovascular Disease

Diabetes is a notable concern for AIANs. Rates of diabetes are higher among AIANs than any other racial group or the U.S. average.[13] Death rates from diabetes are 2.9 times higher in AIANs than the U.S. all-races average, and have increased steadily since 1980.[109] For AIANs with diabetes, compared to their counterparts in the U.S. population, there is a higher risk of comorbid disorders such as hypertension, cerebrovascular disease, mental health disorders, lower-extremity amputations, and liver disease, and these conditions complicate diabetes treatment and self-care, and lead to a higher risk of mortality.[113] Diabetes in AIANs is also strongly linked to renal disease.[110]

One strong contributing factor to AIAN diabetes is a rate of obesity that is greater than the already high U.S. population, starting as early as infancy and early childhood.[114] One contributing factor may be a shift away from a healthier, traditional diet to more processed, fattier foods, combined with a reduction in physical activity.[115] Cardiovascular disease was once rare among AIANs, but has dramatically increased to a rate higher than the national average.[116] Although the rate of hypertension in AIANs is not greater than the U.S. average,[109] it is implicated in the exacerbation of other problems. Glucose-control problems, smoking, and high blood pressure among AIANs are associated with a higher rate of stroke (and higher fatality rate for first stroke) than the U.S. White or African American populations.[117]

Substance Use

Since it was introduced into AIAN populations, alcohol has been a major health concern. According to the Indian Health Service, during the data years 2003 to 2005, AIANs had a 519% greater alcohol-related death rate compared to other U.S. races,[109,118] and AIANs are 4.2 times more likely to die from chronic liver disease and cirrhosis than the U.S. all-races average.[109] Fetal alcohol syndrome is found at some of the highest rates in the nation among certain AIAN tribes.[119]

The rates of any kind of substance dependence or abuse, including alcohol, among AIANs aged 12 or older is extremely high at 21.8%, around three times higher than other racial groups.[120] Additionally, AIANs report higher rates of illicit drug abuse, including marijuana, cocaine, and hallucinogens, than any other single-race group.[118,120] As a result, AIANs are 1.5 times more likely to die from drug-related causes than the U.S. all-races average.[109] The newest drug of greatest concern among AIANs, according to the Indian Health Service (IHS),[118] is methamphetamine, as AIANs have a methamphetamine use rate that is three times the rate of the general population. A complicating factor of drug use in AIANs is a high rate of co-occurring substance abuse and mental health disorders, which can exacerbate each other.[118] Along with Hispanic and African American adults, AIANs have a higher rate of psychological distress, feelings of hopelessness, and feelings of worthlessness than Whites or Asians.[121]

Suicide

The CDC reported in 2012 that suicide was the eighth highest cause of death for AIANs in 2010 (CDC, 2012a), and suicide is the second leading cause of death in both AIAN children aged 5 to 14 years and young adults aged 15 to 24.[109] The IHS reported in 2011 that AIANS have a 73% greater death rate from suicide compared to other races,[118] indicating a significant and understudied health issue affecting AIAN groups. This problem is especially great in Alaska Natives, who commit suicide at rates four times the national average, and teen male Alaska Natives commit suicide at a staggering five to six times the rate of their non-Native peers.[118] Despite recognition of these rates, suicide prevention research in overall AIAN groups (and particularly in rural AIANs residing in a context that dually increases risk of suicide) is severely limited.

Respiratory Health

There are several notable respiratory health characteristics of the AIAN community. Though significant gains have been made since the 1980s, tuberculosis continues to be a health concern for AIANs, and AIANs are 8.5 times more likely to die from tuberculosis than the U.S. all-races average.[109] Additionally, the rates of death from pneumonia, influenza, and asthma for AIANs are around 50% more than the U.S. all-race average.[109] The rate of tobacco use among persons aged 12 or older is much greater in AIANs than the rate from any other racial group, with almost half (48.4%) of AIANs reporting some kind of tobacco use in a 2012 survey.[120] Although the lung cancer rate among AIANs is actually lower than the all-race U.S. average, it has been steadily increasing since 1980.[109] Trachea, bronchus, and lung cancers are the most common type of cancers in the AIAN community for both men and women.[109] Respiratory diseases are some of the most common reasons for hospitalization in AIAN children and the elderly.[109]

Maternal and Child Health

Another notable area of concern is the health of AIAN infants and children. The AIAN population experiences more high birth weights than the average for all races in the United States, which can be a complication of diabetic pregnancies.[109] Low vaccination rates have been reported in AIAN children,[111] and the infant mortality rate in AIAN communities is 20% higher than the national average.[109] The leading causes of infant deaths for AIANs are congenital malformations, deformations, and chromosomal abnormalities, followed by sudden infant death syndrome (SIDS).[109] Additionally, almost three times as many AIAN children aged 1 to 14 years die from unintentional accidents than the national all-races average.[109]

Factors Influencing Health Disparities in AIAN Groups

Both economic and geographic factors influence health disparities in AIANs, who suffer from the highest poverty rate [122] and some of the worst employment statistics[123] of any racial group in the nation. Median household income for AIANs is consistently lower than the national average.[108,124] As a result, AIANs, compared to other racial groups, are highly likely to report having delayed, or completely neglected, receiving medical care due to cost.[111,112] Relatedly, AIANs have the highest rates of being uninsured and the lowest rates of private insurance and insurance provided by employers,[111,112] and cost was cited as the most common response (42.2%) by AIANs for why they did not have health insurance.[112] In the period between 1993 and 2011, the number of AIANs who reported having no usual source of health care increased, with a peak during 2007 to 2008 when 24.4% reported having no usual source of health care.[111]

Recommendations

Targeted health interventions have been found to be effective for various AIAN-specific issues,[116,118,125] and for generally closing the disparity in life expectancies for AIANs.[110] The rising field of telehealth has made improvements to rural AIAN health care, but much work remains in developing the availability and infrastructure needed to make telehealth most effective[126] and to find appropriate ways to navigate licensure portability complications. Community interventions must be evidence based, but more importantly, must be culturally appropriate to be most effective.[118,127]

CONCLUSION

As presented throughout, although significantly understudied, there is consistent evidence that rural minorities face substantial barriers to care ranging from sheer access barriers to underlying cultural factors influencing health care engagement. To truly advance minority health not only in rural areas, but also throughout the entire nation, it is essential that additional research is conducted into ways to promote health and eliminate health disparities within rural minority groups. Innovations such as telehealth and community-based participatory research hold much promise for advancing health within rural minority groups—such initiatives should be encouraged, supported, and appropriately funded to begin to address health inequity in these doubly underserved populations.

REFERENCES

1. Slifkin RT, Goldsmith LJ, Ricketts T. *Race and Place: Urban-Rural Differences in Health for Racial and Ethnic Minorities.* NC Rural Health Research and Practice Working Paper Series, No. 66, 2000.
2. Centers for Disease Control and Prevention. Black or African American Populations. http://www.cdc.gov/minorityhealth/populations/REMP/black.html. Accessed November 5, 2013.
3. US Census Bureau. *Facts for Features, Black (African American) History Month:* February 2013.
4. Centers for Disease Control and Prevention. Health Disparities and Inequalities Report—United States, 2011 (CHDIR). http://www.dcd.gov/nchs/data/hus/hus11/minorityhealth/CHDIReport.html.
5. Housing Assistance Council. *HAC Rural Research Note: Race and Ethnicity in Rural America.* HAC tabulations of 2010 Census of Population and Housing, Summary File 1; 2012.
6. Hueston W, Hubbard E. Preventive services for rural and urban African American adults. *Arch Fam Med.* 2000;9:262–266.
7. Scott A, Wilson R. Social determinants of health among African Americans in a rural community in the Deep South: an ecological exploration. *Rural Remote Health.* 2011;11:1634.
8. Lemacks J, Wells B, Ilich J, Ralston P. Interventions for improving nutrition and physical activity behaviors in African American populations: a systematic review, January 2000 through December 2011. *Prev Chronic Dis.* 2013;10:1–16.
9. South Carolina Rural Health Research Center. Health Disparities: A Rural-Urban Chartbook. 2008. http://rhr.sph.sc.edu.
10. Kochanek K, Xu J, Murphy S, Minino A, Kung H. Deaths: final data for 2009. *Natl Vital Stat Rep.* 2011;60(3).
11. Centers for Disease Control and Prevention. Table 17. *Natl Vital Stat Rep.* 2012;60(3). http://www.cdc.gov/nchc/data/susr60/nvsr60_03.pdf.
12. O'Connor A, Wellenius G. Rural-urban disparities in the prevalence of diabetes and coronary heart disease. *Public Health.* 2012;126:813–820.
13. Centers for Disease Control and Prevention. National diabetes fact sheet, 2011. http://www.cdc.gov/diabetes/pubs/pdf/ndfs_2011.pdf. 2011. Accessed November 6, 2013.
14. Saydan S, Lochner K. Socioeconomic status and risk of diabetes-related mortality in the United States. *Public Health Rep.* 2010;125:377–388.
15. Connolly V, Unwin N, Sherriff P, Belous R, Kelly W. Diabetes prevalence and socioeconomic status: a population based study showing increased prevalence of type 2 diabetes mellitus in deprived areas. *J Epidemiol Community Health.* 2000;54(3):173–177.
16. National Institute of Neurological Disorder and Stroke. What you need to know about stroke. http://www.ninds.nih/gov/disorders/stroke/stroke_needtoknow.htm. 2013.
17. Centers for Disease Control and Prevention. Summary health statistics for U.S. adults: 2010. Table 2. http://www.cdc.gov/nchs/data/series/sr_10/sr10_252.pdf. 2011.
18. Howard G, Labarthe DR, Hu J, Yoon S, Howard VJ. Regional differences in African Americans' high risk for stroke: the remarkable burden of stroke for southern African Americans. *Ann Epidemiol.* 2007;17(9):689–696.

19. Reeves M, Pan W, Smith E, et al. *American Heart Association Rapid Access Journal.* 2010. http://newsroom.heart.org/news/989.
20. Huntley M, Heady C. Barriers to health promotion in African American men with hypertension. *Am J Health Stud.* 2013;28(1):21–26.
21. National Institutes of Health. Researchers uncover genetic variants linked to blood pressure in African Americans. 2009. http://www.nih.gov/news/health/Jul2009/nhgri-16a.htm.
22. Mainous A, King D, Garr D, Pearson W. Race, rural residence, and control of diabetes and hypertension. *Ann Fam Med.* 2004;2(6):563–568.
23. Middleton J. A proposed new model of hypersensitive treatment behavior in African Americans. *J Natl Med Assoc.* 2009;101(1):12–17.
24. Kung H, Hoyert D, Xu J, Murphy S. Deaths: final data for 2005. *Natl Vital Stat Rep.* 2008;56(10).
25. American Cancer Society. *Cancer Facts and Figures for African Americans 2011–2012.* Atlanta, GA: American Cancer Society; 2011.
26. Oliver J, Grindel C. Beliefs and attitudes about prostate cancer and prostate cancer screening practices among rural African American men. *Oncology Nurs Forum.* 2006;33(2):454.
27. Wilson-Anderson K, Williams P, Beacham T, McDonald N. Breast health teaching in predominantly African American rural Mississippi Delta. *ABNF J.* 2013; 24(1):28–33.
28. Frank D, Grubbs L. A faith-based screening and education program for diabetes, CVD, and stroke in rural African Americans. *ABNF J.* 2008;19(3): 96–101.
29. Kennedy B, Paeratakul S, Champagne C, et al. A pilot church-based weight loss program for African American adults using church members as health educators: A comparison of individual and group intervention. *Ethn Dis.* 2005;15(3):373–378.
30. Samuel-Hodge C, Keyserling T, Park S, Johnston L, Gizlice Z, Bangdwala S. A randomized trial of a church-based diabetes self-management program for African Americans with type 2 diabetes. *Diabetes Educ.* 2009;35(3):439–454.
31. United States Department of Agriculture, Economic Research Service. *Rural Hispanics at a Glance.* Economic Information Bulletin Number 8; 2005.
32. Saenz R. *A profile of Latinos in rural America.* Fact Sheet No. 10. Durham, NH: University of New Hampshire, Carsey Institute; 2008.
33. United States Department of Agriculture, Economic Research Service. *Rural Education at a Glance.* Rural Development Research Report Number 98; 2003.
34. Effland AB, Kassel K. *Hispanics in Rural America: The Influence of Immigration and Language on Economic Well-Being.* USDA Economic Research Service; 1998.
35. Mainous AG, Koopman R, Geesey ME. *Diabetes & Hypertension among Rural Hispanics: Disparities in Diagnostics and Disease Management.* South Carolina Rural Health Research Center; 2004.
36. Chang J, Guy MC, Rosales C, et al. Investigating social ecological contributors to diabetes within Hispanics in an underserved U.S.–Mexico border community. *Int J Environ Res Public Health.* 2013;10:3217–3232.
37. Brown SA, Garcia AA, Winter M, Silva L, Brown A, Hanis CL. Integrating education, group support, and case management for diabetic Hispanics. *Ethn Dis.* 2011;21(1):20–26.
38. Mier N, Wang X, Smith ML, et al. Factors influencing health care utilization in older Hispanics with diabetes along the Texas-Mexico border. *Popul Health Manag.* 2012;15(3):149–156.

39. Cohen SJ, Ingram M. Border health strategic initiative: Overview and introduction to a community-based model for diabetes prevention and control. *Prev Chronic Dis.* 2005;2(1):1–5.
40. Ceballos RM, Coronado GD, Thompson B. Having a diagnosis of diabetes is not associated with general diabetes knowledge in rural Hispanics. *J Rural Health.* 2010;26(4):342–351.
41. Coronado GD, Thompson B, Tejeda S, Godina R, Chen L. Sociodemographic factors and self-management practices relates to type 2 diabetes among Hispanics and non-Hispanic Whites in a rural setting. *J Rural Health.* 2007;23(1):49–54.
42. Swenson CJ, Trepka MJ, Rewers MJ, Scarbro S, Hiatt WR, Harmann RF. Cardiovascular disease mortality in Hispanics and non-Hispanic Whites. *Am J Epidemiol.* 2002;156(10):919–928.
43. Agency for Healthcare Research and Quality. *Health Care Disparities in Rural Areas.* AHRX Pub No. 05-P022. 2005.
44. Coughlin SS, Richards TB, Thompson T, et al. Rural and nonrural differences in colorectal cancer incidence in the United States, 1998–2001. *Cancer.* 2006;107(5): 1181–1188.
45. Singh GK. Rural-urban trends and patterns in cervical cancer mortality, incidence, stage, and survival in the United States, 1950–2008. *J Community Health.* 2012;37(1):217–223.
46. Nuno T, Gerald JK, Harris R, Martinez ME, Estrada A, Garcia F. Comparison of breast and cervical cancer screening utilization among rural and urban Hispanic and American Indian women in the southwestern United States. *Cancer Causes Control.* 2012;23(8):1333–1341.
47. Cole AM, Jackson JE, Doescher M. Colorectal cancer screening disparities for rural minorities in the United States. *J Prim Care Community Health.* 2012;4(2):106–111.
48. Bennett KJ, Olatosi B, Probst JC. *Health Disparities: A Rural-Urban Chartbook.* Columbia, SC: South Carolina Rural Health Research Center, University of South Carolina; 2008.
49. Vitale M, Bailey C. Assessing barriers to health care services for Hispanic residents in rural Georgia. *J Rural Soc Sci.* 2012;27(3):17–45.
50. Livaudais JC, Thompson B, Islas I, Ibarra G, Godina R, Coronado GD. Type 2 diabetes among rural Hispanics in Washington State: Perspectives from community stakeholders. *Health Promot Pract.* 2010;11(4):589–599.
51. US Census Bureau. Statesboro, GA Quick Facts. 2010. http://quickfacts.census .gov/qfd/states/13/1373256.html. Accessed March 22, 2013.
52. Bishop B. Finding gay rural America. Daily Yonder. http://www.dailyyonder .com/finding-gay-rural-america/2011/09/26/3536. Accessed September 27, 2011.
53. Round KA. AIDS in rural areas: Challenges to providing care. *Soc Work.* 1988;33: 257–261.
54. Edwards J. Invisibility, safety and psycho-social distress among same-sex attracted women in rural South Australia. *Rural Remote Health.* 2005;5(1):343.
55. Leedy G, Connolly C. Out of the cowboy state: A look at lesbian and gay lives in Wyoming. *J Gay Lesbian Soc Serv: Issues Pract Policy Res.* 2007;19(1):17–34.
56. Swank E, Frost DM, Fahs B. Rural location and exposure to minority stress among sexual minorities in the United States. *Psychol Sexuality.* 2012;3(3):226–243.
57. Brotman S, Ryan B, Jalbert Y, Rowe, B. The impact of coming out on health and health care access: the experiences of gay, lesbian, bisexual and two-spirit people. *J Health Social Policy.* 2002;15(1):1–29.

58. Cochran SD, Mays VM, Alegria M, Ortega AN, Takeuchi D. Mental health and substance use disorders among Latino and Asian American lesbian, gay, and bisexual adults. *J Consult Clin Psychol.* 2007;75(5):785–794.
59. King M, Semlyen J, Tai S, et al. A systematic review of mental disorder, suicide, and deliberate self-harm in lesbian, gay and bisexual people. *BMC Psychiatry.* 2008;8:70.
60. Drabble L, Trocki K. Alcohol consumption, alcohol-related problems, and other substance use among lesbian and bisexual women. *J Lesbian Stud.* 2005;9(3):19–30.
61. Carlo G, Crockett L, Wilkinson J, Beal S. The longitudinal relationships between rural adolescents' prosocial behaviors and young adult substance use. *J Youth Adolescence.* 2011;40(9):1192–1202.
62. Scaramella L, Keyes A. The social contextual approach and rural adolescent substance use: Implications for prevention in rural settings. *Clin Child Fam Psychol Rev.* 2001;4(3):231–251.
63. Austin E, Irwin J. Health behaviors and health care utilization of southern lesbians. *Women's Health Issues.* 2010;20(3):178–184.
64. Rostosky SS, Owens GP, Zimmerman RS, Riggle ED. Associations among sexual attraction status, school belongingness, and alcohol and marijuana use in rural high school students. *J Adolesc.* 2003;26:741–751.
65. Davis JA. HIV and the LGBT community: a medical update. *J Gay Lesbian Ment Health.* 2013;17(1):64–79.
66. Warren JC, Fernández MI, Harper G, Hidalgo M, Jamil O, Torres RS. Predictors of unprotected sex among young sexually active African American, Hispanic, and White MSM: the importance of ethnicity and culture. *AIDS Behav.* 2008;12(3):459–468.
67. Gay and Lesbian Medical Association. *Healthy People 2010: Companion Document for Lesbian, Gay, Bisexual, and Transgender (LGBT) Health.* San Francisco: Gay and Lesbian Medical Association; 2011.
68. Mayer K, Bradford J, Makadon H, Stall R, Goldhammer H, Landers S. Sexual and gender minority health: What we know and what needs to be done. *Am J Public Health.* 2008;98(6):989–995.
69. Bonvicini K, Perlin M. The same but different: clinician-patient communication with gay and lesbian patients. *Patient Educ Couns.* 2003;51(2):115–122.
70. Jones AR, Hoyler CL. HIV/AIDS among women who have sex with women. In: Fernandez F, Ruiz P, eds. *Psychiatric Aspects of HIV/AIDS.* Philadelphia, PA: Lippincott Williams & Wilkins; 2006:299–307.
71. Wainberg ML, Ashley KB. HIV/AIDS among men who have sex with men. In: Fernandez F, Ruiz P, eds. *Psychiatric Aspects of HIV/AIDS.* Philadelphia, PA: Lippincott Williams & Wilkins; 2006:288–298.
72. Preston D, D'Augelli AR, Kassab CD, Starks MT. The relationship of stigma to the sexual risk behavior of rural men who have sex with men. *AIDS Educ Prev.* 2007;19(3):218–230.
73. Centers for Disease Control and Prevention. HIV/AIDS in urban and nonurban areas of the United States. *HIV/AIDS Surveillance Supplemental Report.* 2000;6(2):1–16.
74. Cohn SE. AIDS in rural America. *J Rural Health.* 1997;13:237–239.
75. Steinberg S, Fleming P. The geographic distribution of AIDS in the United States: Is there a rural epidemic? *J Rural Health.* 2000;16(1):11–19.
76. Bostwick WB, Boyd CJ, Hughes TL, McCabe S. Dimensions of sexual orientation and the prevalence of mood and anxiety disorders in the United States. *Am J Public Health.* 2010;100(3):468–475.

77. Cochran SD, Mays VM, Alegria M, Ortega AN, Takeuchi D. Mental health and substance use disorders among Latino and Asian American lesbian, gay, and bisexual adults. *J Consult Clin Psychol.* 2007;75(5):785–794.
78. Gilman SE, Cochran SD, Mays VM, Hughes M, Ostrow D, Kessler RC. Risk of psychiatric disorders among individuals reporting same-sex sexual partners in the National Comorbidity Survey. *Am J Public Health.* 2001;91(6):933–939.
79. Eldridge V, Mack L, Swank E. Explaining comfort with homosexuality in rural America. *J Homosexuality.* 2006;51(2):39–56.
80. Herek GM. Heterosexuals' attitudes toward bisexual men and women in the United States. *J Sex Roles.* 2002;39(4):264–274.
81. Hopwood M, Connors J. Heterosexual attitudes to homosexuality: homophobia at a rural Australian university. *J Gay Lesbian Soc Serv.* 2002;14(2):79–94.
82. Cohn TJ, Leake VS. Affective distress among adolescents who endorse same-sex sexual attraction: Urban versus rural differences and the role of protective factors. *J Gay Lesbian Ment Health.* 2012;16(4):291–305.
83. Boehmer U, Bowen DJ, Bauer GR. Overweight and obesity in sexual-minority women: evidence from population-based data. *Am J Public Health.* 2007; 97(6):1134–1140.
84. Roberts SA, Dibble SL, Nussey B, Casey K. Cardiovascular disease risk in lesbian women. *Women's Health Issues.* 2003;13(4):167–174.
85. Brown J, Tracy J. Lesbians and cancer: an overlooked health disparity. *Cancer Causes Control.* 2008;19(10):1009–1020.
86. Case P, Austin B, Hunter DJ, et al. Sexual orientation, health risk factors, and physical functioning in the Nurses' Health Study II. *J Womens Health.* 2004; 13(9):1033–1047.
87. Gamm L, Hutchison L, Bellamy G, Dabney B. Rural healthy people 2010: Identifying rural health priorities and models for practice. *J Rural Health.* 2002; 18(1):9–14.
88. Southwest Rural Health Research Center. Rural Healthy People 2010: a companion document to Healthy People 2010. http://www.srph.tamhsc.edu/centers/rhp2010
89. Minton H. *Departing from Deviance: A History of Homosexual Rights and Emancipatory Science in America.* Chicago, IL: University of Chicago Press; 2002.
90. Steele LS, Tinmouth JM, Lu A. Regular health care use by lesbians: A path analysis of predictive factors. *Fam Pract.* 2006;23(6):631–636.
91. Pellowski J. Barriers to care for rural people living With HIV: a review of domestic research and health care models. *J Assoc Nurses AIDS Care.* 2013;24(5):422–437.
92. Swank E, Fahs B, Frost DM. Region, social identities, and disclosure practices as predictors of heterosexist discrimination against sexual minorities in the United States: region, social identities, and disclosure practices as predictors of heterosexist discrimination against sexual minorities in the United States. *Sociol Inq.* 2013;83(2):238–258.
93. Boulden WT. Gay men living in a rural environment. *J Gay Lesbian Soc Serv.* 2001;12(3/4):63–75.
94. Lee MG, Quam JK. Comparing supports for LGBT aging in rural versus urban areas. *J Gerontol Soc Work.* 2013;56:112–126.
95. Tiemann KA, Kennedy SA, Haga MP. Rural lesbians' strategies for coming out to health care professionals. *J Lesbian Stud.* 1988;2(1):61–75.
96. Durso LE, Meyer IH. Patterns and predictors of disclosure of sexual orientation to healthcare providers among lesbians, gay men, and bisexuals. *Sexuality Res Soc Policy.* 2013;10(1):35–42.

97. Health Resources and Services Administration. *Mental Health and Rural America: 1994–2005*. Rockville, MD: Office of Rural Health Policy; 2005.
98. Bell D, Valentine G. Queer country: rural lesbian and gay lives. *J Rural Studies*. 1995;11:113–122.
99. Lindhorst T. Lesbians and gay men in the country: practice implications for rural social workers. In: Smith J, Mancoske RJ, Smith J, Mancoske RJ, eds. *Rural Gays and Lesbians: Building on the Strengths of Communities*. Binghamton, NY: Harrington Park Press/The Haworth Press; 1997:1–11.
100. King S, Dabelko-Schoeny H. "Quite frankly, I have doubts about remaining": aging-in-place and health care access for rural midlife and older lesbian, gay, and bisexual individuals. *J LGBT Health Res*. 2009;5(1/2):10–21.
101. Willging CE, Salvador M, Kano M. Pragmatic help seeking: how sexual and gender minority groups access mental health care in a rural state. *Psychiatric Serv*. 2006;57(6): 871–874.
102. Solarz AL. *Lesbian Health: Current Assessment and Directions for the Future*. Washington, DC: Institute of Medicine, National Academies Press; 1999.
103. Eliason M, Hughes T. Treatment counselor's attitudes about lesbian, gay, bisexual, and transgendered clients: Urban vs. rural settings. *Subst Use Misuse*. 2004;39(4): 625–644.
104. Hastings SL, Hoover-Thompson A. Effective support for lesbians in rural communities: the role of psychotherapy. *J Lesbian Stud*. 2011;15(2):197–204.
105. Oswald R, Gebbie E, Culton L. Rainbow Illinois: a survey of non-metropolitan lesbian, gay, bisexual, and transgender people. *J Rural Community Psychol*. 2000;E(5)2. http://www.marshall.edu/jrcp/jrcp%20intro%20glbt/JRCP%20Rainbow/rainbow_illinois.htm
106. Oswald R, Culton LS. Under the rainbow: rural gay life and its relevance for family providers. *Fam Relations*. 2003;52(1):72–81.
107. US Census Bureau. The American Indian and Alaska Native population: 2010. 2012. http://www.census.gov/prod/cen2010/briefs/c2010br-10.pdf. Accessed November 5, 2013.
108. Office of Minority Health. American Indian/Alaska Native profile. 2012. http://minorityhealth.hhs.gov/templates/browse.aspx?lvl=2&lvlid=52. Accessed November 5, 2013.
109. Indian Health Service. *Trends in Indian Health, 2002–2003*. Rockville, MD: Indian Health Service, n.d.
110. Sequist TD, Cullen T, Acton KJ. Indian Health Service innovations have helped reduce health disparities affecting American Indian and Alaska Native people. *Health Affairs*. 2011;30(10):1965–1973.
111. Centers for Disease Control and Prevention. Health, United States, 2012. 2012. http://www.cdc.gov/nchs/data/hus/hus12.pdf#056. Accessed November 5, 2013.
112. Centers for Disease Control and Prevention. Summary health statistics for the U.S. population: National Health Interview Survey, 2011. 2012. http://www.cdc.gov/nchs/data/series/sr_10/sr10_255.pdf. Accessed November 5, 2013.
113. O'Connell J, Yi R, Wilson C, Manson SM, Acton KJ. Racial disparities in health status: a comparison of the morbidity among American Indian and U.S. adults with diabetes. *Diabetes Care*. 2010;33(7):1463–1470.
114. Schell LM, Gallo MV. Overweight and obesity among North American Indian infants, children, and youth. *Am J Hum Biol*. 2012;24:302–313.

115. Eilat-Adar S, Mete M, Fretts A, et al. Dietary patterns and their association with cardiovascular risk factors in a population undergoing lifestyle changes: the Strong Heart Study. *Nutr Met Cardiovasc Dis*. 2013;23:528–535.
116. Brega AG, Pratte KA, Jiang L, et al. Impact of targeted health promotion on cardiovascular knowledge among American Indians and Alaska Natives. *Health Educ Res*. 2013;28(3):437–449.
117. Zhang Y, Galloway JM, Welty TK, et al. Incidence and risk factors for stroke in American Indians: the Strong Heart Study. *Circulation*. 2008;118(15):1577–1584.
118. Indian Health Service. American Indian/Alaska Native National Behavioral Health Strategic Plan: 2011–2015. 2011. http://www.nihb.org/docs/08072012/ AIAN NationalBHStrategicPlan.pdf. Accessed November 5, 2013.
119. Substance Abuse and Mental Health Services Administration. Fetal alcohol spectrum disorders among Native Americans. 2007. http://fasdcenter.samhsa.gov/ documents/WYNK_Native_American_Teal.pdf. Accessed November 6, 2013.
120. Substance Abuse and Mental Health Services Administration. Results from the 2012 National Survey on Drug Use and Health: summary of national findings. 2013. http://www.samhsa.gov/data/NSDUH/2012 SummNatFindDetTables/ NationalFindings/NSDUHresults2012.pdf. Accessed November 6, 2013.
121. Barnes PM, Adams PF, Powell-Griner E. Health characteristics of the American Indian or Alaska Native adult population: United States, 2004–2008. *Natl Health Stat Rep*. 2010;20:1–24.
122. Macartney S, Bishaw A, Fontenot K. U.S. Census Bureau, 2013. Poverty rates for selected detailed race and Hispanic groups by state and place: 2007–2011. 2013. http://www.census.gov/prod/2013pubs/acsbr11-17.pdf. Accessed November 5, 2013.
123. US Department of Labor. Labor force characteristics by race and ethnicity, 2012. 2013. http://www.bls.gov/cps/cpsrace2012.pdf. Accessed November 5, 2013.
124. US Census Bureau. The American Community—American Indians and Alaska Natives: 2004. 2007. http://www.census.gov/prod/2007pubs/acs-07.pdf. Accessed November 5, 2013.
125. Jiang L, Manson SM, Beals J, et al. Translating the Diabetes Prevention Program into American Indian and Alaska Native communities: results from the Special Diabetes Program for Indians Diabetes Prevention demonstration project. *Diabetes Care*. 2013;36(11):2027–2037.
126. Carroll M, Horton MB. Telehealth and Indian healthcare: moving to scale and sustainability. *Telemedicine e-Health*. 2013;19(5):377–379.
127. Gittelsohn J, Rowan M. Preventing diabetes and obesity in American Indian communities: the potential of environmental interventions. *Am J Clin Nutr*. 2011;93(5):1179S–1183S.

CHAPTER 15

Migrant Farmworker Health

Jennie A. McLaurin

Migrant farmworkers are a distinct population within rural public health. A group defined by occupation, mobility, and culture, migrant farmworkers' social determinants of health differ in systematic ways from those of the general rural population of the United States. Poverty, social isolation, immigration status, language, education, housing, regulatory standards, workplace exposures, and frequent mobility all influence access to care and health status. This chapter considers the demographics, health behaviors, health conditions, access barriers, and programs and resources for this mobile poor population. Particular attention is given to issues of occupational and environmental health.

In simplest terms, migrant farmworkers are hired crop laborers who travel from home in order to secure employment. More nuanced definitions are crafted to bound policies and programs directed to this group. References to migrant farmworkers exclude those employed in animal production or fisheries, although parallels can be drawn. Farms and ranches in the United States employ 1.8 to 2.5 million migrant, seasonal, and year-round laborers to assist in plant-based agriculture.[1,2] At least 42 of the 50 states employ migrant farmworkers in their rural locales.[3]

There is a long history of migrant farm labor in the United States, with industrialization in the mid-19th century creating demand for a large number of seasonal workers. Foreign-born workers have always supplied migrant labor, with Asians constituting over 85% of the workforce in the late 1800s.[4] Overfarming, severe drought, and poor land management led to the iconic images of the Dust Bowl era, when many farm owners joined the ranks of migrant workers seeking crop work in California. The Bracero

Agreement of 1942 created a supply of Mexican workers as World War II strained U.S. farmers, and although numerous policies have since replaced that action, Mexican workers remain the chief source of America's rural hired crop workers.[3]

POPULATION CHARACTERISTICS

The migrant and seasonal farmworker population is fluid, with workers regularly leaving and joining this labor pool. Distinctions between seasonal and migrant workers are difficult. Technically, seasonal workers are short-term hired crop laborers who do not move in order to obtain this employment. However, economic and political conditions often affect the mobility of migrants and the stability of seasonal workers. For the purposes of this chapter, health considerations include both seasonal and migrant workers, with exceptions noted as needed.

Over 90% of farmworkers are Hispanic, with the majority foreign-born from landless poor families in Mexico.[3] Although most of the workers are men, women comprise 20% of the labor force and teens represent about 10% of workers. Two thirds of the women are married with children who reside with them even during migration. At least half of the farmworker population is unauthorized to work in the United States. Increasing numbers of indigenous Mexican and Central American workers are part of the migrant population, speaking neither Spanish nor English as their primary language. Further attributes of the indigenous workers will be noted later in the chapter.

A small but important percentage of the migrant crop workers are hired under H-2A legislation. Known as a guestworker program, the Department of Labor grants a specified number of time-limited H2-A visas for U.S. farmers to employ noncitizens in the event of worker shortages. Despite the recent deep recession, demand remains high for foreign workers. Workers under the H-2A program typically travel under the oversight of crew leaders: Families are not allowed to accompany the workers. Supports and protections for the approximately 80,000 H-2A workers include housing, workers' compensation, wage guarantees, and the potential to be remunerated for transportation. Importantly, routine health care is not covered, and ill workers can be abruptly returned home.

Apart from the H-2A program, farmworkers typically migrate in three major patterns. Restricted-circuit migration refers to the practice of traveling for work from a home base, often in groups of a few adults. The distance traveled allows return home and usually repeats seasonally. Point-to-point migration encompasses farther distances and may include the whole family. Often the same farms are worked and migration is to a known workplace. Nomadic migration is the least predictable and secure, typically undertaken by single men in search of work but unsure of their destination. Many of the nomadic workers are trying to support families in their home country and are the most marginalized and isolated of the migrant workers (see Figure 15.1).

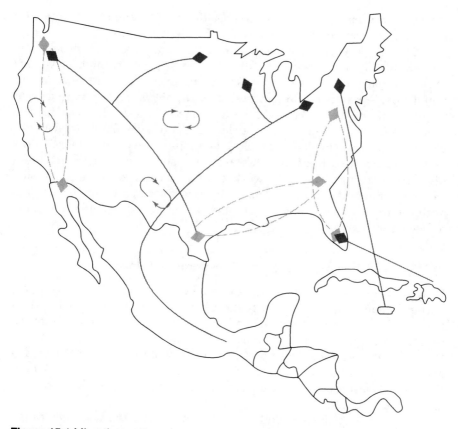

Figure 15.1 Migration patterns.

Farmworkers experience extreme poverty, with individual farmworker earnings ranging from $10,000 to $12,499 annually.[3] Multiple workers may live together in households, with overcrowding common. Adult literacy is limited, with most Mexican farmworkers having received 6 or fewer years of formal education. Indigenous farmworkers may have no written equivalent of their spoken native languages. Health literacy, influenced by cultural understandings as well as communication barriers, may differ markedly in the farmworker population compared to other subsets of the rural poor.[5]

HEALTH ISSUES

Migrant and seasonal farmworker health issues that warrant special consideration include those related to occupational and environmental health, infectious diseases, mental and behavioral health, food insecurity, housing, and oral health. Barriers to health care that influence each of these issues include transportation difficulties, geographic isolation, language and cultural differences, discrimination and anti-immigrant climates, lack of third-party payers, discontinuity of care sites and health records, agricultural regulatory standards and enforcement, poverty, and frequent mobility.

Despite 60 years of government-funded programs and resources to assist health and education of farmworker families, no comprehensive data set exists that provides morbidity and mortality figures particular to this population. A number of research studies supply disease-specific data or regional rates of health access. Mortality related to occupation as a migrant farmworker is unmeasured despite clear and consistent findings that agriculture is one of the most hazardous occupations in the United States.[6] Other mortality indices, such as infant mortality, are also nonexistent. Health issues discussed herein rely then on worker surveys, clinician reports, research studies, farmworker program data, and abstractions made from larger rural health considerations. Limitations of data are discussed as applicable in the following sections.

Occupational and Environmental Health

Injury death rates from agriculture exceed all other industries and continue to rise.[6] Foreign-born workers have the highest risk of death. Nonlethal injuries are most commonly sprains and strains, lacerations, and fractures or dislocations.[7] In addition to injuries, farmworkers are at risk for exposures to toxins, extreme weather, irritants, allergens, violence, and infectious diseases. It can be difficult to separate health effects associated with work from those with housing when housing is included as a benefit and located on or adjacent to a farm field.

Pesticide exposures include those directly associated with application but also with drift, premature re-entry into fields, and paraoccupational exposure in farm residences or with residue on other workers or family members.[8,9] The subpopulations of pregnant women and adolescents are of additional concern. Multiple studies show associations between prenatal pesticide exposure and teratogenic effects, including impaired intellectual development, neural tube defects, and limb anomalies.[10–13] Adolescents are shown to underestimate their exposures risks, which may be heightened by rapid growth and immature nervous systems.[14]

Eye care is an occupational issue as dust, chemicals, sharp objects, and ultraviolet light are all hazardous. Hispanics lack eye care access and understanding at twice the rate of any other racial or ethnic subgroup, with 41% reporting no access.[15] A Florida study of citrus workers found fewer than 2% wore protective eyewear.[16] Similarly, less than 10% of farmworkers in a North Carolina population reported wearing protective eye equipment; discomfort, poor fit, and poor visibility were cited as impediments.[17] Almost half of the North Carolina workers had no history of eye care and 20% had multiple symptoms of eye problems at the time of interview. Only 5% wore corrective lenses but 11% had difficulty recognizing a friend from across a street and 20% had difficulty with vision when reading. Chronic infections and unrecognized eye conditions were common.[17] Citrus workers trained as community health workers for their peers have been shown to positively influence eye preventive health, increasing protective eyewear to 27%.[16]

Workplace violence may affect all farmworkers, but undocumented, female, and adolescent workers are particularly vulnerable. In a 2010 El Paso study, 7% of farmworkers reported experiencing workplace violence, with alcohol an associated factor.[18] In larger studies, up to 80% of women farmworkers reported sexual harassment.[19]

Occupational and environmental health issues of farmworkers are exacerbated by permissive labor regulations for agriculture, lack of enforcement, and immigration fears. Since the passage of the Fair Labor Standards Act of 1938, agriculture has been granted exceptions to workplace health and safety policies present for other industries.[20] Wages are less protected, child labor is permissible at younger ages (12 years) with exposure to more hazards than in other industries, and small farms are exempted from much of the federal oversight on housing and sanitation.[21] Compounding the level of increased risk faced in farm settings, access to care exacerbates any conditions that do arise—at least 70% of farmworkers are uninsured, with most lacking workman's compensation access as well.[3] While this impacts all farmworker groups, undocumented farmworkers are the least likely to seek health services.[3]

Infectious Diseases

Migrant farmworkers are more susceptible to a variety of infectious diseases due to frequent mobility, international travel, poverty, underimmunization, poor sanitation at work and home, cultural practices, and overcrowding. Tropical diseases such as dengue fever, Chagas disease, malaria, and parasitic infections are frequently reported.[22-24] Farmworkers have higher rates of tuberculosis than the general rural population and are at higher risk for HIV infection.[25,26] Cultural risks may include nonsterile use of needles through the practice of "lay injection"; that is, community members serve as medical practitioners and inject medications obtained in Mexico.[27] Depo-Provera, antibiotics, and vitamins are among commonly injected substances.[28] Similarly, amateur tattoo application may also increase infection via needle use.[29] Because these exposures occur outside the context of typical community interventions, there is a great need for the development of culturally tailored approaches to address infectious disease risk in farmworker communities.

Mental and Behavioral Health

Mental and behavioral health needs of migrant farmworkers include conditions related to premigration environments, migration itself, and postmigration situations. High rates of stress, violence exposure, fatigue, overcrowding, fear, bereavement, isolation, and uncertainty contribute to disorders such as anxiety, depression, and posttraumatic stress. Although research in this area of farmworker health is relatively new, rural health practitioners may improve farmworker health by considering the following issues in care planning.

While much has been made of the "healthy immigrant effect,"[30] desperation drives farmworker families to migrate under difficult conditions and to accept a harsh new life. Premigration stressors may include war, civil unrest and violence, natural catastrophes, and extreme poverty. In addition to the stereotypic images of people crossing deserts and rivers at night, migrants entering unlawfully also are more likely to be assaulted, robbed, or held hostage. An estimated 60% of undocumented women experience sexual assault during or after their migration.[19]

In a study of mental health factors specific to farmworkers, Hiott and colleagues found 38% of the participants to have significant stress levels based on several standard tests.[31] Anxiety and depression symptom severity correlated with greater social isolation and difficult working conditions. Over 40% of those studied met screening criteria for clinical depression, over 30% screened as alcohol dependent, and over 20% screened positive for anxiety.[31]

Culture-bound syndromes also occur within migrant farmworker groups. *Coraje, susto,* and *nervios* are three such syndromes associated with mental health symptoms and dysfunction. While no direct translation is fully accurate, emotions of anger, fright, anxiety, and sadness contribute to the conditions. Importantly, these emotions are often thought to be contagious. For example, within these conditions one's anger can be imparted to another and cause that person to be ill from heart disease, asthma, or other diseases.[32] Somatization is common and not associated with patient perceptions of mental health. An Oregon study of farmworkers found 32% of respondents had at least one of the three syndromes mentioned.[32] *Coraje* and *nervios* correlated with significant Patient Health Questionnaire (PHQ-9) scores. Sleep difficulty was associated with *coraje*.

Cultural bereavement is a condition that also applies to many migrant farmworkers. A specific type of grief, it is characterized by a loss of one's social structure and collective cultural identity, in turn associated with underlying perpetual mourning.[33] It can accompany and compound a grief associated with physical death of a loved one. Because grief reactions are culturally shaped, United States rural health practitioners may erroneously label culturally distinct migrants as abnormal if bereavement is misunderstood. Diagnoses of psychosis, depression, and posttraumatic stress have been incorrectly applied to some grieving migrants.[33] Compounding treatment for all these conditions is the fact that Spanish-speaking behavioral and mental health practitioners are in short supply, particularly in rural areas, and indigenous language-speaking migrants may be entirely unable to receive services due to significant associated language barriers.

Positively, immigrant farmworkers do have lower rates of a number of mental health disorders than their American-born counterparts. They have decreased substance abuse, decreased suicide, and decreased risk-taking behaviors in adolescence. The support of a collectivist culture, family identity, and aspirations for work are thought to play a protective role in this relationship.[34]

Food Insecurity and Housing

Multiple studies document food insecurity in the migrant farmworker population with rates higher than others in poverty; over half of farmworker households are estimated to be food insecure.[35–38] Food insecurity is exacerbated by unreliable transportation, inadequate cooking facilities, and insufficient food storage. New immigrants are less likely to seek assistance for food insecurity, fearing government intervention and being unfamiliar with available programs.[37]

Though diverse housing arrangements are made for migrant farmworkers, most studies find housing to be overcrowded, unsanitary, and lacking adequate kitchen and laundry facilities.[39–41] Crowding increases exposures to infectious diseases, stress, injury, and violence. Inability to bathe and launder contributes to increased personal and household exposure to pesticide residue, infectious agents, and other contaminants. Private wells supply most of the water for both the farm worksite and the home. Agrichemicals and animal waste are common contaminants, with numerous studies showing public health risk due to nitrates, heavy metals, and bacteria.[42–45]

Oral Health

Migrant farmworkers have limited experience with preventive dental care and have higher rates of oral health problems than the general population.[1, 2] A survey of farmworkers showed that dental and oral health needs were one of their three most pressing self-reported health needs, diabetes, and hypertension being the other primary concerns.[48] A recent North Carolina study found that many adult farmworkers report chronic pain and functional impairment related to untreated dental disease. Over half of these adults had caries, a third had missing teeth, and only 21% received dental care in the preceding year, with almost all the care delivered in Mexico.[47] It is not uncommon for migrant men to report that they have never seen a dentist.[49]

Although migrant children may receive Medicaid dental coverage, subsidized preventive care is not available to adults. Adult farmworkers typically seek dental care because of pain or infection. Diet, culture, poverty, and access barriers influence knowledge, attitudes, and behaviors of farmworker families toward oral health. Head Start enrollment is shown to improve the oral health status of migrant children and improve the oral health literacy of their parents.[46] Systematic access barriers may still disproportionately exclude migrant families from care even when Medicaid coverage is present.[50]

Maternal and Child Health Concerns

Special concerns of maternal and child health include inadequate prenatal care, sexual violence and infections, delayed cervical and breast cancer screening, fetal and pediatric toxic exposures, childhood educational disruptions, nutritional deficiencies, unmet developmental needs, and inadequate immunizations.[51] Extreme shortages of supervised and subsidized child care contribute to child accompaniment of parents to the fields. Early and prolonged child labor limits educational opportunities and increases adverse influences on healthy growth and development. Migrant children experience the greatest disparities in educational standards of all Title I subcategories of at-risk children.[52,53]

PROGRAMS AND RESOURCES

A number of federally funded programs support migrant farmworker well-being:

* Migrant Health Act—Authorized by Congress as a part of the federally qualified community health center program, the Health Resources and Services Administration (HRSA) oversees approximately 156 migrant health clinics, which serve about 20% of the farmworker population. Primary medical care, dental care, outreach services, and behavioral health care are emphasized.
* Migrant Education—Authorized by Congress and within the Department of Education, this program serves preschool- through high school-age migrant children with supplemental educational services (Title I), including summer programs.
* Migrant Head Start—The U.S. Department of Health and Human Services funds this program for migrant children 6 weeks old to school age. Local grants are awarded to community-based organizations. Approximately 37,000 children are served annually, representing about 25% of the anticipated eligible population.
* Supplemental Food Security—According to the U.S. Department of Agriculture, migrant children are categorically eligible for free and reduced school meals and for Women, Infants, and Children (WIC) services.
* Migrant Clinicians Network (MCN)—This is a private, not-for-profit national organization funded by HRSA as well as by a number of private grants and donations. Dedicated to the promotion of health justice for the nation's mobile poor, MCN provides resources, training, and technical assistance to clinicians serving migrant and seasonal farmworkers. Initiatives include cancer screening and prevention, immunization delivery, lead reduction, occupational and environmental health, adolescent worker safety, family planning, intimate partner violence prevention, care navigation for mobile patients, meaningful use and patient-centered medical homes in the context of migration, and community health worker training.[54]

Successful interventions, whether supported by federal grants or through other means, incorporate culturally appropriate integrated approaches responsive to the barriers already noted. Community health workers, often referred to as *promotores*, are often vital to success. *Promotores* programs have effectively addressed pesticide prevention, eye protection, stress reduction, intimate partner violence, immunization delivery, and cancer screening.[55,56] Partnership with community health workers at Mexican consulates (Ventanillas de Salud) has increased access to health services in a number of rural communities.

Some rural health programs are incorporating occupational and environmental health education into their clinical sites. Through a grant from the Environmental Protection Agency, MCN established 10 Centers of Excellence in Occupational and Environmental Health.[54] Clinicians at these centers are prepared to assess and treat farmworkers in accordance with evidence-based need. Health professions training and postgraduate teaching is another MCN effort to improve care delivery.

A national program resource is Health Network, operated by MCN. It is a form of virtual case management, linking migrant patients to a telephone-based case manager who is able to contact any clinical site within or outside of the United States. Migrant patients are enrolled in the program by their clinician and agree to secure record transfer within the Health Network system. Health Network assists in the provision of a patient-centered medical home for mobile patients, is provided free of charge, and reports data on health outcomes of patients served.

CONCLUSION

In summary, migrant farmworkers in the United States are a young immigrant rural population who experience health access barriers due to frequent mobility, extreme poverty, social isolation, cultural distinctions, immigration concerns, lack of insurance and transportation, communication barriers, and occupational challenges. Despite being a young, strong labor force, they experience disproportionately high rates of injury, disease, and stress. Rural health planning must address occupational and environmental issues, justice concerns, and educational factors as care for this population is designed.

Present programs in health and education available to migrant farmworkers reach only a minority of farmworker families and need expansion as well as enhancement. Primary care services will be most effective when patient-centered care is coupled with outreach efforts and preventive health coverage. Dental care for adults is an urgent need. Behavioral health integration is beginning but requires attention to the workforce and cultural characteristics of this population. Cancer care, palliative care, and end-of-life care are areas in need of thoughtful program implementation. Continuity of care will always be a challenge and is constrained by lack of interstate portability of records and insurance benefits.

In this era of global health meeting rural health, care for migrant farmworkers will be both an international concern and a locally shaped response. Public health practitioners and planners will be assisted by understanding the agricultural labor force in their region of concern, the current regulations affecting that labor, and the available resources for social and health services. A number of organizations have issued recommendations and action steps for addressing disparities in labor and health; familiarity and solidarity with these initiatives are needed.[57–59] Cultural proficiency in population care is an ongoing task and assisted by acquisition of language skills, development of cross-cultural relationships, and global health experience. Advocacy for this marginalized immigrant labor force is an essential public health imperative.

RESOURCES

Migrant Clinicians Network: www.migrantclinician.org
Health Network: http://www.migrantclinician.org/services/network.html
Migrant Health Promotion: www.migranthealth.org
Health Outreach Partners: www.outreach-partners.org
National Center for Farmworker Health: www.ncfh.org
Farmworker Justice: www.farmworkerjustice.org
National Association of Community Health Centers: www.nachc.org
National Farm Worker Ministry: www.nfwm.org

REFERENCES

1. Kandel W. *Profile of Hired Farmworkers: A 2008 Update.* Economic Research Report No. 60. Washington, DC: US Department of Agriculture, Economic Research Service; 2008.
2. Martin P. Immigration reform: implications for agriculture. *Agricultural and Resource Economics Update.* Davis, CA: University of California, Giannini Foundation; 2006.
3. Carroll D, Samardick RM, Bernard S, Gabbard S, Hernandez T. *Findings from the National Agricultural Workers Survey (NAWS) 2001–2002: A demographic and employment profile of the United States farm workers.* Research Report No. 9, US Department of Labor; 2005.
4. National Farmworker Ministry. Timeline of agricultural labor. http://nfwm.org/education-center/farm-worker-issues/timeline-of-agricultural-labor. Accessed June 18, 2012.
5. Arcury TA, Quandt SA. Delivery of health services to migrant and seasonal farmworkers. *Annu Rev Public Health.* 2007;28:345–363.
6. US Bureau of Labor Statistics. National census of fatal occupational injuries in 2009 (preliminary results). 2010. http://www.bls.gov/news.release/pdf/cfoi.pdf. Accessed June 18, 2012.
7. Wang S, Myers JR, Layne LA. Injuries to hired crop workers in the United States—a descriptive analysis of a national probability sample. *Am J Ind Med.* 2011;54(10):734–747.
8. Arcury TA, Grzywacz JG, Davis SW, Barr DB, Quandt SA. Organophosphorus pesticide urinary metabolite levels of children in farmworker households in eastern North Carolina. *Am J Ind Med.* 2006;49:751–760.
9. McCauley LA, Michaels S, Rothlein J, Muniz J, Lasarev M, Ebbert C. Pesticide exposure and self reported home hygiene: practices in agricultural families. *AAOHN J.* 2003;51:113–119.
10. Rull RP, Ritz B, Shaw GM. Neural tube defects and maternal residential proximity to agricultural pesticide applications. *Am J Epidemiol.* 2006;163:743–753.

11. Engel LS, O'Meara ES, Schwartz SM. Maternal occupation in agriculture and risk of limb defects in Washington State, 1980–1993. *Scand J Work Environ Health.* 2000;26:193–198.
12. Bouchard MF, Chevrier J, Harley KG, et al. Prenatal exposure to organophosphate pesticides and IQ in 7-year-old children. *Environ Health Perspect.* 2011;119:1187–1195.
13. Eskenazi B, Huen K, Marks A, et al. PON1 and neurodevelopment in children from the CHAMACOS study exposed to organophosphate pesticides in utero. *Environ Health Perspect.* 2010;118:1775–1781.
14. Salazar MK, Napolitano M, Scherer JA, McCauley LA. Hispanic adolescent farmworkers' perceptions associated with pesticide exposure. *West J Nurs Res.* 2004;26:146–166; discussion 167–175.
15. Primo SA, Wilson R, Hunt JW, et al. Reducing visual health disparities in at-risk community health center populations. *J Public Health Manag Prac.* 2009;15(6): 529–534.
16. Monaghan PF, Forst LS, Tovar-Aguilar JA, et al. Community health worker model helps prevent eye injuries. *Am J Public Health.* 2011;101(12):2269–2274.
17. Quandt SA, Feldman SR, Vallejos QM. Vision problems, eye care history, and ocular protection among migrant farmworkers. *Arch Env Occ Health.* 2008;63(1):13–16.
18. Saenz CD. Health risks and health-seeking behaviors of migrant and seasonal farmworkers on the US-Mexico border. *ETD Collection for University of Texas, El Paso.* 2010; Paper AAI1477825.
19. Bauer M, Ramírez M. *Injustices on Our Plates: Immigrant Women in the U.S. Food Industry.* Montgomery, AL: Southern Poverty Law Center; 2010. http://www .splcenter.org/sites/default/files/downloads/publication/Injustice_on_Our_ Plates.pdf. Accessed June 25, 2012.
20. Fair Labor Standards Act 1938, 29 USC § 203, et seq.
21. Schell G. Farmworker exceptionalism under the law: how the legal system contributes to farmworker poverty and powerlessness. In: Thompson DC Jr, Wiggins MF, eds. *The Human Cost of Food.* Austin, TX: University of Texas Press; 2004:139–166.
22. Villarejo D, Baron SL. The occupational health status of hired farm workers. *Occup Med.* 1999;14(3):613–635.
23. Hansen E, Donohoe M. Health issues of migrant and seasonal farmworkers. *J Health Care Poor Underserved.* 2003;14(2):153–163.
24. Bern C, Montgomery SP. Estimate of the burden of Chagas disease in the United States. *Clin Infect Dis.* 2009;49. http://www.doctorswithoutborders.org/events/ symposiums/2009-dndi-treat-chagas/assets/files/Bern-Montgomery_Chagas-US-burden_CID-090729.pdf. Accessed June 25, 2012.
25. MMWR. Prevention and control of tuberculosis in migrant farm workers. Recommendations of the Advisory Council for the Elimination of Tuberculosis. *MMWR Recomm Rep.* 1992;41(RR-10):1–15. Available at *MMWR Recomm Rep.* Accessed June 25, 2012.
26. Sanchez MA, Lemp GF, Magis-Rodriguez C, Bravo-Garcia E, Carter S, Ruiz JD. Epidemiology of HIV among Mexican migrants and recent immigrants in California and Mexico. *J Acquir Immune Defic Syndr.* 2004;37:S204–S214.
27. McVea KL. Lay injection practices among migrant farmworkers in the age of AIDS: evolution of a biomedical folk practice. *Soc Sci Med.* 1997;45:91–98.
28. Zuroweste E. Clinical alert: Depo parties. Migrant Clinicians network website. http://www.migrantclinician.org/issues/womens-health/discussion.html. Accessed June 25, 2012.

29. Smith SF, Acuña J, Feldman SR, et al. Tattooing practices in the migrant Latino farmworker population: risk for blood-borne disease. *Int J Dermatol.* 2009;48:1397–1403.

30. Vega WA, Sribney WM, Aguilar-Gaxiola S, Kolody B. 12-month prevalence of *DSM-III-R* psychiatric disorders among Mexican Americans: nativity, social assimilation, and age determinants. *J Nerv Ment Dis.* 2004;192: 532–541.

31. Hiott AE, Grzywacz JG, Davis SW, Quandt SA, Arcury TA. Migrant farmworker stress: mental health implications. *J Rural Health.* 2008;24(1):32–39.

32. Donlan W, Lee J. Coraje, nervios, and susto: culture-bound syndromes and mental health among Mexican migrants in the United States. *Adv Mental Health: Migration Mental Health.* 2010;9:288–302.

33. Bhugra D, Becker MA. Migration, cultural bereavement and cultural identity. *World Psychiatry.* 2005;4(1):18–24.

34. Borges G, Breslau J, Su M, Miller M, Medina-Mora ME, Aguilar-Gaxiola S. Immigration and suicidal behavior among Mexicans and Mexican Americans. *Am J Public Health.* 2009;99(4):728–733.

35. Quandt SA, Arcury TA, Early J, Tapia J, Davis JD. Household food security among migrant and seasonal Latino farmworkers in North Carolina. *Public Health Rep.* 2004;19:568–576.

36. Hill BG, Moloney AG, Mize T, Himelick T, Guest JL. Prevalence and predictors of food insecurity in migrant farmworkers in Georgia. *Am J Public Health.* 2011;101:831–833.

37. Quandt SA, Shoaf JI, Tapia J, Hernández-Pelletier M, Clark HM, Arcury TA. Experiences of Latino immigrant families in North Carolina help explain elevated levels of food insecurity and hunger. *J Nutr.* 2006;136:2638–2644.

38. Kilanowski JF, Moore LC. Farmworker children at high risk for food insecurity, inadequate diet. *J Ped Nurs.* 2010;25:360–366.

39. Housing Assistance Council. *No Refuge From the Fields: Findings From a Survey of Farmworker Housing Conditions in the United States.* Washington, DC: Housing Assistance Council; 2001.

40. Gentry AL, Grzywacz JG, Quandt SA, Davis SW, Arcury TA. Housing quality among North Carolina farmworker families. *J Agric Saf Health.* 2007;13:323–337.

41. Early J, Davis SW, Quandt SA, Rao P, Snively BM, Arcury TA. Housing characteristics of farmworker families in North Carolina. *J Immigr Minor Health.* 2006;8:173–184.

42. Center for Watershed Sciences. *Executive Summary: Nitrate in California's groundwater.* Davis, CA: University of California; 2012. groundwaternitrate.ucdavis.edu. Accessed June 22, 2012.

43. Washington State Department of Health. *Drinking Water Serving Temporary Farmworker Facilities: Water System Inspection and Testing Report.* Olympia, WA: Washington State Department of Health; 2000.

44. Nolan BT, Stoner JD. Nutrients in ground waters of the conterminous United States, 1992–1995. *Environ Sci Technol.* 2000;34:1156–1165.

45. Knobeloch L, Salna B, Hogan A, Postle J, Anderson H. Blue babies and nitrate-contaminated water. *Environ Health Perspect.* 2000;108:675–678.

46. Lukes SM. Oral health knowledge attitudes and behaviors of migrant preschooler parents. *J Dent Hyg.* 2010;84(2):87–93.

47. Quandt SA, Hiott AE, Grzywacz JG, Davis SW, Arcury TA. Oral health and quality of life of migrant and seasonal farmworkers in North Carolina. *J Agric Saf Health.* 2007;13:45–55.

48. Health Outreach Partners. *National Needs Assessment on Farmworker Health Outreach: Executive Summary.* Health Outreach Partners; 2010. Available at http://www.outreachpartners.org/docs/FAN%20Exec%20Summary%20Factsheet.pdf. Accessed June 25, 2012.

49. Swan MA, Barker JC, Hoeft KS. Rural Latino farmworker fathers' understanding of children's oral health. *Pediatr Dent.* 2010; 32(5):400–406.

50. Castañeda H, Carrion IV, Kline N, Tyson DM. False hope: effects of social class and health policy on oral health inequalities for migrant farmworker families. *Soc Sci Med.* 2010;71(11):2028–2037.

51. McLaurin JA, Liebman AK. Unique agricultural safety and health issues of migrant and immigrant children. *J Agromedicine.* 2012;17(2):186–196.

52. US Department of Education, Office of the Under Secretary, Policy and Program Studies Service. *A Snapshot of Title I Schools Serving Migrant Students, 2000–2001.* Washington, DC: US Department of Education; 2003.

53. US Department of Education. *School Year 2008–09 Consolidated State Performance Report Parts I and II.* Washington, DC: US Department of Education; 2010.

54. Garcia D, Hopewell J, Liebman AK, Mountain K. Migrant clinicians network: connecting practice to need and patients to care. *J Agromedicine.* 2012;17(1):5–14.

55. Liebman AK, Juárez PM, Leyva C, Corona A. Pilot program using *Promotoras de Salud* to educate farmworker families about the risks from pesticide exposure. *J Agromedicine.* 2007;12(2):33–43.

56. Luque JS, Mason M, Reyes-Garcia C, Hinojosa A, Meade CD. Salud es Vida: development of a cervical cancer education curriculum for promotora outreach with Latina farmworkers in rural southern Georgia. *Am J Public Health.* 2011;101(12):2233–2235.

57. Lee BC, Gallagher SS, Liebman AK, Miller ME, Marlenga B, eds. *Blueprint for Protecting Children in Agriculture: The 2012 National Action Plan.* Marshfield, WI: Marshfield Clinic; 2012.

58. American Public Health Association. *Requiring Clinical Diagnostic Tools and Biomonitoring of Exposures to Pesticides.* Policy Date: 11/9/2010. Policy Number: 20108. http://www.apha.org/advocacy/policy/policysearch/default.htm?id=1400. Accessed June 28, 2012.

59. American Public Health Association. *Ending Agricultural Exceptionalism: Strengthening Worker Protection in Agriculture Through Regulation, Enforcement, Training, and Improved Worksite Health and Safety.* Policy Date: 11/1/2011. Policy Number: 201110. http://www.apha.org/advocacy/policy/policysearch/default.htm?id=1420. Accessed June 28, 2012.

CHAPTER 16

Health and Aging in Rural America

Bret L. Hicken, Derek Smith, Marilyn Luptak,
and Robert D. Hill

To frame the content of this chapter, consider the case example of Richard and Joyce, an aging couple in rural Idaho.

Kootenai County (population 141,132) is located in northern Idaho, about 100 miles south of the Canadian border. It is home to Coeur d'Alene, (population 44,962) and Lake Coeur d'Alene—a well-known summer tourist attraction. Coeur d'Alene provides the services of a large city with a small-town feel. While Kootenai County is designated as a metropolitan county by the U.S. Department of Agriculture (USDA), it supports a large rural population (roughly 30%).

Richard (age 84) and Joyce (age 77) Smith live in a rural part of the county on the east side of Lake Coeur d'Alene. They have lived in the area for 14 years on a 52-acre farm with two residences—their own, and another that belongs to their daughter and her family. They have a few neighbors to the south (mostly of retirement age) and seasonal neighbors that live at the recently developed golf course and resort to their north. The Smiths do not see much of their neighbors; the year-round residents spend most of their time caring for their own property and preparing for the winter months, which are often harsh and can last from October to as late as July.

The nearest services, such as grocery and medical care, are 20 miles away in Coeur d'Alene. Highway 97, the only road to town, has several sharp switchbacks to negotiate before arriving at the interstate. The drive can be treacherous, especially during winter when the roads are ice covered. The trip can be 35 minutes or more in each direction.

Richard was diagnosed with vascular dementia a few years ago and can no longer drive, leaving Joyce as the sole driver in their home. As age has diminished her eyesight and reaction time, she has become uncomfortable with driving. Consequently, they rarely attend church or other social events and only seek medical care when symptoms are unbearable or when their daughter "forces the issue." As Richard's dementia has progressed, Joyce has increasingly assumed a caregiving role. Though she finds fulfillment in taking care of her husband, she feels more stress as she attempts to meet his growing needs. They rely on their daughter and family to run errands and for additional support. Their daughter helps as much as possible, though with a family of her own and full-time employment, she is often unavailable. Richard and Joyce often do not leave their home for several weeks and sometimes go an entire winter without keeping an appointment. As a result, Joyce often feels "trapped" in her home.

AGING RURAL AMERICA

Nationwide, the average life expectancy has been steadily increasing since 1900 and now approaches 80 years of age for men and women.[1,2] This change in life expectancy has brought a concomitant increase in the number of older adults living past age 65. Since 1900, the percentage of Americans 65+ has more than tripled (from 4.1% in 1900 to 13.1% in 2010), with the number of Americans 65+ increasing almost 13 times (from 3.1 million to 40.4 million). The population of the oldest Americans has experienced even more dramatic growth. While the 65 to 74 age group (20.8 million) was 10 times larger in 2010 than in 1900, the 75 to 84 group (13.1 million) was 17 times larger, and the 85+ group (5.5 million) was 45 times larger. The population of persons aged 100 or more in 2010 (53,364) had increased by 53% from 1990 (37,306).[3]

On average, women have a higher life expectancy (81.1 years) than men (76.2 years), though this difference is gradually diminishing.[1,2] This difference in life expectancy means that the oldest age group is predominantly female. In 2000, there were 75 males for every 100 females over age 65, decreasing to 32 males per 100 females after age 85.[4] This has particular ramifications for health and well-being, to be discussed in more detail in the following sections.

The Smith family represents this demographic trend as it plays out in rural communities across the United States. As in urban areas, rural America is aging. However, the growth rate is higher in rural areas compared to urban.[5] In the United States, older adults make up 15% of the rural population and 12% of the urban population. In 2008, older adults accounted for 18% of the population in nonmetropolitan counties.[6]

Two important factors account for this differential. First, many rural communities experience population loss through *out-migration* of young people to urban areas. Young people leave rural communities to pursue education, military service, or employment opportunities. From 1950 to 2000, rural counties experienced net out-migration of young adults ages 20 to 29.[7] Between 1988 and 2008, nearly half of all nonmetropolitan counties in the United States experienced net population loss, a rate exceeding 10% in one third of rural counties.[8] From 1990 to 2000, counties experiencing out-migration population decline lost approximately 6% of their population.[8]

Some rural communities are also experiencing *in-migration* of older adults. Though younger Americans are more likely to relocate than older adults, when older Americans do relocate, they are more likely to choose rural and small-town destinations, especially scenic areas with recreational opportunities[7] or for other quality of life reasons.[9] The USDA classifies nonmetropolitan counties as "retirement destinations" if the population of individuals aged 60 years or older increased by 15% or more between 1980 and 1990 through migration.[4] If past migration patterns hold among aging baby boomers (those born from 1946 to 1964), the rural and small-town population of 55- to 75-year-olds will have increased from 8.6 million in 2000 to 14.2 million in 2020.[10]

Sociodemographic Factors Affecting Older Adults in Rural America

Poverty

On average, older adults in rural areas are more likely to be classified as "poor" or "low income" relative to older adults in urban areas.[6,11] Older women in particular experience higher poverty rates than males, with 14% of older women at the federal poverty level.[12] This socioeconomic trend results from rural employment that is often seasonal in nature, lower wage scales overall, fewer opportunities for part-time work, less lifetime savings, lower education, and less retirement savings. As a result, many rural older adults are not eligible for Social Security (because they lack the required number of quarters of employment) and they receive lower monthly Social Security benefits than those living in urban locations. Despite this lower general payout from Social Security, rural older adults have a higher proportion of their income originating from Social Security.[11,13]

Race

Though rural older adults are predominantly Caucasian, other racial groups are common in certain regions of the United States. Many areas of the Great Plains, Four Corners, and Alaska have large populations of American Indian/ Native Alaskans, many southwestern states have large Hispanic populations, and a high proportion of older adults in the rural South are African American. As in urban areas, many rural communities are also experiencing an influx of immigrants from non–English-speaking countries. Though immigrants are often of working age, many have lower incomes and pay fewer taxes to support public services.[13]

Though Medicare and Medicaid are the principal sources of insurance for rural older minorities, many older immigrants do not qualify for Medicare. While 76% of nonmetropolitan White older adults report having private insurance, only 34% of African Americans, 33% of Hispanics, and 57% of older adults of other races do. Conversely, the proportion of older adults relying on Medicare alone was highest among minorities: 39% of nonmetropolitan African American older adults, 29% of Hispanic older adults, and 28% of older adults of other races have Medicare alone, versus 18% among Whites. The proportion of older adults receiving Medicaid is highest among Hispanics (33%), followed by African Americans (26%) and Whites (6%).[14]

In sum, rural America tends to be older than urban America, a net result of out-migration of young adults and in-migration of retirees. This older population is predominantly female and tends to be poorer than younger adults. Because there are fewer working-age adults per older adult, the tax base is often inadequate to support public services.[8] A lack of public services becomes problematic because, as discussed in the next section, older adults face significant health problems as they age.

PHYSICAL AND MENTAL HEALTH OF RURAL OLDER ADULTS

Physical Health

Aging is associated with the emergence of a variety of chronic physical and/or mental health conditions. Chronic conditions like heart disease and diabetes are highly prevalent and are the most common causes of mortality in older adults in the United States (Tables 16.1 and 16.2).[15,16] In some cases, these conditions are more prevalent among rural older adults relative to their urban counterparts. Note that these conditions are typically progressive and, in many cases, not curable. However, all are generally highly treatable with competent medical care. In their advanced stages, these diseases can create significant disability and disease burden, and growing need for medical care and additional caregiving in-home. However, rurality often makes obtaining care for these health problems especially difficult.

Chronic disease often leads to declines in functioning, but living in a rural area may exacerbate the impact of illness on independence. Age-adjusted rates of activity limitation are highest in rural areas: 15.3% of rural older adults have difficulty performing activities of daily living (ADLs) versus 12.7% of urban older adults. This urban/rural contrast is most apparent in the Northeast and the South.[13] A 2005 report from the National Long-Term Care Survey found that, though rural adults tend to have more disability-free years than urban residents, when they do experience functional decline, they live longer with those disabilities and live a greater proportion of their lives with disability.[17] In 2010, the Centers for Disease Control and Prevention (CDC) reported a greater proportion of rural (relative to urban) older adults

Table 16.1 Mortality and Morbidity Among Adults Aged 65 Years or Older in the United States

Mortality in 2002[15]	White	Non-Hispanic Black	Hispanic
Heart Disease	32.4%	32%	31.8%
Cancer	21.0%	22.7%	21.5%
Stroke	7.4%	8.3%	7.9%
Chronic lower respiratory diseases	3.9%	3.4%	6.4%
Influenza and pneumonia	3.5%	2.7%	3.3%
Alzheimer's disease	2.2%	2.0%	3.4%
Diabetes	6.3%	5.0%	2.6%
All other causes	23.3%	23.9%	23.1%
Prevalence of Chronic Conditions in 2002[15]	**White**	**Non-Hispanic Black**	**Hispanic**
High blood pressure	45.0%	68.4%	49.7%
Arthritis	42.6%	53.4%	48.6%
Coronary heart disease	14.3%	17.4%	21.9%
Any cancer	8.8%	11.2%	22.7%
Diabetes	8.0%	9.6%	8.6%
Stroke	21.9%	24.5%	14.9%

Table 16.2 Chronic Conditions, Ages 65+ (2008–2010)[16]

	Heart Disease	Coronary Heart Disease	Heart Attack	Stroke	Cancer, All	Arthritis	Diabetes
Metropolitan	29.6%	20.4%	9.9%	7.5%	23.4%	50.8%	20.9%
Nonmetropolitan	32.1%	21.8%	12.4%	11.0%	23.8%	53.4%	23.4%

with limitations in their ADLs (44% vs. 37%). More than half of rural African American older adults (55%) and 46% of Hispanic older adults reported functional limitations.[14] Older adults in rural settings are more likely than urban older adults to report being less happy and having worse health. Rural older adults are also more likely to be institutionalized than urban older adults due to an inability to care for themselves at home (Table 16.3).[32,33]

Table 16.3 Difficulty Performing Activities of Daily Living (ADLs) and Instrumental Activities of Daily Living (IADLs) Among Medicare Beneficiaries, Ages 65+: United States 2010[16]

		2010
ADLs	Bathing/showering	9.68%
	Dressing	6.56%
	Eating	2.7%
	Getting in/out of bed/chairs	11.6%
	Walking	24.26%
	Toileting	4.97%
IADLs	Using the telephone	6.84%
	Doing light housework	10.75%
	Doing heavy housework	29.55%
	Preparing meals	8.86%
	Shopping	12.83%
	Managing money	6.78%

Mental Health

Poor physical health can increase risk for mental illness, particularly depression and anxiety, in combined effect with bereavement, poor social support, and functional decline[18]; for rural older adults, these psychiatric comorbidities occur in a context of limited access to care that greatly complicates effective management.

The most common psychiatric diagnoses in older adults are depression, anxiety, substance abuse, and dementia. Depression is not a normal part of aging—the 2006 Behavioral Risk Factor Surveillance System survey found the rate of depression and anxiety among older adults to be approximately 7.7% and 7.6%, respectively.[19] Estimates of mental health problems in rural areas vary. According to a report from the South Carolina Rural Health Research Center, the prevalence of depression is higher (6.11%) among rural populations than it is in urban populations (5.16%).[20] Other reports suggest that the rates of mental illness are similar between urban and rural areas.[6] Suicide rates are also higher in rural areas (17 per 100,000 vs. 12–15 per 100,000 in urban areas).[6] However, the rates of these illnesses increase as other care needs grow.[21] Suicide rates for males are highest among those aged 75 and older (36 per 100,000) and the rate of suicide for adults aged 75 years and older is 16.3 per 100,000.[22]

A 2012 report from the Substance Abuse and Mental Health Services Administration found that rural patients admitted for substance abuse treatment were more likely to use alcohol (49.5% vs. 36.1%) and nonheroin opiates (10.6% vs. 4.0%) as primary drugs of abuse than urban admissions. In contrast, urban patients reported primary abuse of heroin (21.8% vs. 3.1%) or cocaine (11.9% vs. 5.6%). Urban admissions were also almost twice as likely as rural admissions to report daily use of their primary substance (43.1% vs. 23.5%).[23]

Estimates of the prevalence of problem drinking in older adults vary from 1% to 16% depending on how "older adults," "at-risk," and "problem drinking" are defined.[24] The 2010 National Survey on Drug Use and Health found that alcohol use declines with age. Binge-drinking rates among individuals aged 50 to 64 years (part of the baby boom cohort) range from approximately 12% to 20%, while the rate of binge drinking among persons aged 65 or older was 7.6%, down from 9.8% in 2009. The rate of heavy drinking was 1.6% (the National Institute of Alcohol Abuse and Alcoholism recommends no more than 1 drink/day for persons age 65+ [24]).[25]

Up to 5.3 million Americans currently have Alzheimer's disease, the most common type of dementia, the risk for which doubles every 5 years beginning at age 65. By age 85, between 25% and 50% of the population will exhibit signs of the disease. By 2050, the number of individuals with Alzheimer's is expected to more than double. Alzheimer's disease is the sixth leading cause of death in the United States and is the fifth leading cause among persons age 65 and older.[26] Because the population is relatively older in rural areas than urban areas, presumably the prevalence of dementia would also be higher in these areas.

Medication

Older adults are the highest users of prescription medications among all age groups. A Centers for Medicare and Medicaid (CMS) report from 2003 found that 70% of community-dwelling Medicare recipients take at least one prescription medication; 58% take three or more prescription medications.[27] Add to that the many over-the-counter medications and herbal remedies that older adults use and this creates a serious risk for problems related to medication errors and/or side effects. The prevalence of inappropriate medication prescribing (e.g., wrong drug, improper dose, wrong dosing schedule, etc.) is estimated to occur in nearly 8.0% of outpatient office visits,[28] though these estimates vary widely depending on the criteria used to determine "inappropriate"—one recent study found the prevalence of inappropriate prescribing at approximately 23%.[29] The likelihood of adverse drug events increases by 10% for each medication added.[30] Many medications increase risk for problems for which older adults are already at high risk including falls, excessive sedation, increased confusion, urinary retention, decreased food intake, or a general failure to thrive.[31]

ACCESS TO HEALTH CARE

The prevalence and complexity of these health problems in older adults often require primary and specialty care to prevent disease progression and associated functional decline. However, older rural-dwelling adults often downplay pain and other symptoms that indicate illness and may not seek care until illness is at an advanced stage. They may also refrain from seeking preventive care, such as cholesterol tests and mammagrams, that can help detect health problems earlier in their course. Even if they do choose to seek treatment, many rural communities lack sufficient primary care and specialty care to meet the demand. Overall, there are additional specific access barriers faced by rural older adults, including insurance coverage, transportation barriers, specialty care, long-term care, and end-of-life care.

Insurance Coverage

Rural beneficiaries spend an average of 23% of their annual income on health care services compared with 18% spent by urban beneficiaries. Rural older adults are less likely to have supplemental insurance to cover cost sharing for Medicare or prescription drugs. Nearly 10% of older persons living in nonmetropolitan areas adjacent to metropolitan areas are receiving Medicaid or other public assistance versus 5.8% of older adults living in metropolitan areas. Because of insurance and income limitations, rural older adults are more likely to report delays in getting care due to costs.[13] Many older rural residents are classified as poor and rely on Medicare and Medicaid to help pay for their long-term care. However, even with this support, many cannot afford to utilize available services. Some families must pool their funds to help pay for services, which can cause a hardship for families.[32,33]

Assistance in Transportation

A large number of older persons have limited or no driving capability due to poor eyesight, decreased reaction times, limited physical mobility, and other medical conditions. In rural areas, public transportation options are limited or nonexistent, so older adults who cannot drive must rely on family or community members for transportation. As a result, driving to medical appointments can be a significant challenge. In addition to long distances and drive times, rural drivers also face roads that are often narrow, one-lane, and poorly maintained. Adverse weather conditions often add to the challenge of driving in rural areas. When considering emergency transportation, in many cases ambulances cannot make it to rural areas in time to assist in an emergency. Medevac helicopters are often required in emergencies, which can greatly increase the cost of medical care.[34,35]

Specialty Geriatric Care

Despite an aging population, which suggests a need for 30,000 new geriatricians by 2030, current trends in medical school choices indicate that this goal is unrealistic. In 2008, there were 7,012 geriatric physicians in the United States, 90% of whom practiced in urban areas. Despite a 46% increase in geriatricians practicing in rural areas between 2000 and 2008, geriatricians remain concentrated in urban areas, with 1.48 geriatricians per 10,000 older adults in the most urban of counties and 0.80 in the most-rural of counties. There were only 46 geriatricians in the 435 most rural counties in the United States,[36] underscoring the significant lack of access to necessary geriatric-specialty care.

Long-Term Care

A large proportion of those persons in the oldest demographic (over age 85) live in rural areas. This population is more likely to need long-term care and aging services due to the high prevalence of persons within the demographic needing help with activities of daily living (ADLs).[32] However, access to long-term care is limited in rural areas.

Available services include assisted living facilities (ALFs), nursing homes, home health, and home- and community-based services. ALFs in rural areas are usually significantly smaller than urban ALFs and provide minimal services and minimal privacy. Nursing homes are, by far, the most heavily utilized long-term care service outside the home in rural areas. However, they are typically smaller and understaffed relative to urban facilities.[32] Although rural nursing homes have larger populations of patients with dementia and depression, they have fewer specialized services (e.g., Alzheimer's units). Because of these issues, studies have found lower quality of care in rural nursing homes. Home health is an alternative to nursing homes that allows patients to remain in their homes. However, home health and home- and community-based services are severely limited in rural areas. When available, they can only provide a narrow range of services and are usually not as focused on long-term care as they are on post-acute care.[32]

End-of-Life Care

Older rural residents are more likely to die at home than are urban residents. As with long-term care, the provision of end-of-life and palliative care is difficult in rural areas. Doctors and nurses make house calls in rural regions to help informal caregivers care for patients with particularly difficult diseases (e.g., congestive heart failure). Medical professionals have also attempted to develop specialized palliative care services for rural areas. However, house calls are difficult to make due to distance and the lack of available personnel to implement specialized programs. In addition, most medical professionals who provide end-of-life care in rural settings are typically general practitioners and do not have specialized training in palliative care.[32,37,38]

As with nursing homes and ALFs, there are fewer hospices in rural areas than in urban areas. In 1999, more than two thirds of urban counties had a hospice physically located in the county, compared with one third of rural counties.[39] Rural hospices are usually hospital-based, decreasing the availability of choice. Rural residents do not use hospice services as frequently as their urban counterparts do, though the percentage of rural residents in hospice care has gone up in recent years. The rate of hospice use in the most remote rural areas was only 56% of the rate in the most-urban areas.[39] Hospices in rural settings suffer from many of the same issues as other health care facilities. They are frequently understaffed, lack a 24-hour pharmacy, and cover large areas—leading to increased travel distances from patients' homes and for their families.

CAREGIVING IN RURAL AREAS

The health issues described above suggest a population that is sicker and in greater need of caregiving assistance than younger individuals. For many Americans, such caregiving is delivered informally through family and friends. Most dementia care is provided informally through family members.[40] More than 20% of adults provide informal caregiving (i.e., unpaid care) for another adult with chronic illness and disability, which provides $306 billion in economic value to the U.S. economy.[41] Informal care networks are even more essential in rural communities with poor access to health care services. Unfortunately, for many rural older adults, informal care networks are often not available or are significantly stretched.

A 2006 Easter Seals report on rural caregiving noted that rural caregivers spend 21 hours per week in caregiving, with 19% spending more than 40 hours per week caregiving. For many caregivers the demands of caregiving may last for many years. Though 41% of rural caregivers provide care for someone for a year or less, 45% of rural caregivers have provided care between 1 and 9 years and 14% have provided care for 10 years or more.[41] In many cases, caregivers lack the financial resources to fully care for family members—41% of rural caregivers have children or grandchildren living with them, compared to only 28% of urban caregivers. Approximately 62% of rural caregivers report annual incomes under $50,000. Often, the caregivers themselves are older adults and have their own health problems. Indeed, 80% of rural caregivers were 50 and over and 27% were between 75 and 84.[41] This leaves individuals who often need care themselves, assuming a caregiving role for lack of other available options.

Not surprisingly, rurality tends to compound the already significant burden experienced by caregivers. These challenges include limited availability of services in rural areas. Rural caregivers are less likely to use most formal support services such as home health, transportation services, or caregiver support groups. A related issue is the lack of medical providers to offer medical advice and counseling to those providing caregiving services.[41]

Caregiving creates additional pressures on working-age adults who must balance caregiving responsibilities with employment demands—54% of rural caregivers reported working full-time or part-time during the period they were providing care. Fifty-six percent of rural caregivers reported making workplace accommodations, such as taking time off and/or leaving work early, to meet caregiving responsibilities. Eighteen percent took a leave of absence and 8% moved to part-time employment; 4% turned down a promotion; 3% took early retirement; and 5% lost some job benefits. Seven percent gave up work entirely.[41] Such accommodations only serve to further impact the limited financial income of many rural families.

The financial and health burdens noted, in addition to the challenge of providing regular care for a chronically ill or disabled individual, can raise stress levels among caregivers, leading to burnout and poorer health. Rural caregiving is not universally burdensome; however, its effects seem to appear at the "poles" of impact on stress. In the Easter Seals caregiving report, 30% of rural caregivers reported that caregiving was not at all stressful (vs. 25% of urban and 27% of suburban caregivers). However, 21% of rural caregivers reported caregiving to be very stressful while only 18% of their urban and 17% of their suburban counterparts so reported.[41] Caregivers that do experience stress related to caregiving are at risk for higher levels of depressive symptoms and other mental health problems, as well as increased rates of hypertension, cardiovascular disease, and premature mortality compared with noncaregiving peers.[42] Though effective interventions are available to assist caregivers in dealing with their stress, unfortunately, a majority of caregivers do not participate in such support programs.[40] For rural caregivers, the availability of such programs is often nonexistent.

A MODEL OF CARE DELIVERY FOR RURAL CAREGIVERS

In 2010, the Geriatric Research, Education, and Clinical Center in Salt Lake City, Utah, undertook an initiative to provide caregiver support to rural caregivers of veterans with dementia. The project was developed in coordination with the Veterans Rural Health Resource Center–Western Region. Because significant travel distances presented a barrier to caregivers attending in-person sessions, the Supporting Caregivers of Rural Veterans Electronically (SCORE) Project was developed as a remote technology-based intervention. The program provided remote support to caregivers living in rural areas by capitalizing on Internet and telehealth technologies to monitor caregiver status and provide educational content. Details of this program are described elsewhere.[43]

All caregivers were assigned a care manager (licensed clinical social worker) who provided telephone support, assisted with delivery of the educational content, and addressed any questions or concerns over the course of the study. Caregivers could contact their care manager at any point during their participation in the project. Internet-savvy caregivers participated via the Internet while caregivers who were Internet-naïve or who did not have access to the Internet used a simple in-home telehealth device that utilized a telephone line to receive and transmit digital information. Caregivers in this group accessed the intervention content using a very simple touch screen on the telehealth device that guided them through the educational content. The telehealth device also provided reminders, with the use of beeping and a flashing light, when new content was available.

Caregivers accessed the intervention content 3 days per week for approximately 10 to 15 minutes. The intervention content transmitted through both devices was identical and consisted of: (a) weekly video vignettes portraying the progression of dementia and caregiving skills; (b) information about health topics, caregiving skills, and mood management and self-care strategies (2 to 3 times per week); and (c) brief assessments of health and well-being (2 to 3 times per week). Individuals in both technology groups also participated in regular telephone calls with their care manager about the educational content and to address responses to the brief assessments. For example, if a caregiver endorsed severe stress on an assessment question, a care manager could contact the caregiver for additional evaluation and to offer additional stress-reduction strategies. Caregivers could request through the Internet and telehealth device that the care manager call them for additional support.

CONCLUSION

Richard and Joyce Smith in Kootenai County, Idaho, are emblematic of a growing trend in the United States— rural America is aging. Though older adults in rural communities share many challenges in common with younger individuals, the functional declines attendant to age and chronic disease compound the difficulties of living in isolated communities. The care needs of this population may exceed local public services' capacity—if services are even available. Though informal caregivers provide much of the unskilled care required by these individuals, caregiving can be a stressful experience that can take a toll on caregivers' health and well-being.

Telehealth interventions such as SCORE are an emerging method of closing the health care gaps for older adults in rural areas. Though telehealth cannot address every medical need, many health care services can be provided through distance technology. Some telehealth services, such as SCORE, can be delivered in the patient's home, without the help of a technician, reducing the need to travel long distances for care. Federal efforts such as the Recovery Act Broadband Initiatives Program are increasing the penetration of high-speed Internet into rural areas,[44] which will support further dissemination of telehealth to these areas.

REFERENCES

1. National Vital Statistics Reports. *Deaths: Preliminary Data for 2010;* 2010.
2. National Vital Statistics Reports. *Deaths: Final Data for 2009;* 2009.
3. Administration on Aging. Profile of older Americans. http://www.aoa.gov/aoaroot/aging_statistics/Profile/index.aspx. Accessed November 2012.
4. Berry E, Selfa T. Changing face of the rural West: the aging of the West. http://extension.usu.edu/htm/publications/publication=8353. Accessed October 2012.

5. Jones CA, Kandel W, Parker T. Population dynamics are changing the profile of rural areas. http://webarchives.cdlib.org/sw1vh5dg3r/http://ers.usda.gov/AmberWaves/April07/Features/Population.htm. Accessed October 2012.

6. The National Advisory Committee on Rural Health and Human Services. *The 2008 Report to the Secretary: Rural Health and Human Services Issues*. 2008.

7. Johnson K. *Demographic Trends in Rural and Small Town America*. Durham, NH: Carsey Institute; 2006.

8. McGranahan D, Cromartie J, Wojan T. *Nonmetropolitan Outmigration Counties: Some Are Poor, Many Are Prosperous*. United States Department of Agriculture; 2010.

9. Baernholdt M, Yan G, Hinton I, Rose K, Mattos M. Quality of life in rural and urban adults 65 years and older: findings from the National Health and Nutrition Examination Survey. *J Rural Health*. 2012;28(4):339–347.

10. Cromartie J, Nelson P. *Baby Boom Migration and Its Impact on Rural America*. 2011-12-01.

11. Coburn AF, Bolda EJ. Rural elders and long-term care. *West J Med*. 2001;174(3):209–213.

12. Housing Assistance Council. *Poverty in Rural America*. Washington, DC: Housing Assistance Council; 2012.

13. West Virginia University Center on Aging. *Best Practices in Service Delivery to the Rural Elderly*; 2003.

14. Probst JC, Samuels ME, Moore CG, Gdovin J. *Access to Care among Rural Minorities: Older Adults*. South Carolina Rural Health Research Center; 2002.

15. Centers for Disease Control and Prevention. *The State of Aging and Health in America*; 2002.

16. Centers for Disease Control and Prevention. Beyond 20/20 WDS—reports. http://205.207.175.93/HDI/ReportFolders/reportFolders.aspx. Accessed November 2012.

17. South Carolina Rural Health Research Center. *Disability Burdens among Older Americans in Rural and Urban Areas*; 2005.

18. Toner JA, Ferguson KD, Sokal RD. Continuing interprofessional education in geriatrics and gerontology in medically underserved areas. *J Contin Educ Health Prof*. 2009;29(3):157–160.

19. Centers for Disease Control and Prevention. *The State of Mental Health and Aging in America*; 2006.

20. Probst JC, Laditka S, Moore CG, Harun N, Powell P. *Depression in Rural Populations: Prevalence, Effects on Life Quality, and Treatment-Seeking Behavior*. South Carolina Rural Health Research Center; 2005.

21. National Institutes of Mental Health (NIMH). *Older Adults: Depression and Suicide Facts (Fact Sheet)*; 2012.

22. Centers for Disease Control and Prevention. Suicide facts at a glance. http://www.cdc.gov/ViolencePrevention/pdf/Suicide_DataSheet-a.pdf. Accessed December 2012.

23. Center for Behavioral Health Statistics and Quality (Substance Abuse and Mental Health Services Administration). A comparison of rural and urban substance abuse treatment admissions. http://www.samhsa.gov/data/2k12/TEDS_043/TEDSShortReport043UrbanRuralAdmissions2012.htm. Accessed February 2013.

24. Blow FC, Barry KL. Alcohol and substance misuse in older adults. *Curr Psychiatry Rep*. 2012;14(4):310–319.

25. Substance Abuse and Mental Health Services Administration. Results from the 2010 NSDUH: summary of national findings, SAMHSA, CBHSQ. 2010. http://www.samhsa.gov/data/NSDUH/2k10NSDUH/2k10Results.htm#3.1.1., 2012.

26. Centers for Disease Control and Prevention. Dementia/Alzheimer's disease. http://www.cdc.gov/mentalhealth/basics/mental-illness/dementia.htm. Accessed November 2012.

27. Moxey ED, O'Connor JP, Novielli KD, Teutsch S, Nash DB. Prescription drug use in the elderly: a descriptive analysis. *Health Care Financ Rev.* 2003;24(4):127–141.

28. Goulding MR. Inappropriate medication prescribing for elderly ambulatory care patients. *Arch Intern Med.* 2004;164(3):305–312.

29. Buck MD, Atreja A, Brunker CP, et al. Potentially inappropriate medication prescribing in outpatient practices: prevalence and patient characteristics based on electronic health records. *Am J Geriatr Pharmacother.* 2009;7(2):84–92.

30. Gandhi TK, Weingart SN, Borus J, et al. Adverse drug events in ambulatory care. *N Engl J Med.* 2003;348(16):1556–1564.

31. Gray CL, Gardner C. Adverse drug events in the elderly: an ongoing problem. *J Manag Care Pharm.* 2009;15(7):568–571.

32. Hutchison L, Hawes C, Williams L. Access to quality health services in rural areas: long-term care. 2004. http://www.srph.tamhsc.edu/centers/rhp2010/Volume_3/Vol3Ch1OV.htm. Accessed November 2012.

33. Nelson JA, Gingerich BS. Rural health: access to care and services. *Home Health Care Management & Practice.* 2010;22(5):339–343.

34. Arcury TA, Preisser JS, Gesler WM, Powers JM. Access to transportation and health care utilization in a rural region. *J Rural Health.* 2005;21(1):31–38.

35. Goins RT, Williams KA, Carter MW, Spencer M, Solovieva T. Perceived barriers to health care access among rural older adults: a qualitative study. *J Rural Health.* 2005;21(3):206–213.

36. Peterson LE, Bazemore A, Bragg EJ, Xierali I, Warshaw GA. Rural-urban distribution of the U.S. Geriatrics physician workforce. *J Am Geriatr Soc.* 2011;59(4):699–703.

37. Hansen L, Cartwright JC, Craig CE. End-of-life care for rural-dwelling older adults and their primary family caregivers. *Res Gerontol Nurs.* 2012;5(1):6–15.

38. Wilson DM, Justice C, Sheps S, Thomas R, Reid P, Leibovici K. Planning and providing end-of-life care in rural areas. *J Rural Health.* 2006;22(2):174–181.

39. Virnig BA, Moscovice IS, Durham SB, Casey MM. Do rural elders have limited access to Medicare hospice services? *J Am Geriatr Soc.* 2004;52(5):731–735.

40. Podgorski C, King DA. Losing function, staying connected: family dynamics in provision of care for people with dementia. *Generations: J Am Society Aging.* 2009;33:24–29.

41. Easter Seals Disability Services. *Caregiving in Rural America;* 2006.

42. Schulz R, Martire LM. Family caregiving of persons with dementia: prevalence, health effects, and support strategies. *Am J Geriatr Psychiatry.* 2004;12(3):240–249.

43. Daniel CM, Hicken B, Luptak M, Grant M, Rupper R. Using technology to reach caregivers of veterans with dementia. In: Zheng RZ, Hill RD, Gardner MK, eds. *Engaging Older Adults with Modern Technology: Internet Use and Information Access Needs.* Hershey, PA: Information Science Reference/IGI Global Publishing; 2012.

44. US Department of Agriculture. USDA rural development–UTP broadband initiatives program. Main. http://www.rurdev.usda.gov/utp_bip.html. Accessed December 2012.

CHAPTER 17

Future Directions in Rural Public Health

Jacob C. Warren and K. Bryant Smalley

This text has highlighted many of the pressing health challenges and concerns in rural areas, as well as some of the promising practices that are emerging in addressing rural public health issues. As rural health researchers and practitioners look to the future, there are a number of directions and advancements that will help us continue to advance the needs of this particularly underserved group. There are also a number of growth areas, in which a change in the way public health is approached must occur for rural areas to be most benefited.

ADVANCEMENTS IN RURAL PUBLIC HEALTH

Telehealth

The use of technology to address health care access issues has been tied to rural areas almost as long as the field has existed. Because of the unique needs of rural areas to minimize patient transportation burden in a context that simultaneously frequently has too low a demand to justify maintenance of a full-time provider (particularly for specialty care), technology-based or technology-enhanced care delivery (telemedicine) and broader technology-based health promotion and intervention (telehealth) hold much promise in continuing to address health care barriers in rural settings.

Part of the reason that telehealth holds such promise in addressing rural public health problems is that it directly addresses all three of the "traditional" barriers to care encountered in rural settings: accessibility, availability, and acceptability. By allowing for receipt of specialty care in a more familiar, local setting (e.g., primary care office), telehealth directly addresses the accessibility of care. By removing geographic restrictions associated with provision of care, telehealth also addresses availability; even if there is only one specialist in the state, that provider would be able to consult on cases statewide. While telehealth does not necessarily increase the workforce itself, it does maximize the reach of the workforce that is present. It may also encourage providers to expand their traditional services to reach distance patients in order to complement an existing practice. Finally, when structured and designed in a thoughtful manner, telehealth can help address concerns related to acceptability of care as well. By opening the door to more integrated care models (in particular, provision of telehealth-based mental health care services within a primary care/clinic setting), acceptability of these services can be improved. If it is no longer easy to tell that a rural resident is seeking psychological services, for instance, due to its delivery via telehealth in a traditional medical setting, individuals may feel less stigma in seeking those services.

One of the largest barriers to the continued growth of telehealth is the issue of license portability/scope of practice. Currently, nearly all medical and allied health professions hold state-level licenses. Such a licensure system prevents individuals in one state from practicing across state lines. This effectively limits the reach of telehealth providers to their own state. Many times a provider may be geographically closer to a patient population in another state than to potential patients in their own state. This has led to a significant movement toward national licensure to allow for practice across state lines; however, this does represent a significant change in the way that health licensure is accommodated. Such a change is also complicated by variations in scope of practice across states; for instance, Georgia is one of only a few states in which nurse practitioners still cannot practice autonomously. In essence, certain states have effectively "banned" provision of certain services by certain levels of professionals. However, many individuals argue that state lines are relatively arbitrary, as health professionals can already see out-of-state patients as long as they physically enter the state in which the provider practices. The licensure and scope-of-practice debates will likely continue for years to come; we encourage everyone involved to look at the vast potential gain of addressing this core barrier to expansion of telehealth services (which, for the most part, are evidence-based and just as effective as in-person services).

Beyond the provision of clinical care, the Internet and videoconferencing are being increasingly used for the purposes of health promotion and patient education. Again, due to the ability of a centralized "provider" to reach a broad network of individuals needing services, telehealth structures have been used to increase access to diabetes education, smoking cessation, support groups, and even 12-step programs. The evidence base for these services continues to grow, and health-related organizations continue to develop ever-more innovative ways to fund these programs (including insurance bonuses for improved patient outcomes and collaborative funding of positions across formal or informal networks).

The connection between rural health and telehealth has recently become even more officially recognized with the relocation of the federal Office for the Advancement of Telehealth (OAT) within HRSA to now fall under the Office of Rural Health Policy—directly emphasizing the federal connection between telehealth and rural areas. OAT is active in building and supporting telehealth networks that serve rural areas, and is at the forefront of license portability issues. OAT recently competed the Licensure Portability Grant Program (LPGP), which was a competitive grant program designed to provide support to state licensing boards to work together to find ways to address the cross-state practice barriers currently in place that are preventing telehealth from reaching its full potential. The outcome of these grants could provide models for nationwide implementation, and those in the field are closely watching what develops.

Federal Advancements

There are also several advances within the federal government that indicate a growing level of both recognition of and support for rural-focused health research and outreach. Established in 1987, the Office of Rural Health Policy within HRSA is tasked with coordinating activities related to rural health care within the Department of Health and Human Services (DHHS). The office is comprised of five subdivisions focused on border health, community-based work, hospitals, policy research, and telehealth. These divisions operate numerous grant programs spanning the spectrum of outreach and research, including initiatives such as the Rural Healthcare Services Outreach Grant program and the Rural Health Research Center program. These initiatives help with not only creating policy-relevant research focused on rural populations, but also in implementing evidence-based health promotion and intervention practices in rural communities. ORHP plays a very important role in the President's Rural Health Initiative, designed to bring attention and funding to the unique health needs of rural residents.

Another key indication of the increased focus on the needs of rural areas was the formation in June 2011 of the White House Rural Council, created by presidential executive order. In doing so, President Obama stated that "strong rural communities are key to a stronger America . . . that's why I've established the White House Rural Council to make sure we're working across government to strengthen rural communities and promote economic growth."[1] The council is chaired by the Secretary of Agriculture, and includes membership from all cabinet-level agencies and several other relevant federal groups, totaling representation from nearly 30 groups. The council is tasked with coordinating the government's efforts in rural America through three key functions: (a) streamline and improve the effectiveness of federal programs serving rural America; (b) engage stakeholders on issues and solutions in rural communities; and (c) promote and coordinate private-sector partnerships. While the council itself is not exclusively health focused, it does take into consideration health issues, as well as address many of the barriers and socioeconomic factors that influence health outcomes in rural settings. Key health-related agencies represented include the DHHS, the Department of Veterans Affairs, and the Office of National Drug Control Policy. The Council has coordinated several events, including receiving feedback directly from ORHP-funded groups, that have allowed rural practitioners and public health workers to directly interface with the highest levels of government to convey their ideas, concerns, and solutions.

In addition, the recent elevation from center status to institute status for the National Institute on Minority Health and Health Disparities (NIMHD) within the National Institutes of Health has brought renewed focus to rural health (as rural areas are one of the major focus areas of NIMHD). It will be important for this emphasis to continue throughout new appropriation cycles and changes in leadership across these organizations; without continued, focused support, rural health efforts will not be able to adequately address the needs of the more than 30 million Americans who reside in rural areas.

The Affordable Care Act—Good or Bad for Rural?

We would be remiss in not discussing the Affordable Care Act (ACA). This sweeping legislation has the potential to completely transform health care delivery and availability of preventive services throughout the nation, including rural America. While it is difficult to predict the ultimate outcome of this legislation, the National Rural Health Association has released a series of papers examining the positives and potential challenges associated with implementing the ACA.[2] The NRHA identified 21 key provisions within the ACA with strong potential to positively impact health in rural America, and a comprehensive examination of these 21 provisions can be found on their website. Provisions most directly impacting rural areas include: (a) rural physician training grants that will help medical colleges develop specific rural training programs designed to recruit students from rural areas and prepare them for rural practice; (b) expanding area health education centers (AHECs), which have a long-standing role in improving the health care pipeline in rural settings; (c) graduate medical education (GME) improvements that will increase training opportunities in rural health clinics (RHCs) and federally qualified health care centers (FQHCs); (d) protecting rural residency slots from redistribution and prioritizing rural areas for receipt of redistributed slots; (e) National Health Service Corps funding enhancements, which help bring health care providers to underserved rural areas; and (f) increases in funding for community health centers, which form the backbone of the rural safety net not only for medical and psychological care, but also for preventive services and health education programs.

While the ACA did provide many advancements for rural health, there are also concerns. The NRHA identified 22 concerns, discussed in detail on their website. A key concern identified by the NRHA is the proposed development of a council with expanded authority to independently implement payment changes rather than acting in an advisory role to Congress; according to the NRHA, such councils in the past have notoriously underrepresented rural voices, limiting their ability to ensure that rural needs are being met in the Council's recommendations.

As the ACA moves forward in its implementation, other aspects such as the expansion of preventive care services have the potential to dramatically improve public health availability and implementation throughout the nation; however, given the lack of both medical and public health professionals in rural settings, it is unclear how well these new provisions will be able to address the needs of rural groups. Particular attention will have to be paid to creating the pipeline necessary to implement ACA provisions in a way that does not result in a widening of existing rural–urban disparities by only benefiting urban populations.

CHALLENGES IN RURAL PUBLIC HEALTH

Access to Care and Services

While the ACA has been seen by many as the end-all in solving access-to-care issues, many have pointed out the fact that an increase in demand (via coverage) without a corresponding focus on increase in supply (via new providers) will ultimately have limited impact. In fact, given the fact that there are already widespread provider shortages, particularly in rural areas, it is unclear how the increased accessibility of care through insurance coverage will translate to increased availability of care. Without significant progress toward increasing provider supply in rural settings to not only address the current shortages, but also address the new demands for services that will occur with the ACA, the anticipated benefits to health will not occur in rural areas.

Access to care is frequently discussed only in the context of medical services, but access to public health and preventive services is also a critical issue in rural areas. As discussed in Chapter 3, there is a critical and growing shortage of trained public health professionals in general, and this will only continue to restrict the ability of rural areas to attract trained public health workers to their areas. Expansion of a pipeline system such as the National Health Service Corps to more aggressively attract public health professionals focused on prevention could provide a great deal of support to rural areas.

An important component of attracting providers and public health workers to rural areas is mere exposure—incorporating the study of rural populations and health dynamics into training programs not only provides a baseline of knowledge to prevent rural areas from seeming like a "mystery," but it can also serve as recruitment in-and-of itself. Particularly for public health professionals, many health-related workers are drawn to their professions by a desire to make a difference, frequently in areas of most need. By exposing students to the unique needs of rural residents, we can help attract workers to our areas. As discussed in Chapter 3, retention of these workers is an entirely different process, and state and national funders will have to critically examine ways to offer competitive salaries (particularly in underserved rural areas).

Improving the Rural Health Evidence Base

By definition an understudied area, research into rural health needs, dynamics, and solutions has not been able to keep up with demand. By necessity, public health workers frequently find themselves developing and implementing their own programs designed to address the unique needs that they encounter, and as a result methods of improving rural health develop faster than they are able to be evaluated for effectiveness. This does not mean that the programs do not work; however, it severely limits the ability of programs to be both funded and to be disseminated to other rural areas that could benefit from the program.

Unfortunately, research organizations such as universities are rarely located within rural settings. This leaves rural health-focused researchers facing a dilemma—do they live within an urban area and attempt to secure research funding to travel into nearby rural settings (and in the process lose their close integration into the rural community), or do they work in a smaller university within a rural area that is much less likely to receive the types of funding given to researchers at larger, urban universities? This effect can even impact willingness to pursue a rural-health focused career—it is challenging enough to establish an independently funded line of research and outreach—why would new public health researchers take on the additional challenges inherently faced in pursuing a rural health-focused career?

Federal funders increasingly recognize that programs and initiatives springing from within a disparity group have a greatly enhanced potential to be successful and scalable, as evidenced by the ever-increasing emphasis placed upon community-based participatory research strategies in which communities are not just partners but co-leaders in developing, implementing, and evaluating programs. This same view should be applied to rural areas. This requires, however, a comprehensive recognition that, to be maximally effective, rural public health research and innovation should spring from within those rural settings, either through supporting rural-placed researchers or supporting formal collaborations between universities and rural-placed community groups. Without dedicated support and special consideration, university-based researchers focused on rural populations will continue to face substantial barriers in securing support for their work because the research environment is by default less developed than in urban areas.

CONCLUSION

The needs of rural areas are real and present. They have been documented, described, and detailed for decades, yet disparities in incidence, prevalence, and outcomes persist. While there are significant shortages in medical providers, there is also a paucity of public health and prevention-based work that occurs in rural areas. Because of the long-standing shortages in medical care, the need for a focus on prevention and self-maintenance in rural settings is even more crucial; however, the evidence base frequently lags behind the need for such programs. To adequately address the health needs of our rural areas, increased focus on developing and establishing the effectiveness of rural-tailored interventions across the prevention spectrum and varying from individual to community-level impact will be needed.

Despite these challenges, rural areas do offer unique opportunities and strengths to develop such initiatives. The suitability of telehealth to rural needs is nearly unparalleled, and even if current provider restrictions limit its scalability for telemedicine, broader prevention and education programs can capitalize on the strengths of this timely and effective medium. In addition, the close-knit nature of rural areas can be capitalized upon for community-level interventions—if community motivation can be shifted on a particular issue, there is great potential for the community itself to be the change agent that ultimately shifts a health outcome. In addition, the strong presence of churches provides another great avenue for community partnerships to address health in ways that are not necessarily faith based, but faith partnered.

As with any societal issue, addressing the health needs of rural areas requires dedication and determination. There is a growing sense of importance behind improving the lives of rural residents, and the time has never been better for finally achieving dramatic improvements in health. By constantly thinking of the needs of rural areas and how they can be made, we can hope to finally make a difference in the lives of one in five Americans.

REFERENCES

1. http://www.whitehouse.gov/administration/eop/rural-council
2. http://www.ruralhealthweb.org/go/left/government-affairs/health-reform-and-you

Index

AADE. *See* American Association of Diabetes Educators (AADE)
AADE7 Self-Care Behavior model, 159–164
ACA. *See* Affordable Care Act of 2010 (ACA)
access to medical care, 11–25
  assistance in transportation, 248
  barriers to, 12–13
  challenges in, 259–260
  community health centers, 22
  critical access hospitals, 21–22
  defined, 12
  distance programs, 24
  end-of life care, 249–250
  federal programs for, 21
  health insurance coverage, 14–16, 248
  long-term care, 249
  medical professionals, creative deployment of, 23
  mobile services, 24
  needs of rural populations, 13–14
  persons with low socioeconomic status, 19
  primary care, 16–18
  provider availability, 16
  racial and ethnic minority groups, 20–21
  rural health clinics, 21–22
  specialty care, 18–19
  specialty geriatric care, 248–249
  telehealth programs, 24
Access to Recovery (ATR) program, 109
accreditation, of health departments, 32, 33
activities of daily living (ADLs), 122, 244–246, 249
  instrumental, 246
adaptive capacity, defined, 192
adherence to treatment, 23, 70, 163, 164, 176, 180
  barriers to, 162, 205
  HIV/AIDS, 171–172
ADLs. *See* activities of daily living (ADLs)
adolescents
  HIV/AIDS in, 169, 175
  mental health problems in, 87, 88
  obesity of, 139–141
  sexually transmitted diseases in, 61
  smoking, 14
  substance abuse of, 95, 100, 101, 105, 106, 177, 191
adults
  affected by heart attack, 117, 126, 128
  affected by stroke, 119, 128, 129–130
  alcohol abuse of, 97, 99, 100, 102, 105
  cardiovascular diseases in, 115, 125, 130–132, 133
  depression in, 75

diabetes in, 156
dietary intake of, 120
HIV/AIDS in, 169, 175
hypertension in, 116, 117
medical care needs for, 13, 14
mental health problems in, 88
nutrition interventions for, 58
obesity of, 61, 139, 141, 142, 144, 146
older. *See* older adults
primary care for, 16
sedentary lifestyle of, 121
sexually transmitted diseases in, 61
specialty care for, 18
substance abuse of, 95, 98, 99, 103
Affordable Care Act of 2010 (ACA), 22,
    258–259
African Americans
  affected by heart attack, 118
  affected by stroke, 119, 125, 129, 205
  alcohol abuse of, 98
  cancer in, 56–58, 63, 206
  cardiovascular disease in, 59, 115, 121,
      124–125, 128, 131, 133, 134, 204
  diabetes in, 60, 157, 204–205
  dietary intake of, 120
  health disparities prevention,
      recommendations for, 206
  HIV/AIDS in, 173, 174
  hypertension in, 116, 117, 123, 124,
      126, 133, 205
  illicit drug abuse of, 98
  mental health disparities in, 87
  nutrition intake of, 62
  obesity of, 60, 61, 141
  physical activity of, 62
  poverty of, 2
  racism and, 243, 244
  sexually transmitted diseases in, 61
  smoking, 61, 121
Agency for Healthcare Research and
    Quality (AHRQ), 68, 70
aging, 13, 30, 36, 242–244. *See also* older
    adults
agriculture, 6, 22, 145, 230, 231
AHECs. *See* area health education
    centers (AHECs)
AHRQ. *See* Agency for Healthcare
    Research and Quality (AHRQ)
AIAN. *See* American Indians/Alaskan
    Natives (AIAN)

AIDS. *See* HIV prevention and
    treatment, in rural areas
alcohol
  abuse, 7, 87, 95–101, 107, 110, 176, 177,
      179, 231, 247
  dependence, 105, 232
ALFs. *See* assisted living facilities (ALFs)
Alliance of Black Churches Health
    Project, 61
Alzheimer's disease, 247, 249
American Association of Diabetes
    Educators (AADE), 160
American Indians
  access to medical care, 20–21
  chronic vascular disease in, 115
  intensive services and special
      programs for, 105
  obesity of, 141
  racism and, 243
American Indians/Alaskan Natives
    (AIAN), 215–218
  access to medical care, 20–21
  cardiovascular disease, 216
  child health, 217–218
  diabetes, 216
  health disparities
    factors influencing, 218
    prevention, recommendations
        for, 218
  maternal health, 217–218
  racism and, 243
  respiratory health, 217
  substance use, 216–217
  suicide, 217
American Stroke Association
    (ASA), 118
antibiotics, for infectious diseases, 231
antiretroviral therapy, for HIV, 171, 172
Approaches to Take Absolute
    Control through Knowledge
    (ATTACK), 133
area health education centers
    (AHECs), 35, 258
ASA. *See* American Stroke Association
    (ASA)
Asians
  affected by stroke, 125
  cardiovascular disease in, 115
  farmworkers, 227
  substance abuse of, 98

"Ask, Screen, Intervene: Incorporating HIV Prevention into Medical Care of Persons Living with HIV," 178
assisted living facilities (ALFs), 249
ATR program. *See* Access to Recovery (ATR) program
ATTACK. *See* Approaches to Take Absolute Control through Knowledge (ATTACK)
autonomy, 35

Balanced Budget Act, 21
barriers
    to care, LGBT, 212–214
    to care, older Americans, 248–249
    to diabetes prevention, 158
    to HIV prevention and treatment, 170–180
    to integration, 69–70
    to medical care access, 12–13
    to transportation, 248
    to treatment adherence, 162
Barron's magazine, 103
BASIC project. *See* Brain Attack Surveillance in Corpus Christi (BASIC) project
behavioral health (BH)
    Four Quadrant Clinical Integration Model, 69
    integrated programs, barriers to, 69–70
    of migrant farmworkers, 231–232
    settings, primary care integration into, 78
Behavioral Model for Vulnerable Populations, 13
Behavioral Model of Health Services Use, 12–13
    enabling characteristics of, 12
    need characteristics of, 13
    predisposing characteristics of, 12
    revision of, 13
behavioral norms, of rural residents, 7
Behavioral Risk Factor Surveillance System (BRFSS), 119–121, 125, 126, 128, 133, 156, 246
bereavement, cultural, 232
BH. *See* behavioral health (BH)
bioethics, of rural health care, 42–50. *See also* ethics, of rural health care

Black Churches United for Better Health Project, 58
BLESS Project, 59
blood pressure (BP). *See also* hypertension (HTN)
    diastolic, 116
    systolic, 116
Blue Cross of California, 74
BMI. *See* body mass index (BMI)
Board of Medicine, 51
Body and Soul, 58
body mass index (BMI), 60, 78, 124, 133, 156, 159
BPHC. *See* Bureau of Primary Health Care (BPHC)
Bracero Agreement of 1942, 227–228
Brain Attack Surveillance in Corpus Christi (BASIC) project, 125
breast cancer, 12, 57, 58, 63, 129, 191, 233
BRFSS. *See* Behavioral Risk Factor Surveillance System (BRFSS)
brief check-ups, for substance abuse, 108
buprenorphine, for substance abuse, 107
Bureau of Community Health Systems, 36
Bureau of Primary Health Care (BPHC), 76
    New Access Initiative, 68

California Telemedicine and eHealth Center, 74
cancer, 206, 208–209
    breast, 12, 57, 58, 63, 129, 191, 233
    cervical, 12, 233
    church-based interventions for, 56–58
    colorectal, 11, 57, 63
    nutrition and, 58
    screening, 57–58
CARDIAC. *See* Coronary Artery Risk Reduction in Appalachian Communities Project (CARDIAC)
cardiovascular disease (CVD), 204, 208, 216. *See also* coronary heart disease (CHD); heart attack; heart disease, in rural areas; stroke
    church-based interventions for, 58–59
    disparities of, 123–128
        gender, 123
        place of residence, 125–128
        racial and ethnic minorities, 123–125

prevalence of, 115
risk factors of
  contextual factors, 122
  diet, 120
  sedentary lifestyle, 121
  smoking, 121–122
care. *See also* caregiving
  access to medical. *See* access to
    medical care
  delivery model, for rural
    caregivers, 251–252
  end-of life, 249–250
  long-term, 249
  primary, 16–18, 107
  specialty geriatric, 248–249
career and community, connection
  between, 35–36
caregivers
  client–professional conflicts and, 48
  Internet-savvy, 251
  moral distress among, 45, 46
  rural, 250–251
    care delivery model for, 251–252
caregiving, 35, 121, 242, 244, 250–251. *See
  also* care
case finding, 51
case study
  aging, 241–242
  community-based participatory
    research, 189–190
  of rural area integrated care, 73–77
Caucasian, 1–2, 141
  racism and, 243
CBPR. *See* community-based
  participatory research (CBPR)
CDC. *See* Centers for Disease Control
  and Prevention (CDC)
CDE credential. *See* certified diabetes
  educator (CDE) credential
Centers for Disease Control and
  Prevention (CDC), 115, 121, 155,
  204, 205, 215, 217, 244–245
  Division for Heart Disease and Stroke
    Prevention (DHDSP), 119, 132
Centers for Medicaid and Medicare
  (CMS), 247
certified diabetes educator (CDE)
  credential, 164
cervical cancer, 12, 233
Chagas disease, 231

CHD. *See* coronary heart disease (CHD)
CHER. *See* Community Health and
  Environmental Reawakening
  (CHER)
Cherokee Guidance Center, 76
Cherokee Health Systems (CHS),
  73, 76–77, 79
Child Nutrition and WIC
  Reauthorization Act of 2004, 145
children
  American Indians/Alaskan Native,
    217–218
  farmworkers, 233–234
  obesity, 140, 141
Children's Health Insurance Program
  (CHIP), 14
CHIP. *See* Children's Health Insurance
  Program (CHIP)
CHP. *See* Community Health Partners
  (CHP)
CHS. *See* Cherokee Health Systems
  (CHS)
church-based health promotion, in rural
  areas, 55–64. *See also* religion
  cancer, 56–58
  cardiovascular disease, 58–59
  diabetes, 60
  future directions of, 63–64
  general health, 56
  nutrition, 62
  obesity, 60–61
  physical activity, 62
  programs, 62–63
  sexually transmitted diseases, 61
  smoking, 61–62
  success of, 63
Church of Latter Day Saints
  (Mormon), 56
cigarette smoking. *See* smoking
climate change, 191–194
  defined, 192
  impact on mental health, 193–194
  impact on public health, 192–193
clinical health care ethics, 42
CMS. *See* Centers for Medicaid and
  Medicare (CMS)
cocaine abuse, 87, 247
collaborative education, for rural public
  health workforce, 34–35. *See also*
  education

colorectal cancer, 11, 57, 63
Columbia-Union Faith-Based Adolescent STI/HIV Prevention Project, 61
Commission on Accreditation of Rehabilitation Services, 108
Community Dimensions of Practice, 31
Community Health and Environmental Reawakening (CHER), 189–190
Community Health Partners (CHP), 73–74
Community Trials Intervention to Reduce High-Risk Drinking, 102
community(ies)
    -based programs and interventions, for cardiovascular disease, 130–133
    -based services, in rural areas, 249
    and career, connection between, 35–36
    engagement, 122
    erosion, 194
    factors associated with obesity, 144–145
    food environment, 122
    frontier, 4, 23, 159
    health centers, 22, 71, 74
    levels and policies, for obesity reduction, 147–148
    rural, 4, 98–100, 102
    substance use issues in, 98–100, 102
community-based participatory research (CBPR), 188–190
    case study, 189–190
    defined, 188
competency
    development, 31, 33, 36, 37
    tracking of, 33
confidentiality, 51, 63, 106, 107, 110
    barriers to, 108
    HIV testing, 170, 178
    threats to, 46–47
contextual factors, of cardiovascular disease, 122
continuing care, for substance abuse, 108–109
Coordinating Center for the Substance Abuse and Mental Health Services Administration Primary Care-Mental Health Initiative, 78
coraje, 232
Coronary Artery Risk Reduction in Appalachian Communities Project (CARDIAC), 133

coronary heart disease (CHD), 117, 118. See also cardiovascular disease (CVD); heart attack; heart disease, in rural areas; stroke
costs, of obesity, 139–140
counseling, for substance abuse
    group, 108
    peer, 108
    telephone-based, 108
critical access hospitals, 21–22, 49, 52
cultural barriers to integration, 70
cultural bereavement, 232
cultural health care ethics, 42
CVD. See cardiovascular disease (CVD)

DARE. See Drug Abuse Resistance Education (DARE)
DBP. See diastolic blood pressure (DBP)
dengue fever, 231
Department of Education, 234
Department of Health and Human Services (DHHS), 234, 257, 258
Department of Labor, 228
Department of Veterans Affairs, 258
Depo-Provera, for infectious diseases, 231
depression, 23, 72–76, 88, 140, 231, 246, 249. See also isolation; loneliness
    comorbid, 163
    distance and telehealth programs for, 24
    HIV/AIDS and, 180
    obesity and, 141–142
    PHQ-9, 72, 74, 75, 232
detoxification (detox) services, 104–105, 106, 107
DHHS. See Department of Health and Human Services (DHHS)
diabetes, 13, 14, 24, 155–164, 204–205, 207–208, 216
    belt, 155
    and cardiovascular disease, 126, 133
    church-based interventions for, 60
    mobile services for, 24
    in rural areas, 155–164
        AADE7 Self-Care Behavior model, 159–164
        barriers/challenges to, 158
        disparity sources of, 157

prevention/control practices,
158–159
recommendations for, 164
in rural older adults, 244
sedentary lifestyle and, 121
type 2, 60, 133, 155
diabetes self-management education
(DSME)
AADE7 Self-Care Behaviors
model, 159–164
DIAMOND (Depression Improvement
Across Minnesota Offering a
New Direction) Program, 73,
75–76
diastolic blood pressure (DBP), 116
dietary intake, and cardiovascular
disease, 120. See also food
discrimination. See also stigma
HIV/AIDS patients, 170, 171
LGBQ individuals, 88
disparities
of cardiovascular disease, 123–128
gender, 123
place of residence, 125–128
racial and ethnic minorities, 123–125
in rural mental health, 86–89
sources of diabetes, 157
Division for Heart Disease and Stroke
Prevention (DHDSP) (CDC),
119, 132
Drug Abuse Resistance Education
(DARE), 100
Drug Free Communities
program, 109
DSME. See diabetes self-management
education (DSME)

e-mail, medical consultation
through, 24, 176
eating patterns, and
obesity, 142–143
education
collaborative, 34–35
diabetes self-management, 159–164
graduate medical, 258
for rural public health
workforce, 33–34
EFNEP. See Expanded Food and
Nutrition Education Program
(EFNEP)

elderly, 49, 80, 88
cardiovascular disease in, 130
climate change impact on, 193
health care resources for, 44
medical care needs of, 13
mental health problems in, 88
embolic stroke, 118
end-of life care, 249–250
enumeration, of rural public health
workforce, 30–31
environmental health
of migrant farmworkers, 230–231
in rural areas, 187–195
climate change impact on, 191–194
community-based participatory
research, 188–190
gene–environment
interactions, 190–191
environmental justice, 188–190
Environmental Protection Agency, 235
ethical standards of practice, 42
ethics, of rural health care, 41–53
bioethics, 42–50
clinical, 42
considerations for, 50–53
cultural, 42
ethical standards of, 42
limited resources for, 51–53
professional codes of, 42
regulatory and policy, 42
theoretical, 42
ethnic minorities. See racial and ethnic
minorities
evidence base of rural health,
improving, 260
Expanded Food and Nutrition
Education Program
(EFNEP), 146–147
expectations, of rural public health
workforce, 32–33

Fair Labor Standards Act
of 1938, 231
family(ies)
effects, of methamphetamine
abuse, 98–99
factors associated with
obesity, 142–143
strategies for reducing, 146–148
planning clinics, 47

federal advancements, for rural public
    health, 257–258
Federal School Meal Programs, 145
Federally Qualified Health Centers
    (FQHCs), 22, 71, 73, 74, 258
financial constraints, and
    obesity, 142–143
Flex. *See* State Medicare Rural Hospital
    Flexibility (Flex) Grant Program
food. *See also* dietary intake, and
    cardiovascular disease
  access, and obesity, 144
  insecurity
    of migrant farmworkers, 233
    and obesity, 142
Four Quadrant Clinical Integration
    Model, 69
FQHCs. *See* Federally Qualified Health
    Centers (FQHCs)
frontier communities, 4. *See also*
    community(ies)
  Improving Health Among Rural
    Montanans program, 23
  Montana Diabetes Control
    Program, 158–159
  rural communities versus, 4
FTE. *See* full-time equivalent (FTE)
full-time equivalent (FTE), 74
future directions, in rural public
    health, 255–261

gateway hypothesis, 101
gender. *See also* men, in rural areas;
    women, in rural areas
  disparities in mental health, 88
  and heart attack, 123
  and hypertension, 123
  and obesity, 140–141
  and stroke, 123
gene–environment
    interactions, 190–191
general health, church-based
    interventions for, 56
general practitioner, 49, 249
Georgia Southern University
  Rural Health Research Institute, 160
Geriatric Research, Education, and
    Clinical Center, 251
GME. *See* graduate medical
    education (GME)

Governor's Mental Health Initiative
    (Minnesota), 75
graduate medical education
    (GME), 258
group counseling, for substance
    abuse, 108
Guide to Health, 62

H-2A legislation, 228
hallucinogens, 98
HARP. *See* Health and Religion Project
    (HARP)
Health and Religion Project (HARP), 59
Health Care for the Homeless
    Programs, 74
health care providers
  availability of, 16
  distribution and characteristics
    of, 104–105
  incompetent, 51
  role in obesity
    reduction, 147–148
  treatment models with relevance
    for, 106–108
health care resources, and moral
    distress, 44–45
Health Center Act, 22
Health Center Program, 22
health insurance
  coverage, 14–16, 248
  Medi-Cal, 74
  Medicaid. *See* Medicaid
  Medicare. *See* Medicare
  TennCare, 76
Health Network, 235
health professional shortage areas
    (HPSAs), 16, 31
Health Resources and Services
    Administration (HRSA), 2, 4,
    234, 257
  Cherokee Health Systems, 76
  funding to Migrant Clinicians
    Network, 234
  funding to Open Door Community
    Health Centers, 75
  Health Center Program, 21
  Office for the Advancement of
    Telehealth, 257
  Office of Rural Health
    Policy, 85, 257

rural public health workforce,
    enumeration of, 30
health status, and moral distress,
    44–45
Health Underserved Rural Areas
    grants, 70–71
HealthSource, 76
Healthy Hunger-Free Kids Act of
    2010, 145, 146
heart attack, 117–118. *See also*
    cardiovascular disease (CVD);
    coronary heart disease (CHD);
    heart disease, in rural areas;
    stroke
    changes in rates over time, 118
    gender and, 123
    knowledge and awareness of, 128
    mortality rates associated with, 118
    place of residence and, 126–127
    prevalence of, 117–118
heart disease, in rural areas, 115–134.
    See also cardiovascular disease
    (CVD); coronary heart disease
    (CHD); heart attack; stroke
    cardiovascular disease
        disparities, 123–128
    cardiovascular disease risk
        factors, 120–122
    community-based programs and
        interventions for, 130–133
    heart attack, 117–118, 123, 126–127, 128
    hypertension and, 116–117,
        123–124, 126
    knowledge and awareness of, 128–129
    stroke, 118–120, 123, 125, 127–128,
        129–130
hemorrhagic stroke, 118
heroin abuse, 105, 107, 247
heterosexism, 88
Hispanics
    affected by stroke, 125, 208
    alcohol abuse of, 98
    cancer in, 208–209
    cardiovascular disease in, 115,
        121, 208
    diabetes in, 158, 207–208
    health disparities
        factors contributing to, 209
        prevention, recommendations for,
            209–210

hypertension in, 124, 208
illicit drug abuse of, 98
racism and, 243, 244
HIV prevention and treatment, in rural
    areas, 47, 169–180
    barriers to, 170–180
    future of, 178–180
    regional differences in, 172–178
home-based services, in rural
    areas, 249
home health, in rural areas, 249
housing issues, of migrant
    farmworkers, 233
HPSAs. *See* health professional shortage
    areas (HPSAs)
HRSA. *See* Health Resources and
    Services Administration (HRSA)
human ecological theory, for
    understanding obesity
    community factors, 144–145
    family and household factors, 142–143
    individual factors, 140–142
Hurricane Katrina, 192
hypertension (HTN), 116–117, 205, 208.
    See also blood pressure (BP)
    changes in rates over time, 117
    defined, 116
    gender and, 123
    mortality rates associated
        with, 116
    place of residence and, 126
    prehypertension, 116
    prevalence of, 116, 117
    in racial and ethnic
        minorities, 123–124

IHS. *See* Indian Health Service (IHS)
ILOs. *See* intensive livestock operations
    (ILOs)
immunization clinics, 47
Improving Health Among Rural
    Montanans program, 23
income, and obesity, 142
incompetent providers, 51
Indian Health Service (IHS), 20
infectious diseases, migrant
    farmworkers affected by, 231
inhalants, 87, 95, 98
Institute of Medicine, 32, 68
institutional review board (IRB), 50, 52

instrumental activities of daily living
(IADLs), 246. *See also* activities of
daily living (ADLs)
insurance. *See* health insurance
integrated care, in rural areas, 67, 70–81,
89. *See also* integration
case studies of, 73–77
in changing policy environment,
77–79
current and best practices in, 72–73
practical steps to, 79–81
state fiscal pressures, 77–78
integration. *See also* integrated care, in
rural areas
background of, 68
barriers to, 69–70
classification of, 69
defined, 68
evidence for, 70
models of, 69
reverse, 78, 89
intensive livestock operations
(ILOs), 189, 190
intensive services for substance abuse
treatment, lack of, 105
Intergovernmental Panel of Climate
Change (IPCC), 192
Internet interventions, 24, 108, 176,
179, 251, 256
for HIV/AIDS, 178, 179
men who have sex with men, 180
for obesity, 147–148
IPCC. *See* Intergovernmental Panel of
Climate Change (IPCC)
IRB. *See* institutional review
board (IRB)
ischemic stroke, 118–119, 127
Islam, 56
isolation, 5–6, 23, 31, 68, 86–88, 98,
179, 180. *See also* depression;
loneliness
geographic, 4–6, 86, 87, 141, 194, 229
professional, 35, 49
social, 87, 141, 148, 171, 227, 232, 235

Judaism, 55–56

Ka lei mano'olana (KLM), 58
Kansas Association of Local Health
Departments, 36

Kansas Public Health Association
(KPHA), 36
Kansas Public Health Leadership
Institute, 33
KLM. See ka lei mano'olana (KLM)
KPHA. *See* Kansas Public Health
Association (KPHA)

Latinos, 20
access to medical care, 24
HIV/AIDS in, 173, 175–176
lay injection, 231
leadership training, 33, 34
lesbian, gay, bisexual, and questioning
(LGBQ) individuals, 87–88
lesbian, gay, bisexual, and transgender
(LGBT), 210–215
barriers to care, 212–214
health disparities prevention,
recommendations for, 214–215
mental health, 211–212
risk-taking behaviors, 211
substance use, 210–211
women's health, 212
LGBQ individuals. *See* lesbian, gay,
bisexual, and questioning (LGBQ)
individuals
LGBT. *See* lesbian, gay, bisexual, and
transgender (LGBT)
LHDs. *See* local health departments
(LHDs)
licensure portability, 256
Licensure Portability Grant Program
(LPGP), 257
Life Skills Training model, 101
Linkage Initiative Program, 71
Livingston Help for Seniors program, 23
local health departments (LHDs), 30, 31
Kansas Association of Local Health
Departments, 36
loneliness, 86, 88, 141, 180. *See also*
depression; isolation
long-term care, 249
long-term support, for substance abuse
treatment, 108–109
LPGP. *See* Licensure Portability Grant
Program (LPGP)

Maine Rural Health Research Center, 71
malaria, 231

marijuana abuse, 87, 97, 107
maternal health
    American Indians/Alaskan Native,
        217–218
    of migrant farmworkers, 233–234
MCN. *See* Migrant Clinicians Network
    (MCN)
Medi-Cal (California's Medicaid
    program), 74
media campaigns, for HIV prevention
    and treatment, 179, 180
Medicaid, 14, 15, 71, 73, 74, 76–78,
    248. *See also* health insurance;
    TennCare
    cancer screening, 57
    critical access hospitals, 21
    for older adults, 244, 248
    oral health, 233
    persons with low socioeconomic
        status, 19
    rural health clinics, 22
    school environment, 145
    state fiscal pressures and, 77, 78
    Western region, 176
Medical Expenditures Panel Survey
    (MEPS), 156
Medicare, 14, 15, 71, 74, 247, 248. *See also*
    health insurance
    critical access hospitals, 21
    for older adults, 244, 246
    rural health clinics, 22
    State Medicare Rural Hospital
        Flexibility Program, 21
    Western region, 176
men, in rural areas. *See also* gender;
    women, in rural areas
    affected by heart attack, 117, 123, 128
    affected by stroke, 123, 125
    cardiovascular disease in, 115, 125, 131
    heart disease in, 124, 129
    HIV/AIDS in, 169–180
    hypertension in, 116, 117, 126
    mental health disparities in, 88
    obesity, 139, 140, 141
    substance abuse, 98, 176
men who have sex with men (MSM),
    170, 173, 178, 179–180
mental health
    climate change impact on, 193–194
    LGBT, 211–212

of migrant farmworkers, 231–232
of older adults, 246–247
professionals, shortage of, 16, 21
in rural areas, 7–8, 85–90
    acceptability of, 86
    accessibility of, 86
    availability of, 86
    disparities in, 86–89
    problems in, addressing, 89
Mental Health Parity and Addiction
    Equity Act of 2008, 77
Mental Health Professional Shortage
    Areas (MHPSAs), 86
MEPS. *See* Medical Expenditures Panel
    Survey (MEPS)
Mercer University
    Center for Rural Health and Health
        Disparities, 160
methadone use, 105
methamphetamine (meth) abuse, 87, 95,
    97–99, 101, 177
MHPSAs. *See* Mental Health
    Professional Shortage Areas
    (MHPSAs)
Midwest
    HIV prevention and treatment, 172,
        173, 175–176
    primary care professionals, shortages
        of, 16
    public health workforce,
        enumeration of, 30
Migrant Clinicians Network
    (MCN), 234, 235
Migrant Education, 234
migrant farmworkers' health, 227–236
    behavioral health, 231–232
    child health, 233–234
    environmental health, 230–231
    food insecurity, 233
    housing, 233
    infectious diseases, 231
    maternal health, 233–234
    mental health, 231–232
    occupational health, 230–231
    oral health, 233
    population characteristics of, 228–229
    programs and resources, 234–235
Migrant Head Start, 234
Migrant Health Act, 234
Migrant Health Centers, 74

migration
nomadic, 228
point-to-point, 228
restricted-circuit, 228
Minnesota Council of Health, 75
Minnesota Department of Human
Services, 73, 75
Minnesota Mental Health Action Group
(MMHAG), 75
MMHAG. See Minnesota Mental Health
Action Group (MMHAG)
mobile services, 24. See also telephones
Montana Diabetes Control
Program, 158–159
Montana Meth Project, 103
moral distress, in health
professionals, 43–50
health care resources, 44–45
health status, 44–45
personal–professional boundaries,
overlapping, 46
professional–client cultural
perspectives, variance in, 47–48
professional practice
expectations, 49–50
threats to confidentiality and
privacy, 46–47
morbidity
asthma, 191
cardiovascular disease, 134
diabetes, 155
HIV/AIDS, 169, 171
of older adults, 245
stroke, 123, 130
mortality
cardiovascular disease, 134
diabetes, 155
heart attack, 118
HIV/AIDS, 169, 171
hypertension, 116
of older adults, 245
stroke, 123, 130
motivational interviewing, 74
MSM. See men who have sex with men
(MSM)
myocardial infarction. See heart attack

National Council for Community
Behavioral Healthcare
(NCCBH), 69, 78

National Health and Nutrition
Examination Survey (NHANES),
116, 123, 133
National Health Interview Survey
(NHIS), 124, 126, 133
National Health Service Corps, 35,
258, 259
National Heart, Lung, and Blood
Institute (NHLBI), 118, 119
National Institute of Alcohol Abuse and
Alcoholism, 247
National Institute of Environmental
Health Sciences (NIEHS), 187, 189
National Institute on Minority
Health and Health Disparities
(NIMHD), 258
National Institutes of Health, 258
national-level barriers to integration, 69
National Long-Term Care Survey
2005, 244
National Rural Health Advisory
Committee, 85
National Rural Health Association
(NRHA), 71, 258–259
NRHA Connect, 36
National Survey on Drug Use and
Health 2002–2004, 96, 101
National Survey on Drug Use and
Health 2010, 247
National Youth Anti-Drug Media
Campaign, 105
Native Americans
alcohol abuse of, 98
cancer screening, 58
cardiovascular disease in, 124
illicit drug abuse of, 98
substance abuse of, 95
NCCBH. See National Council for
Community Behavioral
Healthcare (NCCBH)
nervios, 232
A New DAWN: Diabetes Awareness and
Wellness Network, 60
NHANES. See National Health and
Nutrition Examination Survey
(NHANES)
NHIS. See National Health Interview
Survey (NHIS)
NHLBI. See National Heart, Lung, and
Blood Institute (NHLBI)

NIEHS. *See* National Institute of
   Environmental Health Sciences
   (NIEHS)
NIMHD. *See* National Institute on
   Minority Health and Health
   Disparities (NIMHD)
Northeast region, HIV prevention and
   treatment in, 177–178
NRHA. *See* National Rural Health
   Association (NRHA)
nursing homes, in rural areas, 249
nutrition
   and cancer, 58
   intake, church-based interventions
      for, 62

OAT. *See* Office for the Advancement of
   Telehealth (OAT)
Obama, Barack, 257
obesity, in rural America, 14, 139–148.
      See also overweight
   church-based interventions
      for, 60–61
   costs of, 139–140
   ecological approach to understanding
      community factors, 144–145
      family and household factors,
         142–143
      individual factors, 140–142
   prevalence of, 139
   strategies for reducing
      community level and
         policies, 147–148
      individual and family
         levels, 146–147
occupational health
   of migrant farmworkers, 230–231
   in rural areas, 187–195
      climate change impact on, 191–194
      community-based participatory
         research, 188–190
      gene–environment
         interactions, 190–191
Office for the Advancement of
   Telehealth (OAT), 257
Office of Management and Budget
   (OMB), 2
   defining rurality, 3, 4
Office of National Drug Control Policy,
   105, 258

Office of Rural Health Policy (ORHP),
   85, 257
Ohio Department of Drug Addiction
   Services, 108
older adults. *See also* adults
   access to health care, 248–250
   medication for, 247
   mental health of, 246–247
   physical health of, 244–246
   sociodemographic factors
      affecting, 243–244
OMB. *See* Office of Management and
   Budget (OMB)
Open Door Community Health Centers,
   73, 74–75
Opiate Medication Initiative for Rural
   Oregon Residents, 107
opiates abuse, 105, 107, 247
opioid treatment programs (OTPs), 105
oral health, of migrant farmworkers, 233
ORHP. *See* Office of Rural Health Policy
   (ORHP)
OTPs. *See* opioid treatment programs
   (OTPs)
overweight, 139–145, 147. *See also*
   obesity, in rural America
oxycodone abuse, 95
OxyContin abuse, 95, 98, 99

Pacific Islanders
   affected by stroke, 125
   alcohol abuse of, 98
   cardiovascular disease in, 115
   illicit drug abuse of, 98
Paint-the-State campaign, 103
parasitic infections, 231
Park County Diabetes Project, 158
The Partnership for Health, 178
patient-centered medical homes
   (PCMHs), 68, 69, 78, 79, 234, 235
Patient Health Questionnaire-9 (PHQ-9),
   72, 74, 75, 232
patient-level barriers to integration, 70
Patient Protection and Affordable Care
   Act, 77, 78
Pawtucket Heart Health Program, 59
PCMHs. *See* patient-centered medical
   homes (PCMHs)
peer counseling, for substance
   abuse, 108

people living with HIV/AIDS (PLWHA), 171, 173–174, 175, 177–180
personal–professional boundaries, overlapping, 46
PH. *See* physical health (PH)
physical activity, 7, 56, 57, 59
  for cardiovascular health, 121, 130, 133
  church-based interventions for, 62
  and diabetes, 158, 159, 161
  and obesity, 141, 144–145
  school environment, 145
physical health (PH)
  Four Quadrant Clinical Integration Model, 69
  of older adults, 244–246
place of residence, disparities associated with, 125–128
  heart attack, 126–127
  hypertension, 126
  stroke, 127–128
PLWHA. *See* people living with HIV/AIDS (PLWHA)
population characteristics, of migrant farmworkers, 228–229
posttraumatic stress disorder (PTSD), 88, 194, 231, 232
poverty, 6
  and obesity, 142
  of older adults, 243
practice barriers to integration, 70
prehypertension, 116. *See also* hypertension (HTN)
prenatal or family planning clinics, 47
prescription drugs, 87
President's New Freedom Commission on Mental Health, 68, 89
President's Rural Health Initiative, 257
Prevention IS Care, 178
primary care
  access to, 16–18
  role in substance abuse treatment, 107
Primary Care-Mental Health Initiative, 78
privacy
  HIV testing, 170
  threats to, 46–47
professional codes of ethics, 42
professional practice expectations, and moral distress, 49–50

professional–client cultural perspectives, variance in, 47–48
professional–personal boundaries, overlapping, 46
Project Venture, 101
promotores, 234–235
psychoterratic illness, defined, 194
PTSD. *See* posttraumatic stress disorder (PTSD)
Public Health Accreditation Board, 32
public health, climate change impact on, 192–193
Public Health Service Act, 22, 74
Public Housing Primary Care Programs, 74

racial and ethnic minorities, 123–125
  access to medical care, 20–21
  affected by stroke, 125
  heart disease in, 124–125
  hypertension in, 123–124
  obesity of, 141
  older adults, 243–244
RCAP. *See* Rural Center for AIDS/STD Prevention (RCAP)
Recovery Act Broadband Initiatives Program, 252
Recovery Month Toolkit, 109
recruitment, of public health workers, 31–32
regionalization, 32
regulatory and policy health care ethics, 42
regulatory barriers to integration, 70
reimbursement, 76, 77, 79, 80, 107
  barriers to integration, 70
  Medi-Cal, 74
  Medicaid, 22
  Medicare, 22, 74
  telehealth, 75, 108
  tuition, 32
religion, 6–7, 55. *See also* church-based health promotion, in rural areas
remoteness, in rurality, 5–6
residential service options, in substance abuse treatment, 108
respiratory health, of American Indians/Alaskan Native, 217
retention, of public health workers, 31–32

reverse integration, 78, 89
RHCs. *See* rural health clinics (RHCs)
risk-taking behavior, of LGBT, 211
role diffusion, 31, 35
RUCAs. *See* Rural-Urban Community
    Areas (RUCAs)
RUCCs. *See* Rural-Urban Continuum
    Codes (RUCCs)
Rural Center for AIDS/STD Prevention
    (RCAP), 178
rural communities. *See also*
    community(ies)
  versus urban communities, 3
  substance use issues in, 98–100, 102
Rural Health Clinic Program,
    21, 22
rural health clinics (RHCs), 21–22, 258
Rural Health Initiative, 70
Rural Health Outreach grant
    (2002), 76
Rural Health Research Center
    program, 257
Rural Healthcare Services Outreach
    Grant program, 257
Rural Healthy People 2010, 156, 157,
    176, 188
Rural Healthy People 2020, 156
rural medical professionals, shortage
    of, 16
Rural Mental Health Demonstration
    Program, 71
rural minority health, 203–218
  African Americans, 204–206
  American Indians or Alaska
    Native, 215–218
  Hispanics, 207–210
  LGBT, 210–215
Rural Murals, 103
rural providers. *See also* health care
    providers
  distribution and characteristics
    of, 104–105
  treatment models with relevance
    for, 106–108
Rural Research Agenda, 42–43
Rural-Urban Community Areas
    (RUCAs), 3
Rural-Urban Continuum Codes
    (RUCCs), 3, 4

rural veterans, mental health problems
    in, 88–89
Rural Women's Recovery Program, 108
rurality, 2–8. *See also individual entries*
  agriculture, 6
  behavioral norms, 7
  defined, 2–4
  isolation, 5–6
  poverty, 6
  religion, 6–7
  remoteness, 5–6
  stigma, 7–8

"safety net," for medical care, 16, 17
SAMHSA. *See* Substance Abuse
    and Mental Health Services
    Administration (SAMHSA)
SBP. *See* systolic blood pressure (SBP)
scarce resources, allocation of, 50
school environment, impact on
    obesity, 145
SCORE Project. *See* Supporting
    Caregivers of Rural Veterans
    Electronically (SCORE) Project
screening, 51
  of cancer, 57–58
SCRHRC. *See* South Carolina Rural
    Health Research Center
    (SCRHRC)
sedentary lifestyle, and cardiovascular
    disease, 121
self-help groups
  role in substance abuse treatment, 108
Seventh-Day Adventists, 56
sexually transmitted diseases (STD)
  church-based interventions for, 61
  clinics, 47
sexually transmitted infections
    (STIs), 180
smoking, 7, 8, 14, 101, 188, 189
  and cardiovascular disease,
    121–122, 131
  cessation, 59, 61, 74, 130, 163, 256
  church-based interventions
    for, 61–62
  rural–urban disparity in, 14
SNAP-Ed, 146, 147
social capital, 33–34, 37
social cohesion, defined, 122

social home environment, and obesity, 143
Social Security Act, 22
South Carolina Rural Health Research Center (SCRHRC), 246
Southern region, HIV prevention and treatment in, 173–175
Southern Rural Access Program, 36
specialty care services, 18–19
specialty geriatric care, 248–249
state fiscal pressures, 77–78
State Medicare Rural Hospital Flexibility (Flex) Grant Program, 21
STD. *See* sexually transmitted diseases (STD)
stigma, 5, 7–8, 18, 43, 51, 63, 70, 86, 87, 89, 107, 164, 256. *See also* discrimination
  HIV-related, 169–171, 174, 179, 180
  seeking public assistance, 6
STIs. *See* sexually transmitted infections (STIs)
stoicism, 88
stress
  obesity and, 141–142
  posttraumatic, 88, 194, 231, 232
stroke, 118–120, 205, 208. *See also* cardiovascular disease (CVD); coronary heart disease (CHD); heart attack; heart disease, in rural areas
  changes in rates over time, 120
  gender and, 123
  knowledge and awareness of, 129–130
  mortality rates associated with, 119
  place of residence and, 127–128
  prevalence of, 119
  in racial and ethnic minorities, 125
  types of, 118
Stroke Belt, 119, 127
"Stroke Buckle," 127
Strosahl's model of integration, 69, 73, 74
Substance Abuse and Mental Health Services Administration (SAMHSA), 109, 247
  Recovery Month Toolkit, 109

substance abuse, in rural America, 7, 95–110
  continuing care, 108–109
  long-term support, 108–109
  patterns of, 96–98
  prevalence of, 96–100
  prevention of, 100–104
    applying theory and practice, 102–104
    reviewing theory and practice, 100–102
  treatment for
    challenges to accessibility, 106
    detoxification (detox) services, 104–105, 106
    lack of intensive services, 105
    primary care, role of, 107
    residential service options, 108
    rural providers, distribution and characteristics of, 104–105
    telehealth, 108
substance use, in rural America, 87, 95–110
  American Indians/Alaskan Native, 216–217
  issues in rural communities, 98–100
  LGBT, 210–211
  patterns of, 96–98
  prevalence of, 96–100
suicide
  American Indians/Alaskan Native, 217
  in rural areas, 87
Supplemental Food Security, 234
Supporting Caregivers of Rural Veterans Electronically (SCORE) Project, 251, 252
Surgeon General's Report on Mental Health, 68
sustainment, of rural public health workforce, 34
susto, 232
system-level barriers to integration, 69
systolic blood pressure (SBP), 116

teleconferencing, for HIV prevention and treatment, 179

telehealth, 89
    advancements in, 255–257
    programs, to promoting rural medical
        access, 24
    treatment
        for HIV, 176
        for substance abuse, 108
Telehealth and Visiting Specialist Center
    (TVSC), 75
telemedicine, 24, 255, 261
telephones. *See also* mobile services
    based counseling, for substance
        abuse, 108
    medical consultation through, 24
TennCare, 76. *See also* health insurance;
    Medicaid
Tepeyac Project, 57
theoretical health care ethics, 42
threats to confidentiality and
        privacy, 46–47
340B Drug Pricing Program, 77
tobacco use, 87, 101, 103, 110, 188
training
    interdisciplinary, 34
    leadership, 33, 34
    rural public health workforce, 33–34
tranquilizers abuse, 107
transportation barriers, 248
travel distance/hours of operation, as
        barrier to medical care, 17–18
TVSC. *See* Telehealth and Visiting
    Specialist Center (TVSC)

unemployment, 6
United States Department of
        Agriculture, 234
U.S. Census Bureau, 3, 4, 56
U.S. Department of Agriculture
        (USDA), 145, 241, 243
    defining rurality, 3–4
    Economic Research Service, 2
USDA. *See* U.S. Department of
    Agriculture (USDA)

Veterans Affairs (VA)
    system, 88–89
Veterans Rural Health Resource
    Center–Western Region, 251
victimization, of LGBQ
    individuals, 88

videoconferencing, medical consultation
        through, 24, 176, 256
vitamins, for infectious diseases, 231
vulnerable rural populations, access to
        medical care by, 19
    people with low socioeconomic
        status, 19
    racial and ethnic minority
        groups, 20–21

Wagner's Chronic Care Model, 69
WATCH Project. *See* Wellness for
    African Americans Through
    Churches (WATCH) Project
Weight Watchers®, 59
Wellness for African Americans Through
    Churches (WATCH) Project, 57
Western region, HIV prevention and
    treatment in, 176–177
White House Rural Council, 257–258
WHO. *See* World Health Organization
    (WHO)
Wholeness, Oneness, Righteousness,
    Deliverance (WORD) project, 61, 62
WIC (Special Supplemental Nutrition
    Program for Women, Infants and
    Children), 47, 48, 50, 146–147
Wing, Steve, 189
WISEWOMAN (Well-Integrated
    Screening and Evaluation
    for Women across the
    Nation), 132–133
Witness Project, 57–58
women, in rural areas. *See also* gender;
        men, in rural areas
    affected by heart attack, 118, 120, 121,
        123, 128
    affected by stroke, 123, 125, 129–133
    cancer in, 57, 58
    cardiovascular disease in, 115, 124,
        128–129
    dietary intake of, 120
    HIV/AIDS in, 172, 174, 175
    hypertension in, 116, 117, 123, 126
    LGBT, 212
    mental health disparities in, 88
    obesity of, 139, 140, 141
    participation behavioral weight loss
        programs, 24
    substance abuse of, 98, 105, 106

WORD project. *See* Wholeness, Oneness, Righteousness, Deliverance (WORD) project
workforce issues, in rural public health, 29–37
    career and community, connection between, 35–36
    challenges to, 29–32
    characteristics of, 31
    collaborative education, 34–35
    educating, 33–34
    enumerating, 30–31
    expectations of, 32–33
    overview of, 29–32
    sustaining, 34
    training, 33–34
    workers, recruiting and retaining, 31–32
workplace daycare, 32
World Health Organization (WHO), 191, 193